Advances in Infection Control and Prevention

Advances in Infection Control and Prevention

Editor: Tiffany Donnelly

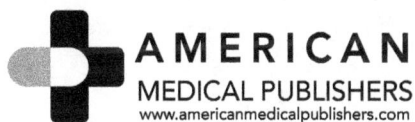

AMERICAN
MEDICAL PUBLISHERS
www.americanmedicalpublishers.com

AMERICAN
MEDICAL PUBLISHERS
www.americanmedicalpublishers.com

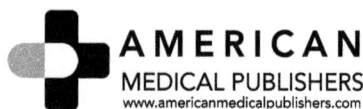

Cataloging-in-Publication Data

Advances in infection control and prevention / edited by Tiffany Donnelly
   p. cm.
Includes bibliographical references and index.
ISBN 978-1-63927-216-7
1. Infection--Control. 2. Communicable diseases--Prevention. 3. Infection--Prevention.
4. Nosocomial infections--Prevention. I. Donnelly, Tiffany.
RC112 .A38 2022
616.9--dc23

American Medical Publishers,
41 Flatbush Avenue,
1st Floor, New York,
NY 11217, USA

ISBN978-1-63927-216-7 (Hardback)

Contents

Preface

The world is advancing at a fast pace like never before. Therefore, the need is to keep up with the latest developments. This book was an idea that came to fruition when the specialists in the area realized the need to coordinate together and document essential themes in the subject. That's when I was requested to be the editor. Editing this book has been an honour as it brings together diverse authors researching on different streams of the field. The book collates essential materials contributed by veterans in the area which can be utilized by students and researchers alike.

Infection control is the discipline that deals with the prevention of nosocomial or healthcare-related infections. It is an important part of the health care infrastructure. It is similar to public health practice and uses anti-infective agents such as antibiotics, antifungals, antiprotozoals, antibacterials and antivirals for infection prevention and control. Infection control also focuses on the factors related to the infections that spread within the healthcare settings such as patient to patient or among staff. It also takes care of prevention against these infections by taking care of hand hygiene, disinfection, sterilization or vaccination. It monitors the suspected spread of infection and its management. This book is a valuable compilation of topics, ranging from the basic to the most complex advancements in the field of infection control and prevention. It strives to provide a fair idea about this discipline and to help develop a better understanding of the latest advances within this field. It is appropriate for students seeking detailed information in this area as well as for experts.

Each chapter is a sole-standing publication that reflects each author's interpretation. Thus, the book displays a multi-facetted picture of our current understanding of application, resources and aspects of the field. I would like to thank the contributors of this book and my family for their endless support.

Editor

Implementation of the WHO multimodal Hand Hygiene Improvement Strategy in a University Hospital in Central Ethiopia

Frieder Pfäfflin[1,2,3]* , Tafese Beyene Tufa[2,4], Million Getachew[2,4], Tsehaynesh Nigussie[2,4], Andreas Schönfeld[1,2], Dieter Häussinger[1,2], Torsten Feldt[1,2] and Nicole Schmidt[5,6]

Abstract

Background: The burden of health-care associated infections in low-income countries is high. Adequate hand hygiene is considered the most effective measure to reduce the transmission of nosocomial pathogens. We aimed to assess compliance with hand hygiene and perception and knowledge about hand hygiene before and after the implementation of a multimodal hand hygiene campaign designed by the World Health Organization.

Methods: The study was carried out at Asella Teaching Hospital, a university hospital and referral centre for a population of about 3.5 million in Arsi Zone, Central Ethiopia. Compliance with hand hygiene during routine patient care was measured by direct observation before and starting from six weeks after the intervention, which consisted of a four day workshop accompanied by training sessions and the provision of locally produced alcohol-based handrub and posters emphasizing the importance of hand hygiene. A second follow up was conducted three months after handing over project responsibility to the Ethiopian partners. Health-care workers' perception and knowledge about hand hygiene were assessed before and after the intervention.

Results: At baseline, first, and second follow up we observed a total of 2888, 2865, and 2244 hand hygiene opportunities, respectively. Compliance with hand hygiene was 1.4% at baseline and increased to 11.7% and 13.1% in the first and second follow up, respectively (p < 0.001). The increase in compliance with hand hygiene was consistent across professional categories and all participating wards and was independently associated with the intervention (adjusted odds ratio, 9.18; 95% confidence interval 6.61-12.76; p < 0.001). After the training, locally produced alcohol-based handrub was used in 98.4% of all hand hygiene actions. The median hand hygiene knowledge score overall was 13 (interquartile range 11–15) at baseline and increased to 17 (15–18) after training (p < 0.001). Health-care workers' perception surveys revealed high appreciation of the different strategy components.

Conclusion: Promotion of hand hygiene is feasible and sustainable in a resource-constrained setting using a multimodal improvement strategy. However, absolute compliance remained low. Strong and long-term commitment by hospital management and health-care workers may be needed for further improvement.

Keywords: Hand hygiene, Ethiopia, World Health Organization, Infection control, Health-care worker, Alcohol-based handrub

* Correspondence: frieder.pfaefflin@charite.de
[1]Department of Gastroenterology, Hepatology and Infectious Diseases (DGHID), Heinrich Heine University, Düsseldorf, Germany
[2]Hirsch Institute of Tropical Medicine, research and training centre of DGHID, operated in cooperation with Arsi University, Asella, Ethiopia
Full list of author information is available at the end of the article

Background

Hand hygiene is referred to as either hand washing with soap and water or hand disinfection. Important benefits of proper hand hygiene include reduction of nosocomial infections [1], reduced transmission of multi-drug resistant pathogens [2, 3], and cost effectiveness [4, 5]. Alcoholic handrub is regarded to be superior to washing hands with soap and water. It has greater activity against microorganisms, less time constraints, and better skin tolerability [5–7]. Furthermore, alcoholic handrub is better accessible in most settings as it can be provided in pocket bottles and may thus be available at any time at the point of care. The World Health Organization (WHO) has identified formulations for the local preparation of alcohol-based handrubs with substantially lower costs compared to commercial products [8].

Compliance with hand hygiene varies greatly between countries and settings but is globally low [5]. Several factors have been shown to be related to low compliance with hand hygiene in developed countries [9]. In low-income countries the major reason for non-compliance with hand hygiene may be lack of adequate facilities [10]. The burden of health-care associated infections (HAIs) is high in developing countries [11]. WHO has established a multimodal implementation strategy to improve compliance with hand hygiene [12]. Furthermore, the concept "my five moments for hand hygiene" was developed to perform hand hygiene in key moments [13]. Allegranzi et al. found that the implementation of WHO's hand-hygiene strategy is feasible and sustainable in different settings and countries and leads to significant compliance and knowledge improvement in health-care workers (HCWs) [14]. There are, however, few data on the implementation of the WHO multimodal hand hygiene improvement strategy in Ethiopia, a country with high rates of nosocomial infections [15].

The main objective for this study was to assess compliance with hand hygiene in selected wards of the Asella Teaching Hospital (ATH) before and after the implementation of the hand hygiene campaign. The secondary objectives were to assess compliance with hand hygiene for the different professional categories and the different wards and to assess perception and knowledge for the different professional categories before and after the implementation of the hand hygiene campaign.

Methods
Study setting

The study was carried out in selected wards of ATH in the Arsi Zone, Oromia Region, Central Ethiopia. The ATH is the university hospital of the Arsi University and serves as a referral centre for a population of roughly 3.5 million in the Arsi and neighbouring zones. Hirsch Institute of Tropical Medicine (HITM) is a research and training centre of the Department of Gastroenterology, Hepatology and Infectious Diseases (DGHID) of Heinrich Heine University Düsseldorf, Germany, operated in cooperation with the Arsi University on the campus of ATH. All wards involved in perinatal and maternal care were included. These comprised gynaecology, obstetrics, paediatrics, and neonatology. The study was funded by the European ESTHER alliance (*Ensemble pour une Solidarité Thérapeutique Hospitalière en Réseau*) within a hospital partnership project to reduce perinatal and maternal morbidity and mortality due to infectious diseases.

Study design

Ethics approval was obtained from College of Health Arsi University Ethical Review Committee (reference number A/U/H/C/120/10407/07). Additionally, written support from hospital leaders was obtained before starting project activities.

Activities consisted of three different phases in an uncontrolled before-and-after design.

Phase 1 is referred to as baseline assessment. It comprised a ward infrastructure survey, a HCWs' perception survey, a hand hygiene knowledge questionnaire, and the observation of HCWs' hand hygiene practices. The ward infrastructure survey was carried out involving senior members of the hospital management, the respective wards, and the study team. Within this survey, the availability of functional sinks was assessed and locations were identified where wall-fixed alcoholic handrub dispensers should be mounted. The HCWs' perception survey, the hand hygiene knowledge questionnaire, and the observation form for hand hygiene practices were all designed by WHO [16]. Minor changes were made to the hand hygiene knowledge questionnaire to adapt to the local situation. English was the only language used in presentations as this is the language of medical education in Ethiopia. Question and answer sessions were held in English and Amharic. The observation of HCWs' hand hygiene practices was carried out by two trained HCWs. Observations were performed only during day shifts for logistical reasons. The observers came to the wards at random times without prior announcement. They acted as unobtrusively as possible but disclosed their task readily on enquiry. Observation sessions lasted about 20 (±10) minutes. The purpose of breaking down the observation into sessions was to acquire an overview of practices [17]. Potential opportunities for hand hygiene according to the "my 5 moments of hand hygiene" were recorded and the actual number of episodes of hand hygiene. Hand washing referred to washing hands with either water alone or with soap and water, hand disinfection referred to the use of alcohol-based hand rub. Compliance with hand hygiene was calculated by the number of occasions when hand hygiene was performed divided by the number of total hand hygiene opportunities. All professional health care providers and students who were working in the selected wards were included in the study. HCWs were divided into two broad professional categories: (1) nurse/midwife/health officer/emergency surgeon (nurse with training in emergency surgery)/nurse student/midwife student/health officer student, (2) medical doctor/intern/medical student. The other two professional categories foreseen by WHO (auxiliary and other HCW) were not considered as they play a negligible role during patient care at ATH.

Phase 2 was the intervention. A four-day workshop was conducted with lectures on cultural aspects and scientific evidence of hand hygiene, and nosocomial infections in neonatology. Practical issues of the implementation of the multimodal hand hygiene improvement strategy were explained and baseline results of the HCWs' perception survey and the hand hygiene knowledge questionnaire were presented. The workshop addressed hospital management, department heads, head nurses, focal persons for hygiene in the selected wards, and all interested staff of ATH. Four further half-day trainings were conducted to specifically address HCWs who could not attend the workshop. Additionally, all interns of ATH were explicitly invited to attend the trainings as they undergo rotations within the different wards and it was anticipated that some of them would be assigned to work on the wards where study activities were undertaken. HCWs who could not attend any training session were handed a pocket bottle with alcohol-based handrub after a short explanation of the concept "my five moments in hand hygiene". Posters emphasizing the importance of hand hygiene were placed at strategic sites within ATH. WHO-recommended handrub formulations were produced according to WHO guidelines [8]. Demonstrations of the production were given by HITM staff during the workshop. Each HCW working in the pre-selected wards received a 100 ml pocket bottle filled with alcoholic handrub. A sticker on the pocket bottle indicated that once empty, refill for the bottle would be available at HITM. Wall-fixed hand disinfectant dispensers were mounted prior to the workshop and were filled immediately after the workshop with alcoholic handrub. Stickers on the containers indicated that refill would be available at HITM.

Phase 3 was the follow up assessment. The hand hygiene knowledge questionnaire was repeated immediately after the workshop or the training sessions, respectively. Starting from six weeks after the intervention, the HCWs' perception survey and the observation of hand hygiene activities were repeated as described above. Study results were presented to hospital management and all concerned HCWs. An award was issued to the ward, which reached highest compliance with hand hygiene in the first follow up. Responsibility for the hand hygiene project was gradually transferred to ATH. A second follow up assessment was performed by only one observer (TN) starting from three months after the first follow up additionally recording the use of gloves but not recording the type of ward (Fig. 1).

Statistical analysis

To detect a difference of 10% between rates of hand hygiene compliance before and after the implementation, 286 opportunities for hand hygiene had to be observed at baseline and follow up for each category [17]. Compliance at baseline and at follow up overall and for the different professional categories was compared with χ^2 tests. Multivariable logistic regression was used with the observation period (before or after the intervention) as the main independent variable. Type of ward and professional category were included as potential confounders. These confounders were chosen as in most studies it has been shown that compliance with hand hygiene varied by hospital ward and professional category, with higher compliance among nurses compared to doctors [18].

Hand hygiene knowledge questionnaire scores were calculated for each participant as the sum of all correct

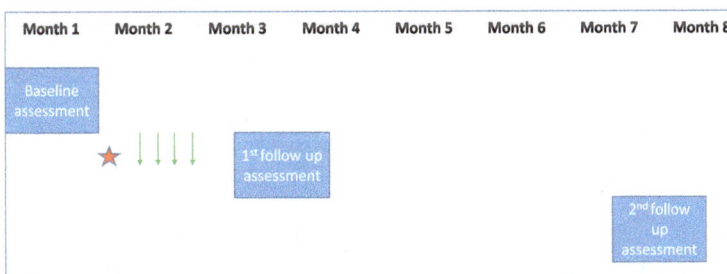

Fig. 1 Time axis of study procedures. NOTE: Red star denotes workshop accompanied by placement of posters, filling of wall-fixed handrub dispensers, and distribution of pocket bottle hand disinfectants; thin green arrows denote half-day trainings for HCWs who could not attend the workshop. The HCWs' perception survey was performed at baseline and at first follow up but not at second follow up

answers (each correct answer equalling 1 point). Results are expressed as medians and interquartile ranges (IQRs). Statistical significance was assessed by Wilcoxon rank-sum test, as participants were anonymous and pairing was therefore impossible. Results from the HCWs' perception survey are shown as medians and IQRs of points given by participants on the 7-point Likert scale and were assessed by Wilcoxon rank-sum test. Data analysis was performed using EpiInfo, version 3.5.4 and SPSS, version 20. Two-tailed p values of less than 0.05 were considered to indicate statistical significance.

Results

Observation of compliance with hand hygiene

At baseline, first, and second follow up 146, 167, and 212 observation sessions were conducted, respectively. The median observation time per session was 22 (IQR 15–26) and 20 (IQR 16–25) minutes at baseline and first

follow up, respectively. The duration of the observation sessions was not recorded during the second follow up.

Education

A total of 164 HCWs participated in the trainings. All participants were listed and cross matched with registration lists. Due to intense staff rotation and unclear spelling of names we cannot give an exact number of how many HCWs were assigned to work in the respective wards during our study activities. We estimate, however, that at least 90% of the targeted HCWs were trained.

Compliance with hand hygiene

A total of 7997 hand hygiene opportunities were assessed at baseline and follow up. Compliance with hand hygiene was 1.4% at baseline and rose to 11.7% and 13.1% in the first and second follow up, respectively. A significant increase in compliance with hand hygiene was seen across both professional categories and in all

Table 1 Compliance with hand hygiene at baseline and at follow up

Variable	Baseline			First follow up				Second follow up			
	No of HH actions	No of HH opportunities	Compliance (%)	No of HH actions	No of HH opportunities	Compliance (%)	P value[1]	No of HH actions	No of HH opportunities	Compliance (%)	P value[1]
Over all	41	2888	1.4	335	2865	11.7	<0.001	294	2244	13.1	<0.001
Professional category											
Category I	25	1470	1.7	157	1387	11.3	<0.001	73	678	10.8	<0.001
Category II	16	1418	1.1	178	1478	12.0	<0.001	221	1566	14.1	<0.001
Nurse	14	516	2.7	103	986	10.4	<0.001	63	461	13.7	<0.001
Midwife	6	284	2.1	46	324	14.2	<0.001	5	61	8.2	0.029
Medical doctor	9	285	3.2	27	275	9.8	0.002	70	306	22.9	<0.001
Intern	7	1109	0.6	151	1205	12.5	<0.001	151	1265	11.9	<0.001
Ward											
Paediatrics	9	882	1.0	50	807	6.2	<0.001	ND	ND		
Neonatology	24	672	3.6	166	677	24.5	<0.001	ND	ND		
Gynaecology	3	651	0.5	17	664	2.6	0.002	ND	ND		
Obstetrics	5	683	0.7	102	717	14.2	<0.001	ND	ND		
Indication											
b. p. c.	8	550	1.5	40	459	8.7	<0.001	10	86	11.6	<0.001
b. a. p.	2	275	0.7	5	305	1.6	0.455	20	422	4.7	0.003
a. b. f. e.	10	258	3.9	113	398	28.4	<0.001	5	10	50.0	<0.001
a. p. c.	15	1208	1.2	149	923	16.1	<0.001	130	924	14.1	<0.001
a. c. p. s.	6	597	1.0	28	780	3.6	0.002	129	804	16.0	<0.001

Only the major professional categories are displayed. Therefore, the sum of opportunities for these categories does not equal the total number of opportunities. Category I: nurse/midwife/health officer/emergency surgeon/nurse, midwife, health officer student; Category II: medical doctor/intern/medical student. NOTE: HH, hand hygiene; b.p.c., before patient contact; b.a.p., before aseptic procedure; a.b.f.e., after body fluid exposure; a.p.c., after patient contact; a.c.p.s., after contact with patient surroundings; ND, no data. [1]Detemined by χ^2 tests with compliance at baseline as the reference.

indications except for "before aseptic procedures" in the first follow up (Table 1). The increase in compliance with hand hygiene was associated with the intervention (crude odds ratio, 9.19: 95% confidence interval (CI) 6.62-12.77; p < 0.001). This association remained significant after adjustment for the potential confounders 'type of ward' and 'professional category' (adjusted odds ratio, 9.18; 95% CI 6.61-12.76; p < 0.001). Compliance with hand hygiene in the neonatology ward was higher compared to the paediatric ward as a reference at baseline (3.6% vs. 1.0%, p = 0.001) and at first follow up (24.5% vs. 6.2%, p < 0.001). Out of 41 hand hygiene actions at baseline 23 (56.1%) were handrub and 18 (43.9%) were hand washing, whereas at follow up handrub accounted for 619 (98.4%) and hand washing for 10 (1.6%) out of 629 hand hygiene actions, respectively.

The use of gloves was solely assessed during the second follow up. Gloves were used in 393 out of the 422 (93.1%) indications before aseptic procedures whereas gloves were used in 76 out of 1822 (4.2%) indications in the remaining four indications.

Hand hygiene knowledge questionnaire

The hand hygiene knowledge questionnaire was distributed before and immediately after the training sessions. A total of 141 HCWs filled the questionnaire before the training. Out of these, 70 HCWs belonged to category I and 61 HCWs belonged to category II. The remaining 10 participants did not belong to either of the predefined

categories. After the training, the questionnaire was filled by a total of 139 HCWs (category I: 67; category II 63; neither category 9). The median knowledge score for all participants was 13 (IQR 11–15) at baseline and increased to 17 (IQR 15–18) after training (p < 0.001). Knowledge scores for category I and II at baseline were 12 (IQR 9–14) and 15 (IQR 12–17) and increased to 16 (IQR 12–18) (p < 0.001) and 18 (IQR 16–19) (p < 0.001), respectively (Fig. 2).

Health-care workers' perception of the strategy

At baseline and at first follow up, 100 HCWs' perception surveys were handed to focal persons for hygiene for further distribution among HCWs. The return rates at baseline and follow up were 61% and 53%, respectively (Table 2).

Before the training and at first follow up, the effectiveness of hand hygiene was judged to be high or very high by more than 90% of the HCWs. Self-assessment of compliance with hand hygiene revealed high estimates (70% compliance with hand hygiene at baseline and follow up) that did not match with observation results (see Additional file 1).

After the training, HCWs perceived the impact and different elements of the multimodal hand hygiene campaign to be very positive. All questions asked in the HCWs perception survey received median scores of 7 on the 7-point Likert scale, thus indicating maximum agreement (Table 3).

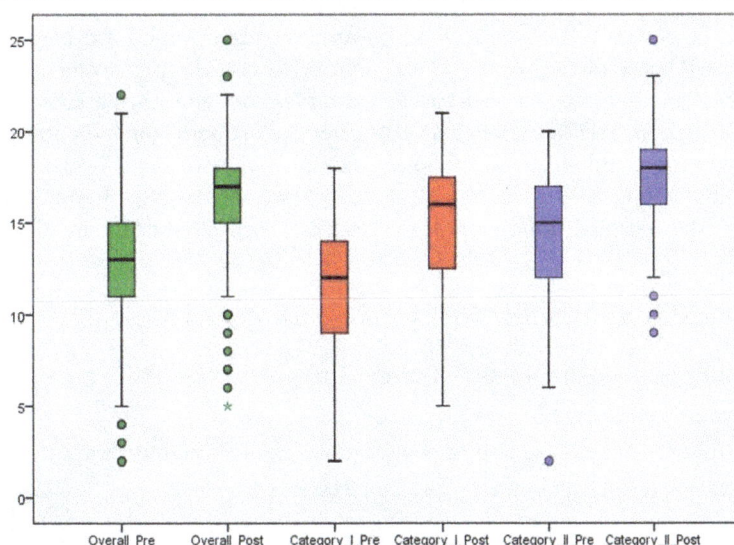

Fig. 2 Knowledge of hand hygiene before and after the training. Box plot of overall scores (maximum score 25); 5%, 25%, 50%, 75%, 95% percentiles and outliers (circles); asterix denotes two outliers with equal scores. NOTE: Pre, before the intervention; post, after the intervention. Category I: nurse/midwife/health officer/emergency surgeon/nurse, midwife, health officer student; Category II: medical doctor/intern/medical student

Table 2 HCWs' perception of the 5 components of the WHO multimodal hand hygiene improvement strategy

	Baseline	Follow up	P value[a]
No of respondents	61	53	
Category I	42	20	
Category II	19	33	
Strategy Component[b]			
System change:			
The healthcare facility makes alcohol-based handrub available at each point of care	6 (1–7)	6 (3–7)	0.359
Education:			
Clear and simple instructions for hand hygiene are made visible for every HCW	6 (3–7)	6 (4–7)	0.138
Each HCW is trained in hand hygiene	5 (3–7)	6 (3–7)	0.165
Feedback:			
HCWs regularly receive the results of their hand hygiene performance	4 (2–7)	5 (2–7)	0.969
Workplace reminders:			
Hand hygiene posters are displayed at point of care as reminders	3 (2–7)	6 (5–7)	<0.001
Patient safety climate:			
Leaders at your institution support and openly promote hand hygiene	5 (2–7)	6 (4–7)	0.062
Patients are invited to remind HCWs to perform hand hygiene	4 (1–7)	2 (1–7)	0.719

Category I: nurse/midwife/health officer/emergency surgeon/nurse, midwife, health officer student; Category II: medical doctor/intern/medical student. NOTE: HCW, health-care worker; WHO, World Health Organization. HCWs were asked to respond to the listed statements following the introductory question: "In your opinion, how effective would the following actions be to increase hand hygiene permanently in your institution?" [a]Determined by Wilcoxon rank-sum test. [b]Data show median scores (IQR) on a 7-point Likert scale (with extremes labelled as "not effective" at the lower and "very effective" at the higher end)

Consumption of alcohol-based hand rub

The consumption of locally produced alcohol-based handrub was solely recorded at HITM. It increased steadily after the training until the end of the first follow up (Fig. 3). Before the intervention, alcohol-based solutions were produced in the hospital pharmacy and responsibility for production of alcoholic handrub was transferred to ATH after the first follow up. Therefore, the consumption of alcohol-based disinfectants can only be indicated as shown.

Discussion

In our study, we found a very low compliance with hand hygiene at baseline. Compliance at baseline was similar to two studies that had been undertaken in Ethiopia [19, 20] but was lower compared to a study from Bamako, Mali [21]. The main reason for the low baseline compliance appears obvious: hand hygiene products and facilities were not available on the wards. Alcoholic disinfectants were only used for disinfection of patients' skin prior to aseptic procedures. For this purpose, usually one bottle of gentian violet-stained alcoholic solution was provided on each ward. The accessibility of soap and water was similarly difficult. The majority of sinks were non-functional for different reasons. Furthermore, the water supply of ATH was limited. This was especially true during the dry season when water supply was completely cut for several days in a row on various occasions.

In addition to the lack of alcoholic handrub and water – although presumably less important – compliance with hand hygiene at baseline may have been low for social reasons. One senior physician mentioned that he was reluctant to use his own pocket bottle hand disinfectant in order not to create envy and shame among other HCWs.

Observation at follow up showed a significant increase of compliance with hand hygiene. This increase was consistent across both predefined professional categories and in all four wards and persisted in the second follow up after responsibility for hand hygiene had been transferred to ATH. Improvement was associated with the intervention and this association remained significant after adjustment for potential confounders. However, compliance with hand hygiene remained low compared to data from developed countries. In a landmark study, which was conducted in the University of Geneva

Table 3 HCWs' perception about impact and different elements of the multimodal hand hygiene improvement strategy

	Median (IQR)
Has the use of alcohol-based handrub made hand hygiene easier to practice in your daily work?	7 (6–7)
Is the use of alcohol-based handrub well tolerated by your hands?	7 (6–7)
Did knowing the results of hand hygiene observation in your ward help you to improve your hand hygiene practices?	7 (5–7)
Has the fact of being observed made you paying more attention to your hand hygiene practices?	7 (4–7)
Were the educational activities that you participated in important to improve your hand hygiene practices?	7 (6–7)
Has your awareness of your role in preventing HAIs by improving your hand hygiene practices increased during the current hand hygiene promotional campaign?	7 (6–7)

NOTE: IQR, interquartile range; HAI, health-care associated infection. Results are shown as median scores on a 7-point Likert scale (with extremes labelled as "not at all" at the lower end and "very important" or "very much" at the higher end)

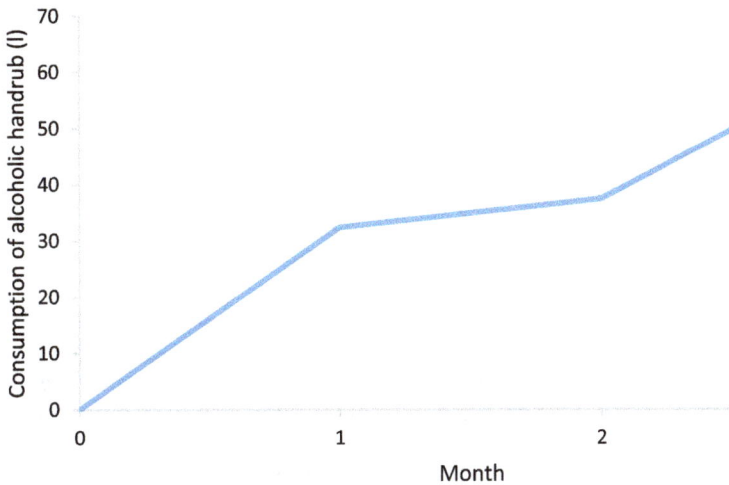

Fig. 3 Consumption of alcohol-based handrub. Consumption of alcohol-based handrub in selected wards of Asella Teaching Hospital from the intervention (month 0) until the end of the first follow up. Display of total monthly consumption in litres

Hospitals, compliance with hand hygiene rose from 47.6% at baseline to 66.2% over a four-year period [3]. Particularly high rates of compliance with hand hygiene were observed in selected sites with vulnerable patients like intensive-care units after the implementation of a hand hygiene campaign [22, 23]. It must be considered, however, that in these studies only specific indications for hand hygiene were assessed (e.g. after completion of patient contact, on entrance into the unit). The concept "my five moments in hand hygiene" was not applied. One important study assessed the implementation of WHO's hand hygiene improvement strategy in five countries with different socio-economic background [14]. Overall compliance before the intervention was significantly lower in low-income and middle-income countries than in high-income countries.

Compliance with hand hygiene improved across all indications except for "before aseptic procedures" in the first follow up. To our knowledge, this finding was not reported from previous studies. After having noticed preferential use of gloves before aseptic procedures at baseline and at first follow up, the use of gloves was systematically assessed during the second follow up. Observation revealed a high percentage of use of gloves (>90%) solely in the indication 'before aseptic procedures'. The failure to change or remove contaminated gloves has been identified as major component of inadequate infection control practices [24]. We had emphasized the need for hand hygiene regardless of the use of gloves in our trainings. However, data show that this imperative was not understood and must be stressed further. Compliance with hand hygiene was highest after body fluid exposure and after patient contact. This possibly reflects the HCWs' priority for self-protection rather than for protection of the patients. Self-protection

has been shown to be the engine for hand hygiene adherence in several studies [5, 14, 25].

Interestingly, compliance with hand hygiene was similar in HCWs from category I and category II. This is in contrast to many studies, which found lower compliance in doctors than in nurses [5, 9], although Allegranzi et al. observed better compliance with hand hygiene in doctors than in nurses in Mali [21]. They hypothesized that the better compliance with hand hygiene in doctors could be due to a higher level of education and a stronger perception of their professional role [14]. The compliance with hand hygiene was higher in the neonatology ward when compared to the paediatrics ward as a reference. One possible reason for this – apart from the presumptions that hygiene is of critical importance in neonatology and many HCWs in neonatology may be particularly dedicated to their work - may have been the presence of a professor who emphasized a lot the importance of hand hygiene in routine patient care. It has been shown that role models may influence compliance with hand hygiene [26]. In our case the professor was a person that many HCWs looked up to and thus at least some HCWs may have tried to copy his behavior.

We produced alcohol-based handrub locally. Costs of local production were less than one fifth compared to commercially bought products. The skin tolerability of the handrub was perceived to be very good. After the intervention, hand hygiene actions were almost exclusively performed with handrub indicating high acceptance. The consumption of alcohol-based handrub increased steadily from the intervention until the end of the first follow up. The amount of alcohol-based handrub used was selected as indirect marker for compliance with hand hygiene in many settings although assessment based on product consumption cannot determine whether hand hygiene actions are performed in the right indications [5].

There were several challenges in our setting, which may have hampered achievement of better compliance with hand hygiene. First, we faced intense staff rotation on all levels within ATH. Since the beginning of the planning process until the end of the second follow up assessment, the position of medical director of ATH changed three times. Staff rotation on the wards resulted in observation of entirely different teams at baseline and follow up. Second, during the follow up assessment we were frequently shown empty wall-fixed alcoholic handrub dispensers and empty private pocket bottle hand disinfectants. Refill of alcoholic hand-rub had occasionally been fetched at HITM but then no further distribution among HCWs of the respective ward had been undertaken. On one ward, alcoholic handrub had been locked and was only accessible for one HCW. Third, although we did not measure the consumption of alcoholic handrub from wall-fixed dispensers and from pocket bottles independently, we felt that wall-fixed dispensers were used preferentially. According to our ward infrastructure, wall-fixed dispensers were mounted in selected sites with intense patient care. It seems obvious that the provision of wall-fixed dispensers to every room where patient care is performed would have been preferable. The concentration solely on the provision of alcohol-based handrub was regarded as a limitation by many HCWs and parts of the management of ATH. Whitby and McLaws demonstrated, however, that improved accessibility to sinks does not lead to improvement in compliance with hand hygiene [27]. In addition, WHO recommends the combined provision of pocket bottles and wall-fixed dispensers filled with alcohol-based handrub without focusing on water supply [5]. Just before the end of this study, management of ATH implemented a hygiene committee. The committee took over responsibilities like identification of further structural necessities. It has been shown that designated staff is one major critical component of an effective infection control program [28].

Results of the hand hygiene knowledge questionnaire were significantly better after the training than before the training. The improvement was seen in both professional categories and was similar to the improvement detected in a study from Bamako, Mali [21]. It may seem surprising that even immediately after the training the median scores reached were still far below the possible maximum score. We found that the way several questions should have been answered was not understood by many examinees (e.g. in some questions it is stated "tick one answer only" whereas in others there is no such statement. Many examinees wrongly only ticked one answer in these questions, too and therefore lost the

chance to reach higher scores). We had already adapted the questionnaire to the local situation in accordance with WHO recommendations. However, some structural modifications may be necessary especially for HCWs who are not used to multiple choice exams and may be confused by the changing design of the questions. In further studies, current tools could be compared with adapted tools to confirm or refute our concern.

In contrast to Allegranzi et al., who detected significant increases in median perception scores for all five components of the multimodal WHO hand hygiene improvement strategy, we only found increased median scores in the component "reminders at the workplace" [21]. This may be explained by the high baseline scores in our study. HCWs estimated their compliance with hand hygiene and the compliance of their co-workers to be high. Estimates differed greatly from our observation findings. This is in line with various studies, which reported that the correlation between self-assessment and observation findings is low [29, 30]. The acceptance of the different elements of the hand hygiene campaign and the perceived impact of hand hygiene were very high as indicated by maximum scores after the training. This finding supports the multimodal approach recommended by WHO. We cannot know, however, which element was most important for the observed outcomes and how the outcomes would have been if one or several elements had been omitted.

Our study has several limitations. First, although English is the official language of medical education in Ethiopia, not all HCWs have good English language skills. HCWs insisted on English presentations and WHO could not provide working materials in Amharic. We managed to establish question and answer sessions in Amharic after each training but we cannot exclude that outcomes would have been better if Amharic had been used preferentially.

Second, it seems logical that HCWs are reminded of performing hand hygiene actions in the presence of an observer. Observation at second follow up was entirely performed by local staff (TN), whereas international staff (NS) did most of the observation at baseline and at first follow up. Assessments of different observers may vary. However, all observers were well trained in WHO hand hygiene observation methods, and criteria defined by WHO are straightforward to minimize inter-observer differences [17].

Third, the hospital management addressed the wish of extension of our hygiene activities to the entire hospital arguing that all HCWs and patients should benefit from the positive effects of proper hand hygiene. We felt that our approach was adequate as pilot project to demonstrate feasibility and efficacy. Hospital management was in charge of ensuring sustainability of the project and of extending activities to the ward that had not yet been covered.

Fourth, we performed two follow up assessments in relatively short time intervals after the intervention. It would have been preferable to perform a time series analysis with several follow ups to longitudinally assess compliance with hand hygiene.

Last but not least, the clinical relevance of our intervention remains unclear in the light of compliance rates that were still low at follow up. To assess the rates of HAIs in ATH surveillance activities would have to be implemented. Surveillance is essential to record the burden of infectious diseases and the effect of interventions. Moreover, by itself, surveillance can lead to reduction in HAIs [31]. The most widely used surveillance definitions for HAIs come from the Centers for Disease Control and Prevention (CDC) and the National Healthcare Safety Network [32]. They are rarely applied in low-income countries as strict criteria have to be used including bacterial culture in most settings. Future research may help to develop criteria, which are adapted to the settings in resource-constrained countries. Ideally, prospective investigations should assess both compliance with hand hygiene and rates of HAIs.

Conclusion

We successfully implemented the WHO multimodal hand hygiene improvement strategy in selected wards of ATH. The intervention was highly appreciated by participating HCWs. The increase in compliance with hand hygiene persisted after responsibility for the project had been transferred to ATH. A time series analysis should be performed to further assess the longitudinal evolution of compliance with hand hygiene. Compliance with hand hygiene was low compared to similar projects. Simultaneous surveillance of HAIs could help to assess the clinical impact of such interventions.

Abbreviations

ATH: Asella Teaching Hospital; CDC: Centers for Disease Control and Prevention; CI: Confidence interval; DGHID: Department of Gastroenterology, Hepatology and Infectious Diseases; ESTHER: Ensemble pour une Solidarité Thérapeutique Hospitalière en Réseau; HAI: Health-care associated infection; HCW: Health-care worker; HITM: Hirsch Institute of Tropical Medicine; IQR: Interquartile range; WHO: World Health Organization

Acknowledgements

Not applicable.

Funding

The study was funded by the European ESTHER alliance, award number LSC-2013-83152725. The funder had no role in conception of the study, data collection, data analysis, and writing of the manuscript.

Authors' contribution

FP: study design, facilitation of contacts, provision of trainings, data analysis, writing of manuscript; TBT: study design, facilitation of contacts, provision of trainings; MG: production of alcohol-based handrub, provision of trainings, statistical analysis; TN: provision of trainings, data collection; AS: responsibility for second follow up; DH: facilitation of contacts, facilitation of infrastructure, study coordination; TF: facilitation of contacts, provision of training, drafting of manuscript; NS: provision of trainings, data collection, data entry, writing of manuscript. All authors read and approved the final manuscript.

Competing interests

The authors declare that they have no competing interests.

Consent for publication

Not applicable.

Author details

[1]Department of Gastroenterology, Hepatology and Infectious Diseases (DGHID), Heinrich Heine University, Düsseldorf, Germany. [2]Hirsch Institute of Tropical Medicine, research and training centre of DGHID, operated in cooperation with Arsi University, Asella, Ethiopia. [3]Department of Infectious Diseases and Pulmonary Medicine, Charité – Universitätsmedizin Berlin, Augustenburger Platz 1, 13353 Berlin, Germany. [4]Arsi University, Asella, Ethiopia. [5]Institute of Tropical Medicine and International Health, Charité – Universitätsmedizin Berlin, Berlin, Germany. [6]Department for Infectious Disease Epidemiology, Robert Koch Institute, Berlin, Germany.

References

1. Harbarth S, Sax H, Gastmeier P. The preventable proportion of nosocomial infections: an overview of published reports'. J Hosp Infect. 2003;54(4):258–66.
2. 'MDRO_literature-review.pdf'. [Online]. Available: http://www.who.int/gpsc/5may/MDRO_literature-review.pdf. Accessed 6 Nov 2016.
3. Pittet D, et al. Effectiveness of a hospital-wide programme to improve compliance with hand hygiene. Infection Control Programme'. Lancet. 2000;356(9238):1307–12.
4. Pittet D, Sax H, Hugonnet S, Harbarth S. Cost Implications of Successful Hand Hygiene Promotion'. Infect Control Hosp Epidemiol. 2004;25(03):264–6.
5. 'World Health Organization, WHO Guidelines on Hand Hygiene in Health Care. First Global Patient Safety Challenge Clean Care is Safer Care.' [Online]. Available: http://apps.who.int/iris/bitstream/10665/44102/1/9789241597906_eng.pdf. Accessed 7 Nov 2016.
6. Kampf G, Löffler H, Gastmeier P. Hand hygiene for the prevention of nosocomial infections'. Dtsch Arztebl Int. 2009;106(40):649–55.
7. Löffler H, Kampf G, Schmermund D, Maibach HI. How irritant is alcohol?'. Br J Dermatol. 2007;157(1):74–81.
8. 'Guide_to_Local_Production.pdf'. [Online]. Available: http://www.who.int/gpsc/5may/Guide_to_Local_Production.pdf. Accessed 7 Nov 2016.
9. Pittet D, Mourouga P, Perneger TV. Compliance with handwashing in a teaching hospital. Infection Control Program'. Ann Intern Med. Jan. 1999;130(2):126–30.
10. Uneke CJ, Ndukwe CD, Oyibo PG, Nwakpu KO, Nnabu RC, Prasopa-Plaizier N. Promotion of hand hygiene strengthening initiative in a Nigerian teaching hospital: implication for improved patient safety in low-income health facilities'. Braz J Infect Dis Off Publ Braz Soc Infect Dis. 2014;18(1):21–7.
11. Allegranzi B, et al. Burden of endemic health-care-associated infection in developing countries: systematic review and meta-analysis'. Lancet. 2011;377(9761):228–41.
12. 'Guide_to_Implementation.pdf'. [Online]. Available: http://www.who.int/gpsc/5may/Guide_to_Implementation.pdf. Accessed 7 Nov 2016.
13. Sax H, Allegranzi B, Uçkay I, Larson E, Boyce J, Pittet D. "My five moments for hand hygiene": a user-centred design approach to understand, train, monitor and report hand hygiene'. J Hosp Infect. 2007;67(1):9–21.
14. Allegranzi B, et al. Global implementation of WHO's multimodal strategy for improvement of hand hygiene: a quasi-experimental study'. Lancet Infect Dis. 2013;13(10):843–51.
15. Kotisso B, Aseffa A. Surgical wound infection in a teaching hospital in Ethiopia'. East Afr Med J. 1998;75(7):402–5.
16. 'WHO | Tools for evaluation and feedback'. [Online]. Available: http://www.

who.int/gpsc/5may/tools/evaluation_feedback/en/. Accessed 1 July 2016.

17. Sax H, Allegranzi B, Chraïti M-N, Boyce J, Larson E, Pittet D. The World Health Organization hand hygiene observation method'. Am J Infect Control. 2009;37(10):827–34.

18. Pittet D, Boyce JM. Hand hygiene and patient care: pursuing the Semmelweis legacy'. Lancet Infect Dis. 2001;1(Supplement 1):9–20.

19. Schmitz K, et al. Effectiveness of a multimodal hand hygiene campaign and obstacles to success in Addis Ababa, Ethiopia'. Antimicrob Resist Infect Control. 2014;3(1):8.

20. Feyissa GT, Gomersall JCS, Robertson-Malt S. Compliance to Hand Hygiene Practice among Nurses in Jimma University Specialized Hospital in Ethiopia: a best practice implementation project'. JBI Database Syst Rev Implement Rep. 2014;12(1):318–37.

21. Allegranzi B, et al. Successful implementation of the World Health Organization hand hygiene improvement strategy in a referral hospital in Mali, Africa'. Infect Control Hosp Epidemiol. 2010;31(2):133–41.

22. Mayer JA, Dubbert PM, Miller M, Burkett PA, Chapman SW. Increasing handwashing in an intensive care unit'. Infect Control IC. 1986;7(5):259–62.

23. Raskind CH, Worley S, Vinski J, Goldfarb J. Hand hygiene compliance rates after an educational intervention in a neonatal intensive care unit'. Infect Control Hosp Epidemiol. 2007;28(9):1096–8.

24. Thompson BL, Dwyer DM, Ussery XT, Denman S, Vacek P, Schwartz B. Handwashing and Glove Use in a Long-Term-Care Facility'. Infect Control Hosp Epidemiol. 1997;18(2):97–103.

25. Borg MA, et al. Self-protection as a driver for hand hygiene among healthcare workers'. Infect Control Hosp Epidemiol. 2009;30(6):578–80.

26. Schneider J, et al. Hand hygiene adherence is influenced by the behavior of role models'. Pediatr Crit Care Med J Soc Crit Care Med World Fed Pediatr Intensive Crit Care Soc. 2009;10(3):360–3.

27. Whitby M, McLaws M-L. Handwashing in healthcare workers: accessibility of sink location does not improve compliance'. J Hosp Infect. 2004;58(4):247–53.

28. Hughes JM. Study on the efficacy of nosocomial infection control (SENIC Project): results and implications for the future'. Chemotherapy. 1988;34(6):553–61.

29. O'Boyle CA, Henly SJ, Larson E. Understanding adherence to hand hygiene recommendations: the theory of planned behavior'. Am J Infect Control. 2001;29(6):352–60.

30. Jenner EA, Fletcher BC, Watson P, Jones FA, Miller L, Scott GM. Discrepancy between self-reported and observed hand hygiene behaviour in healthcare professionals'. J Hosp Infect. 2006;63(4):418–22.

31. Gastmeier P, et al. Effectiveness of a nationwide nosocomial infection surveillance system for reducing nosocomial infections'. J Hosp Infect. 2006;64(1):16–22.

32. 'CDC/NHSN Surveillance Definitions for Specific Types of Infections - 17pscnosinfdef_current.pdf'. [Online]. Available: http://www.cdc.gov/nhsn/pdfs/pscmanual/17pscnosinfdef_current.pdf. Accessed 7 Nov 2016.

2

Healthcare associated infection and its risk factors among patients admitted to a tertiary hospital

Solomon Ali[1,9*†] [iD], Melkamu Birhane[2†], Sisay Bekele[3], Gebre Kibru[1], Lule Teshager[1], Yonas Yilma[4], Yesuf Ahmed[5], Netsanet Fentahun[6], Henok Assefa[7], Mulatu Gashaw[1] and Esayas Kebede Gudina[8†]

Abstract

Background: Healthcare associated infection (HAI) is alarmingly increasing in low income settings. In Ethiopia, the burden of HAI is still not well described.

Methods: Longitudinal study was conducted from May to September, 2016. All wards of Jimma University Medical Centre were included. The incidence, prevalence and risk factors of healthcare associated infection were determined. A total of 1015 admitted patients were followed throughout their hospital stay. Biological specimens were collected from all patients suspected to have hospital aquired infection. The specimens were processed by standard microbiological methods to isolate and identify bacteria etiology. Clinical and laboratory data were collected using structured case report formats.

Results: The incidence rate of hospital acquired infection was 28.15 [95% C.I:24.40,32.30] per 1000 patient days while the overall prevalence was 19.41% (95% C.I: (16.97–21.85). The highest incidence of HAI was seen in intensive care unit [207.55 (95% C.I:133.40,309.1) per 1000 patient days] and the lowest incidence was reported from ophthalmology ward [0.98 (95% C.I: 0.05,4.90) per 1000patient days]. Among patients who underwent surgical procedure, the risk of HAI was found to be high in those with history of previous hospitalization (ARR = 1.65, 95% C.I:1.07, 2.54). On the other hand, young adults (18 to 30-year-old) had lower risk of developing HAI (ARR = 0.54 95% C.I: 0.32,0.93) Likewise, among non-surgical care groups, the risk of HAI was found to be high in patients with chest tube (ARR = 4.14, 95% C.I: 2.30,7.46), on mechanical ventilation (ARR = 1.99, 95% C.I: 1.06,3.74) and with underlying disease (ARR = 2.01, 95% C.I: 1. 33,3.04). Furthermore, hospital aquired infection at the hosoital was associated with prolonged hospital stay [6.3 more days, 95% C.I: (5.16,7.48), t = 0.000] and increased in hospital mortality (AOR, 2.23, 95% CI:1.15,4.29).

Conclusion: This study revealed high burden and poor discharge outcomes of healthcare associated infection at Jimma University Medical Centre. There is a difference in risk factors between patients with and without surgery. Hence, any effort to control the observed high burden of HAI at the hospital should consider these differences for better positive out put.

Keywords: Health-care associated infection, Nosocomial infection, Jimma, Ethiopia, Africa

* Correspondence: solali2005@gmail.com; Solomon.ali@ju.edu.et
†Equal contributors
[1]School of Medical laboratory Science, Institute of Health, School of Medical laboratory Science, Jimma University, P.O. Box 1368, Jimma, Ethiopia
[9]WHO-TDR clinical research former fellow at AERAS Africa and Rockville, Rockville, MD, USA
Full list of author information is available at the end of the article

Background

Healthcare associated infection (HAI) is localized or systemic condition resulting from adverse reaction to the presence of infectious agent or its toxins acquired from health care settings that was not incubating or symptomatic at the time of admission to the healthcare facility [1]. It accounts for a large proportion of damages caused by healthcare processes in both developed countries and low income settings [2–4]. HAI is increasingly becoming a major global public health problem posing great threat to patient safety and wellbeing of healthcare providers [5, 6].

HAIs contribute to increased morbidity and mortality [7, 8], excess health care cost [9, 10] and prolonged hospital stay [11]. It has a far reaching consequence to the public resulting in widespread occurrence of multidrug resistant pathogens in hospital settings [12, 13] and dissemination of emerging and re-emerging infections to healthcare providers and the community [14, 15].

HAI affects about 7.6% of patients in regular wards [16] and at least half of those admitted to intensive care units (ICU) [17] in developed countries. The magnitude of the problem in the low-income settings remains largely unknown and in most cases underestimated due to the complex nature of its diagnosis and lack of proper surveillance [18, 19]. Studies conducted in low-income settings showed that hospital-wide prevalence of HAI is about 15.5 per 100 patients [18] which is much higher than reports from Europe [20] and North America [21]. As a matter of fact, most of the global reports of HAIs are focused on prevalence and there are only very few reports about the incidence rate of HAIs.

In Ethiopia, few HAIs studies focused on point prevalence are available since 1988 [22, 23]. Many of these were limited to postoperative HAIs [22–25] with estimated prevalence of 11% to 36% [24–27]. Surgical site, urinary tract and blood stream infections were found to be commonest forms [24–26]. The type of surgery, patients' underlying medical conditions and the type of the ward were found to be important factors associated with increased risk of HAI in Ethiopia [22, 23, 28, 29].

At least 50% of HAIs are preventable with current evidence based interventions [19, 30]. Despite this fact, they remain great threat to quality of healthcare delivery system worldwide and even more so in low-income settings. Overcrowding and limited number of health task force in hospitals result in inadequate infection control practices. On top of these, lack of infection control policies, guidelines and trained professionals make the problem even worse [18, 19].

To the best of our knowledge, there is no single report about the incidence rate of HAIs from Ethiopia before. All previously published studies were estimted the point prevalence of HAIs based on a data collected from one or two wards of respective hospitals [22–27]. In the current study, we tried to estimate the incidence rate of HAI at tertiary hospital in southwest Ethiopia. The study also aimed to provide a comprhensive hospital level prevalence data to overcome the limitations in the previous reports from the country as most of them were limited to few wards and units.

Methods

Setting

The study was conducted at Jimma University Medical Centre (JUMC) in southwest Ethiopia. It is the only referral and teaching medical centre in the region serving over 15 million people. The annual average admission of the centre is over 15,000 patients (https://www.ju.edu.et/jimma-university-specialized-hospital-jush).

Study design and study population

A hospital based longitudinal study design was conducted from May 1 to September 30, 2016. All patients admitted to ICU, gynaecology & obstetrics, paediatrics, surgical, ophthalmology, and medical wards with no evidence of bacterial infections at admission were included in the study.

Data collection procedures

Written consent was obtained from each participant prior to commencing any study procedures. For pediatric participants consent from the parents/ legal gardians together with an assent from the child was obtained. For patients in comma, their closest relatives were consented. Socio-demographic and clinical data were collected by structured questioner (Additional file 1). They were followed first for 48 h. Patients who have developed any form of infection within 48 h of admission and/or had asymptomatic bacteriuria were excluded. All the rest of the patients were followed until discharge for the occurrence of HAI, progress or death by attending physician and research staffs. Occurance of HAI was confirmed by sinior specilsts of this research team members working in respective wards. All clinical data from all participants were registered on case report form (CRF).

Biological specimens were collected from those participants suspected to have HAI. The specimens were investigated by microbiological methods following WHO manual to isolate the culprit bacteria [31]. Furthermore, blood culture was done by using BD BACTEC™ FX40 blood culture system as per manufacturers' instruction.

Definition of outcome variables

The primary outcome variable was occurrence of infection after 48 h of hospitalization in a patient otherwise not having symptomatic or incubating infection on hospital admission. The following are definitions used in this study for specific type of HAI (*Adopted from* Centre for disease control/National Health care Safety Network (*CDC/NHSN*) *surveillance definition for health care–associated infection* [1] with slight modification):

Blood stream infection

Patient with any of the following signs and symptoms: fever (>38 °C), Chills/rigours or hypotension and at least one positive blood culture not related to contamination.

Healthcare associated pneumonia

Respiratory symptoms with at least two of the following signs and symptoms appearing during hospitalization: cough, purulent sputum, new infiltrate on chest radiograph consistent with infection.

Surgical site infection

Any purulent discharge, abscess, or spreading cellulitis at the surgical site during the month after the operation.

Urinary tract infection

Mid-stream urine cultures with $\geq 10^5$ colony forming units (CFU) and catheter urine with $\geq 10^2$ CFU/ml with no more than 2 species of microorganisms isolated OR positive dipstick for leukocyte esterase OR pyuria (≥ 10 white blood cells /high power field) of clean catch urine in a patients with or without signs and symptoms in the presence or absence of recent urinary catheterization.

Data management and analysis

The collected data were checked for completeness and then entered to EpiData version 3.1. Then, it was exported to STATA® version 10.0. (College Station, TX: StataCorp LP) and SPSS® Statistics for Windows, Version 20.0 (Armonk, NY: IBM Corp) for analysis. Incidence and prevalence of nosocomial infection was determined at the confidence interval of 95%. Chi-square test was done to identify factors associated with HAIs first. Then bi-variate and multivariate logistic regression was used to depict the risk ratio (RR) and adjusted risk ratio (ARR) to identify factors with increased risk of HAIs. A *p*-value of <0.05 was used as level of statistical significance.

Data quality control

All data collectors were trained on basic procedures of data collection. Data collection was closely supervised by principal investigators. To ensure quality of clinical data and specimen, all clinical information were collected by trained treating physicians and research nurses in each ward. Clinical specimens were collected and processed as per Standard Operating procedures (SOPs) for isolation and identification of bacteria. Qualities of prepared culture plates and broth were checked for their sterility and performance as per the SOP. All laboratory tests were performed by qualified laboratory professionals after one day orientation training.

Results

Socio-demographic characteristics of the participants

A total of 1069 hospitalized patients were enrolled in this study. However, 54 participants showed signs of infection and/or asymptomatic bacteriuria within the first 48 h and were excluded from the study. The rest 1015 were followed for the occurrence of hospital acquired infection until discharge or death. From these, 23 participants were excluded from final analysis due to incomplete data set. A total of 992 participants were included in the final analysis.

About 55% of the participants were female. The mean age in years was 34.12 (SD ± 16.86). Almost half (49.20%) of the participants were younger than 30 years of age (Table 1). Obstetrics and gynaecology, surgical, and medical wards constituted for around a quarter of participants each. Furthermore, 22 (2.22%) of the participants were included from intensive care unit (ICU) (Table 1). More than half, 510 (51.41%) of the participants underwent surgical procedures during the current admission. From these, 244 (47.94%) had emergency surgical procedures of which majority, 149 (61.07%), had Caesarean section.

Underlying chronic medical conditions were reported by 263 (26.54%) participants. Cardiovascular diseases was the most common co-morbidity identified in 67 (25.48%) participants followed by hypertension, 57 (21.67%) and diabetes mellitus (DM) 39 (14.83%). Severe acute malnutrition, mainly among paediatric patients and HIV infection were also reported in 23 (8.75%) participants each. Twenty (7.60%) of participants were already diagnosed with different forms of cancer and tuberculosis each. Chronic renal failure was also reported from 14 (5.32%) participants, Overall, 76 (7.66%) patients have also reported history of prior hospitalization for either the same as current reason of admission or other ailments.

Incidence, prevalence and type of health care associated infection

The mean onset of HAI is 4.64 (95% C.I:4.42, 8.86) patient days. The overall incidence rate of HAI at JUMC was 28.15 (95% C.I 24.40, 32.30) per 1000 patient days while the prevalence was 19.41% (195/992) (95% C.I: 16.97, 21.85). Stratification of the incidence by ward of admission revealed significant variability. The highest incidence rate was seen in ICU (207.60, 95% C.I:133.40, 309.10) per 1000 patient days. Conversely, the lowest incidence rate of HAIs was seen in ophthalmology ward (0.98, 95% C.I: 0.05, 4.90) per 1000 patient days. The incidence rate of HAIs in paediatrics and surgical wards were 69.16 (95% C.I:45.30,101.30) and 29.55 (95% C.I: 23.1,37.2) per 1000 patient days respectively (Fig. 1).

Table 1 Background characteristics of the patients admitted to Jimma University Medical Centre, Ethiopia

Characteristic	Frequency	Proportion in % (95% CI)
Sex		
Male	443	44.66 (41.41.56–47.76)
Female	549	55.34 (52.24–58.44)
Age in Years		
< 18	147	14.82 (12.60–17.03)
18–30	341	34.38 (31.41–37.33)
31–45	269	27.12 (24.35–29.88)
> 45	235	23.69 (21.04–26.34)
Residency		
Urban	361	36.39 (33.39–39.39)
Rural	631	63.861 (60.61–66.61)
Occupation[a]		
Farmer	371	37.40 (34.38–40.41)
Employed	148	14.92 (12.70–17.14)
Student	108	10.89 (8.95–12.82)
Merchant	102	10.28 (8.39–12.18)
Daily labourer	84	8.47 (6.73–10.20)
Others	179	18.08 (15.65–20.44)
Marital Status[b]		
Married	700	70.56 (67.72–73.41)
Single	180	24.09 (21.43–26.76)
Divorced	27	2.72 (1.71–3.74)
Widowed	26	2.62 (1.63–3.62)
Education		
Illiterate	448	45.16 (42.06–48.26)
Read & write	127	12.80(10.72–14.89)
Elementary school	151	15.22 (12.98–17.46)
High school	93	9.38 (7.56–11.19)
Diploma	81	8.17 (6.46–9.87)
First degree	70	7.06 (5.46–8.65)
Above first degree	22	2.22 (1.30–3.14)
Ward of admission		
Obstetrics and Gynaecology	282	28.43 (25.62–31.24)
Surgical	253	25.50 (22.79–28.22
Medical	223	22.48 (19.88–25.08)
Ophthalmology	153	15.42 (13.17–17.67)
Paediatrics	59	5.95 (4.47–7.42)
ICU	22	2.22 (1.23–3.14)

[a]Parental occupation and education in case of paediatrics, *ICU* intensive care unit

[b]59 paediatrics participants were excluded

The most frequently observed type of hospital acquired infection was UTI reported in 68.71% of the cases (alone and in combination with other infections) followed by surgical site infection (SSI), 28.72% (alone and in combination with other infections). It is observed that 27.69% of the participants had developed two types of HAI at the same time (Fig. 2).

Clinical samples were collected from 192 (97.46%) participants with HAI to identify causative microorganism. Three requested specimens were missed because participants were not able to give the specimen. Overall, 22 species of bacteria were isolated from 118 specimen which gives 118/192 (61.46%) culture positivity rate. Of these, 16 (72.73%) were Gram negative and (27.27%) were Gram positive bacteria. The most common isolated bacteria were *Escherichia coli* (26.27%), *Klebsella species* (24.58%) and *Staphylococcus aureus* (17.80%).

Comparison of participants with HAI and without HAI

From the total enrolled 992 participants, 22 of them were admitted to ICU. Furthermore, 50 patients had cataract surgery and were admitted to ophthalmology ward. Most patients admitted to ICU were younger than 24 years of age (59.09%), on mechanical ventilator (57.14%), on NG tube (54.55%), on peripheral IV line (72.73%) and had indwelling urinary catheter (59.09%). However, statistical analysis could not be applied for analysis of risks since all patients admitted to ICU had developed HAIs. On the other hand, only 1 participant with cataract surgery had developed HAI. Again, it is not possible to apply statistical test to analyse risks of HAIs in this ward. Thus, 22 participants admitted to ICU and 50 participants who had cataract surgery were excluded from risk factor analysis.

We have stratified the rest 920 participants in to two groups based on whether they had surgical procedures or not to precisely identify risk factors for those with and without surgery. Accordingly, 450 participants had surgery and grouped as "Surgical care". The rest 470 participants didn't have any surgery and grouped as "Non-surgical care". The demographic and baseline clinical characteristics were compared between patients who developed HAIs and those who did not in each specific group (Table 2).

Among surgical care participants, bi-variate analysis of risk ratio has indicated that male gender, having elective surgery, clean contaminated wound and history of previous hospitalization to predispose for HAIs (Table 2). However, the adjusted risk ratio analysis controlled for cofounders, stratified by age and gender has indicated that only participants with history of previous hospitalization had higher risk of developing HAIs (ARR = 1.65, 95% C.I:1.07, 2.54) (Table 2).

The mean age of participants with HAIs grouped under surgical care was 35.11 ± 20.07SD. This value is significantly higher than the mean age of the participants with no HAIs (31.09 ± 13.76SD, $t = 0.022$) in the same group. On the other hand multivariate adjusted risk ratio

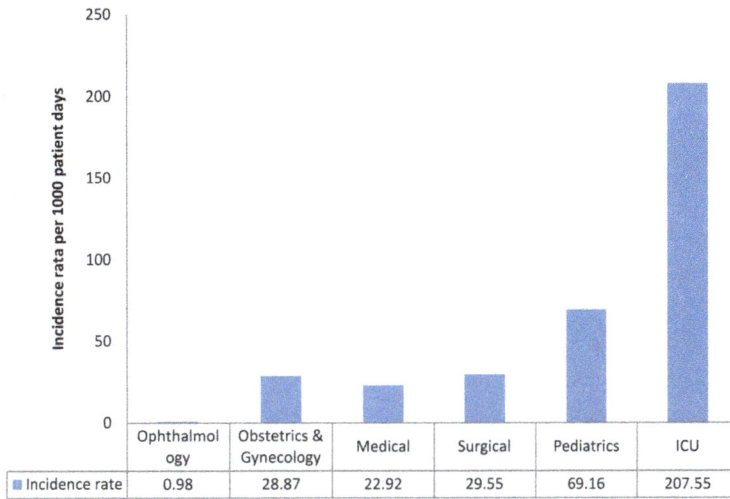

Fig. 1 Incidence rate of healthcare associated infection in different wards of admission at Jimma University Medical Centre, Ethiopia

analysis has indicated that age group between 18 and 30 years had lower risk of developing HAIs (ARR = 0.54 95% C.I: 0.32,0.93)(Table 2).

Among non-surgical patients, bi-variate analysis of risk ratio has indicated that chest tube, indwelling urinary catheter, mechanical ventilation and underlying disease were the risk factors for HAIs. However, the multivariate analysis to depict adjusted risk ratio (ARR) indicated that chest tube (ARR = 4.14, 95% C.I: 2.30,7.46), mechanical ventilation (ARR = 1.99, 95% C.I: 1.06,3.74) and underlying diseases (ARR = 2.01, 95% C.I: 1.33,3.04) were only the risk factors for developing HAI (Table 2). The mean age of non surgical patients with HAI was $27.96 \pm 16.44SD$

which is significantly lower than the mean age of participants with no HAI 36.52 ± 17.17, $t = 0.0001$. However, the risk of HAI is low between age 30 and 45 (ARR = 0.54, 95% C.I: 0.31,0.93), and among participants older than 45 years of age (ARR = 0.22, 95% C.I:0.10,0.48).

HAI and discharge outcome
The mean duration of hospital stay for HAI patients was 13.95 days (SD ± 8.99) while that of patients without HAI was 7.63 days (SD ± 6.86). There is a significant mean difference of 6.32 days [(SE of difference = 0.59), 95% C.I: (5.16, 7.48), t = 0.000] between the two groups.

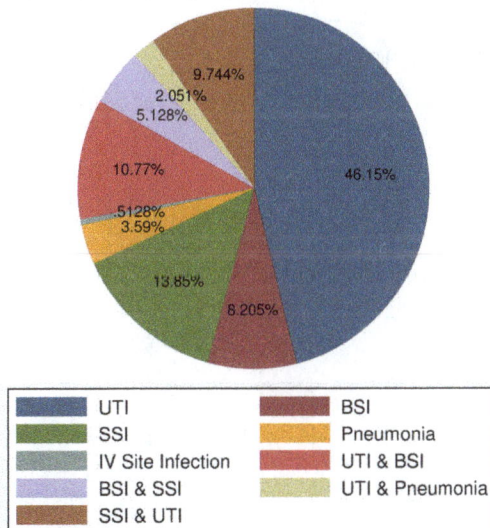

Fig. 2 Type of Healthcare associated infection at Jimma University Medical Centre, Ethiopia, where BSI – blood stream infection, IV – intravenous, SSI – surgical site infection, UTI – urinary tract infection

Table 2 Risk of HAI in relation to age, sex, underlying disease and healthcare risk factors among patients with surgical care and without

Variable	Surgical care ($n = 450$)				Non-surgical care ($n = 470$)			
	HAI (%/)***	Total	RR (95% CI)	ARR(95% CI)	HAI (%)	Total	RR(95%CI)	ARR(95% CI)
Age in years								
< 18	20(33.33)	60			20(27.40)	73		
18–30	28(13.53)	207	0.41(0.25,0.67)*	0.54(0.32,0.93)*	19(15,45)	123	0.56(0.32,0.98)	0.61(0.34,1.07)
31–45	25(22.94)	109	0.69(0.42,1.13)	0.94(0.56,1.55)	27(18.24)	148	0.67(0.40,1.10)	0.54(0.31,0.93)
> 45	26(35.14)	74	1.05(0.66,1.69)	1.07(0.66,1.46)	7(5.56)	126	0.20(0.09,0.46)	0.22(0.10,0.48)
Gender								
Male	52(30.95)	168	1.85 (1.32,2.62)*	1.44(0.97,2.14)	32(13.79)	232	0.80, (0.52,1.22)	0.97(0.64,1.49)
Female	47(16.67)	282			41(17.23)	238		
Previous hospitalization###								
Yes	20(44.44)	45	2.28(1.56,3.34)*	1.65(1.07,2.54)	6(23.08)	26	1.53(0.73,3.19)	
No	79(19.51)	405			67(15.09)	444		
Type of surgery					NA			
Elective	60(27.03)	222	1.58 (1.10, 2.26)*	0.98(0.65,1.46)				
Emergency	39(17.11)	228						
Type of wound #					NA			
Contaminated/ dirty	13(23.64)	55	1.30(0.77,2.22)	0.81(0.47,1.42)				
Clean contaminated	28(35.90)	78	1.98(1.35,2.89)*	1.28(0.85,1.94)				
Clean	56 (18.12)	309						
Recent endotracheal intubation								
Yes	24(19.83)	121	0.87(0.58,1.31)		2(40)	5	2.62(0.87,7.82)	
No	75(22.80)	329			71(15.27)	465		
Chest tube								
Yes	2(16.67)	12	0.75(0.21,2.70)		3(75.00)	4	5.05(2.75,9.26)*	4.14(2.30,7.46)
No	97(22.15)	438			69(14.84)	465		
Mechanical ventilator								
Yes	3(37.50)	8	1.72(0.69,4.29)		12(35.29)	34	2.52(1.51,4.20)*	1.99(1.06,3.74)
No	96(21.72)	442			61(13.99)	436		
Indwelling urinary catheter								
Yes	48(19.12)	251	0.74(0.53,1.05)		17(28.33)	60	2.07(1.29,3.32)*	1.28(0.76,2.14)
No	51(25.63)	199			56(13.66)	410		
IV line								
Yes	80(21.45)	373	0.87(0.56,1.34)		30(20.13)	149	1.50(0.98,2.29)	
No	19(24.68)	77			43(13.40)	321		
Naso-gastric tube								
Yes	3(9.68)	31	0.42(0.14,1.25)		5(25.00)	20	1.67(0.76,3.69)	
No	96(22.91)	419			67(14.32)	449		
Preoperative prophylaxis#					NA			
Given	88(22.11)	398	0.98(0.56,1.71)					
Not given	11(22.45)	49						
Underlying disease								
Yes	9(13.85)	65	0.59(0.31,1.11)		44(24.58)	179	2.54(1.64,3.93)*	2.01(1.33,3.04)
No	90(23.38)	385			28(9.66)	290		

*** Percentage was calculated from row total, *RR* relative risk, *ARR* Adjusted relative risk, *CI* – confidence interval, * Statistically significant # please note missing participant, ### participants who had history of hospital admission in the past five years

Overall, there were 44 deaths (in hospital mortality rate of 4.3%). The mortality rate in those with hospital acquired infection was 7.5%. Patients who developed HAI had 2.24 times increased risk of dying in the hospital (COR = 2.24, 95% CI:1.18–4.27, $P = 0.014$) than those who did not have it. This association persisted even after controlling for age, sex and underlying medical condition (AOR = 2.23, 95% CI: (1.15–4.29, $p = .017$).

Discussion

The over all incidence rate of healthcare associated infection at JUMC is 28.15 per 1000 patient days. This is the first report for incidence rate of HAI from Ethiopia. It is higher than finding from Europe [32]. Our study also revealed an overall prevalence rate of HAI of 19.41%; a finding which is again much higher than most reports from high income settings [16, 20, 21]. It is also higher than the reported prevalence from some of the studies done in the country [25, 26]. This might be associated with the comprehensive nature of this study which involved all admitted patients including those in intensive care and those with debilitating medical conditions. These might have contributed for the observed higher prevalence.

When compared with other similar studies done in Africa, the finding of this study is higher than reports from Nigeria (2.6%), Morocco (10.3%) and Tanzania (14.8%) [33–35]. This could be explained by the high patient load, overcrowding, poor infrastructure and design of the hospital layout. On the other hand, the observed prevalence of HAI in this study is lower than reported prevalence from Addis Ababa (35.8%) and Mekelle (27.6%) [24, 27].

The incidence rate of HAI at different wards indicated a large variability that ranges from 0.98 per 1000 patient days at ophthalmology ward to 207.55 per 1000 patient days at Intensive care unit (ICU). It is not surprising to see such high incidence of HAI at ICU given that most of the patients admitted to ICU are debilitated, critical and subjected to insertion of different medical devices. Such patients are at high risk of developing any infection especially in facilities with substandard infection prevention practice [36]. Studies in both low-and-middle, and high income countries also revealed the highest rates of HAI in ICU. Even in settings with better standards of care, HAI may affect up to half of patients in ICU [17]. Findings from other settings also revealed high prevalence of HAI in intensive care setting, 34.5% in Morocco and 46.7% from Saudi Arabia [34, 37].

In addition to patient and healthcare setting related factors, HAI is often related to surgical wounds and presence of indwelling devises [16]. As a result, urinary tract and surgical site infections remain the commonest forms [16, 24, 33]. In our study, UTI was found to be the commonest form of HAI followed by surgical site infection. Even though this is consistent with findings in different settings, the proportion of UTI in this study (68.71%) is higher than findings in the other studies [34, 38]. This might be associated with the diverse nature of our participants and high rate of urinary catheterization. Moreover, 50.85% of UTI were associated with indwelling urinary catheter.

Our finding has also revealed that the observed HAI infections are more of systemic infection than localized wound or soft tissue infection as evidenced by 27.69% of them developing two or more types of HAIs at the same time. Nevertheless, the overlap of multiple HAI in such patients deserves utmost attention due to the magnitude of the problem and threat to patient population getting service at the hospital. In line with this, the two most frequently isolated bacteria were *E.coli and Klebsella species.* These bacteria are known to cause community acquired UTI in Ethiopia [39, 40]. This finding suggests that these bacteria are also the main etiologist of nosocomial UTI and they might have colonized the medical devices or the hospital environment.

This study has indicated that among surgical care group the risk of HAI is higher on patients with history of previous hospitalization and lower in young adults (18–30 years). It is possible to speculate that patients who did visit hospitals frequently might have some chronic underlying disease which potentially expose them for HAIs. Furthermore, the possibility of colonozation by drug resistant bacteria in those with previous hospitalization might have also contributed to the occurrence of HAI in the current admission. On the other hand, the fact that young adults have better overall health status may expalin the lower risk of HAI in this group of patients.

The risk of HAI among non-surgical patients were higher on patients with chest tube, mechanical ventilator and those with underlying diseases. This result suggests most of HAIs in this group of patients related to contamination of the medical devices by bacteria. This can be due to improper handling and storage, and/or substandard application of aseptic procedures during handling, insertion and removal of the medical devices. This situation might also be further fueled by the existance of one or more underlying medical conditions.

Our study revealed a twofold increment in mortality in patients who developed HAI. Besides, six additional days of hospital stay in patients with HAI in this study is already a huge healthcare cost in any setting and deserves emergency action. As some of these patients might have also left the hospital setting without proper treatment, they risk potential dreadful outcome to themselves and dissemination of multidrug resistant strains to the community. This, in places where antibiotic choices are limited and health care seeking behaviour is low, may perpetuate a vicious circle that may affect the whole healthcare system unless kept in check urgently.

The strength of this study is that it included patients admitted to all wards of the hospital; prospectively followed them until discharge implementing proper technique for identification and susceptibility testing of causative bacteria. However, the full burden of HAI could not be captured as our study was limited to in hospital assessment leaving out patients who may potentially develop HAI after discharge. The second limitation is associated with failure to include neonatal ICU which may portray different nature of HAI to other types reported here. It should also be noted that our microbiological assessment was limited to bacterial HAI without considering other causes such as fungal infection. As this is the first comprehensive assessment to report incidence and prevalence of HAI at the hospital, we strongly believe that this finding may provide valuable imput to plan for proper intervention.

Conclusion and recommendations

Hospital acquired infection is a significant problem at Jimma University Medical Centre. The problem is immense at ICU, Paediatrics and Surgical wards. Risk factors for HAI among patients who had surgery is different from those patients who did not have surgical intervention. Previous hospitalization history was the main independent risk factor for patients who had surgery. Whereas, insertion of medical devices and underlying diseases were the main risk factors for patients who did not have surgery. HAI was also associated with increased mortality and prolonged hospital stay. Hence, any prospective effort to control HAI at JUMC should consider this risk factor differences to tackle the problem with maximum positive outcome.

Abbreviations

BSI: Blood stream infection; HAI: Health care associated infection; ICU: Intensive care unit; JUMC: Jimma University Medical Center; NI: Nosocomial infection; SSI: Surgical site infection; UTI: Urinary tract infection

Acknowledgements
We would like to thank Jimma University for the financial support. Jimma University Medical Centre for the support during data collection and the participants for giving us all information we needed unreservedly.

Funding
This project was funded by Jimma University through institute of Health, Research and publication office.

Authors' contributions
SA, MB and EKG equality contributed in study design, instrument development, supervision of data collection, analysis and manuscript writing. SB, GK, LT, YY, YA, NF, HA, MG participated in study design, development of instruments, supervision of data collection and writing of the manuscript. All the authors have read the manuscript and have approved it.

Consent for publication
Not applicable – This manuscript does not contain any individual person's data.

Competing interests
The authors declare that they have no competing interests.

Author details
[1]School of Medical laboratory Science, Institute of Health, School of Medical laboratory Science, Jimma University, P.O. Box 1368, Jimma, Ethiopia. [2]Department of paediatrics and child health, Jimma University, Jimma, Ethiopia. [3]Department of ophthalmology, Jimma University, Jimma, Ethiopia. [4]Department of Surgery, Jimma University, Jimma, Ethiopia. [5]Department of Obstetrics and Gynaecology, Jimma University, Jimma, Ethiopia. [6]Department of Health education and behavioural health, Jimma University, Jimma, Ethiopia. [7]Department of Epidemiology, Jimma University, Jimma, Ethiopia. [8]Department of Internal Medicine, Jimma University, Jimma, Ethiopia. [9]WHO-TDR clinical research former fellow at AERAS Africa and Rockville, Rockville, MD, USA.

References
1. Horan TC, Andrus M, Dudeck MA. CDC/NHSN surveillance definition of health care-associated infection and criteria for specific types of infections in the acute care setting. Am J Infect Control. 2008;36(5):309–32.
2. Leape LL, Brennan TA, Laird N, et al. The nature of adverse events in hospitalized patients. Results of the Harvard medical practice study II. N Engl J Med. 1991;324(6):377–84.
3. Hauri AM, Armstrong GL, Hutin YJ. The global burden of disease attributable to contaminated injections given in health care settings. Int J STD AIDS. 2004;15(1):7–16.
4. Feinmann J. Unsafe surgery: make it zero. BMJ. 2011;343:d7773.
5. Rosenthal VD, Maki DG, Mehta Y, et al. International Nosocomial infection control consortium (INICC) report, data summary of 43 countries for 2007-2012. Device-associated module. Am J Infect Control. 2014;42(9):942–56.
6. Allegranzi B, Storr J, Dziekan G, Leotsakos A, Donaldson L, Pittet D. The first global patient safety challenge "clean care is safer care": from launch to current progress and achievements. J Hosp Infect. 2007;65(Suppl 2):115–23.
7. Schumacher M, Wangler M, Wolkewitz M, Beyersmann J. Attributable mortality due to nosocomial infections. A simple and useful application of multistate models. Methods Inf Med. 2007;46(5):595–600.
8. Dramowski A, Whitelaw A, Cotton MF. Burden, spectrum, and impact of healthcare-associated infection at a south African children's hospital. J Hosp Infect. 2016;94(4):364–72.
9. Nero DC, Lipp MJ, Callahan MA. The financial impact of hospital-acquired conditions. J Health Care Finance. 2012;38(3):40–9.
10. Fuller RL, McCullough EC, Bao MZ, Averill RF. Estimating the costs of potentially preventable hospital acquired complications. Health Care Financ Rev. 2009;30(4):17–32.
11. Forster AJ, Taljaard M, Oake N, Wilson K, Roth V, van Walraven C. The effect of hospital-acquired infection with Clostridium Difficile on length of stay in hospital. CMAJ. 2012;184(1):37–42.
12. Gandhi NR, Weissman D, Moodley P, et al. Nosocomial transmission of extensively drug-resistant tuberculosis in a rural hospital in South Africa. J Infect Dis. 2013;207(1):9–17.
13. Struelens MJ. The epidemiology of antimicrobial resistance in hospital acquired infections: problems and possible solutions. BMJ. 1998;317(7159):652–4.
14. Shears P, O'Dempsey TJ. Ebola virus disease in Africa: epidemiology and nosocomial transmission. J Hosp Infect. 2015;90(1):1–9.
15. Fu C, Wang S. Nosocomial infection control in healthcare settings: protection against emerging infectious diseases. Infect Dis Poverty. 2016;5:30.
16. Allegranzi B, Nejad SB, Castillejos GG, Kilpatrick C, Kelley E, Mathai E. Report on the burden of endemic health care–associated infection worldwide. Geneva, Switzerland: World Health Organization; 2011.

17. Vincent JL, Rello J, Marshall J, et al. International study of the prevalence and outcomes of infection in intensive care units. JAMA. 2009;302(21):2323–9.

18. Allegranzi B, Bagheri Nejad S, et al. Burden of endemic health-care-associated infection in developing countries: systematic review and meta-analysis. Lancet. 2011;377(9761):228–41.

19. Bagheri Nejad S, Allegranzi B, Syed SB, Ellis B, Pittet D. Health-care-associated infection in Africa: a systematic review. Bull World Health Organ. 2011;89(10):757–65.

20. Marschang S, Bernardo G. Prevention and control of healthcare-associated infection in Europe: a review of patients' perspectives and existing differences. J Hosp Infect. 2015;89(4):357–62.

21. Klevens RM, Edwards JR, Richards CL, et al. Estimating health care-associated infections and deaths in U.S. hospitals, 2002. Public Health Rep. 2007;122(2):160–6.

22. Gedebou M, Habte-Gabr E, Kronvall G, Yoseph S. Hospital-acquired infections among obstetric and gynaecological patients at Tikur Anbessa hospital, Addis Ababa. J Hosp Infect. 1988;11(1):50–9.

23. Habte-Gabr E, Gedebou M, Kronvall G. Hospital-acquired infections among surgical patients in Tikur Anbessa hospital, Addis Ababa, Ethiopia. Am J Infect Control. 1988;16(1):7–13.

24. Endalafer N, Gebre-Selassie S, Kotiso B. Nosocomial bacterial infections in a tertiary hospital in Ethiopia. J Infect Prev. 2011;12(1):38–43.

25. Mulu W, Kibru G, Beyene G, Damtie M. Postoperative Nosocomial infections and antimicrobial resistance pattern of bacteria isolates among patients admitted at Felege Hiwot referral hospital, Bahirdar, Ethiopia. Ethiop J Health Sci. 2012;22(1):7–18.

26. Yallew WW, Kumie A, Yehuala FM. Point prevalence of hospital-acquired infections in two teaching hospitals of Amhara region in Ethiopia. Drug Healthc Patient Saf. 2016;8:71–6.

27. Tesfahunegn Z, Asrat D, Woldeamanuel Y, Estifanos K. Bacteriology of surgical site and catheter related urinary tract infections among patients admitted in Mekelle hospital, Mekelle, Tigray. Ethiopia Ethiop Med J. 2009; 47(2):117–27.

28. Melaku S, Gebre-Selassie S, Damtie M, Alamrew K. Hospital acquired infections among surgical, gynaecology and obstetrics patients in Felege-Hiwot referral hospital, Bahir Dar, northwest Ethiopia. Ethiop Med J. 2012; 50(2):135–44.

29. Amenu D, Belachew T, Araya F. Surgical site infection rate and risk factors among obstetric cases of jimma university specialized hospital, southwest ethiopia. Ethiop J Health Sci. 2011;21(2):91–100.

30. Zimlichman E, Henderson D, Tamir O, et al. Health care–associated infections:AMeta-analysis of costs and financial impact on the US health care system. JAMA Intern Med. 2013;173(22):2039–46.

31. Vandepitte J, Verhaegen J, Engbaek K, Rohner P, Piot P, Heuck CC. Basic laboratory procedures in clinical bacteriology. Second ed. Geneva, Switzerland: World Health Organization; 2003.

32. Petersen MH, Holm MO, Pedersen SS, Lassen AT, Pedersen C. Incidence and prevalence of hospital-acquired infections in a cohort of patients admitted to medical departments. Dan Med Bul. 2010;57(11):A4210.

33. Ige OK, Adesanmi AA, Asuzu MC. Hospital-acquired infections in a Nigerian tertiary health facility: an audit of surveillance reports. Niger Med J. 2011; 52(4):239–43.

34. Razine R, Azzouzi A, Barkat A, et al. Prevalence of hospital-acquired infections in the university medical center of Rabat. Morocco Int Arch Med. 2012;5(1):26.

35. Gosling R, Mbatia R, Savage A, Mulligan JA, Reyburn H. Prevalence of hospital-acquired infections in a tertiary referral hospital in northern Tanzania. Ann Trop Med Parasitol. 2003;97(1):69–73.

36. Halle TG, Engeda EH, Abdo AA. Compliance with standard precautions and associated factors among healthcare Workers in Gondar University Comprehensive Specialized Hospital, Northwest Ethiopia. J Environ Public Health. 2017;2017:2050635.

37. Balkhy HH, Cunningham G, Chew FK, et al. Hospital- and community-acquired infections: a point prevalence and risk factors survey in a tertiary care center in Saudi Arabia. Int J Infect Dis. 2006;10(4):326–33.

38. Durando P, Bassetti M, Orengo G, et al. Hospital-acquired infections and leading pathogens detected in a regional university adult acute-care hospital in Genoa, Liguria, Italy: results from a prevalence study. J Prev Med Hyg. 2010;51(2):80–6.

39. Kibret M, Abera B. Prevalence and antibiogram of bacterial isolates from urinary tract infections at Dessie Health Research Laboratory, Ethiopia. Asian Pac J Trop Biomed. 2014;4(2):164–8.

34. Razine R, Azzouzi A, Barkat A, et al. Prevalence of hospital-acquired infections in the university medical center of Rabat. Morocco Int Arch Med. 2012;5(1):26.

35. Gosling R, Mbatia R, Savage A, Mulligan JA, Reyburn H. Prevalence of hospital-acquired infections in a tertiary referral hospital in northern Tanzania. Ann Trop Med Parasitol. 2003;97(1):69–73.

36. Haile TG, Engeda EH, Abdo AA. Compliance with standard precautions and associated factors among healthcare Workers in Gondar University Comprehensive Specialized Hospital, Northwest Ethiopia. J Environ Public Health. 2017;2017:2050635.

37. Balkhy HH, Cunningham G, Chew FK, et al. Hospital- and community-acquired infections: a point prevalence and risk factors survey in a tertiary care center in Saudi Arabia. Int J Infect Dis. 2006;10(4):326–33.

38. Durando P, Bassetti M, Orengo G, et al. Hospital-acquired infections and leading pathogens detected in a regional university adult acute-care hospital in Genoa, Liguria, Italy: results from a prevalence study. J Prev Med Hyg. 2010;51(2):80–6.

39. Kibret M, Abera B. Prevalence and antibiogram of bacterial isolates from urinary tract infections at Dessie Health Research Laboratory, Ethiopia. Asian Pac J Trop Biomed. 2014;4(2):164–8.

3

Reduced rate of intensive care unit acquired gram-negative bacilli after removal of sinks and introduction of 'water-free' patient care

Joost Hopman[1*†], Alma Tostmann[1†], Heiman Wertheim[1], Maria Bos[1], Eva Kolwijck[1], Reinier Akkermans[3], Patrick Sturm[1,4], Andreas Voss[1,2], Peter Pickkers[5] and Hans vd Hoeven[5]

Abstract

Background: Sinks in patient rooms are associated with hospital-acquired infections. The aim of this study was to evaluate the effect of removal of sinks from the Intensive Care Unit (ICU) patient rooms and the introduction of 'water-free' patient care on gram-negative bacilli colonization rates.

Methods: We conducted a 2-year pre/post quasi-experimental study that compared monthly gram-negative bacilli colonization rates pre- and post-intervention using segmented regression analysis of interrupted time series data. Five ICUs of a tertiary care medical center were included. Participants were all patients of 18 years and older admitted to our ICUs for at least 48 h who also received selective digestive tract decontamination during the twelve month pre-intervention or the twelve month post-intervention period. The effect of sink removal and the introduction of 'water-free' patient care on colonization rates with gram-negative bacilli was evaluated. The main outcome of this study was the monthly colonization rate with gram-negative bacilli (GNB). Yeast colonization rates were used as a 'negative control'. In addition, colonization rates were calculated for first positive culture results from cultures taken ≥3, ≥5, ≥7, ≥10 and ≥14 days after ICU-admission, rate ratios (RR) were calculated and differences tested with chi-squared tests.

Results: In the pre-intervention period, 1496 patients (9153 admission days) and in the post-intervention period 1444 patients (9044 admission days) were included. Segmented regression analysis showed that the intervention was followed by a statistically significant immediate reduction in GNB colonization in absence of a pre or post intervention trend in GNB colonization. The overall GNB colonization rate dropped from 26.3 to 21.6 GNB/1000 ICU admission days (colonization rate ratio 0.82; 95%CI 0.67–0.99; $P = 0.02$). The reduction in GNB colonization rate became more pronounced in patients with a longer ICU-Length of Stay (LOS): from a 1.22-fold reduction (≥2 days), to a 1.6-fold (≥5 days; $P = 0.002$), 2.5-fold (for ≥10 days; $P < 0.001$) to a 3.6-fold (≥14 days; $P < 0.001$) reduction.

Conclusions: Removal of sinks from patient rooms and introduction of a method of 'water-free' patient care is associated with a significant reduction of patient colonization with GNB, especially in patients with a longer ICU length of stay.

Keywords: Intensive care unit, Sinks, Gram-negative bacilli, Multidrug resistance, 'Water-free' patient care, Length of stay, Colonization

* Correspondence: Joost.Hopman@Radboudumc.nl
P. Pickkers and Hans vd Hoeven share senior authorship.
†Equal contributors
[1]Department of Medical Microbiology, Radboud university medical center, Geert Grooteplein 10, Postbus 9101, 6500, HB, Nijmegen, The Netherlands
Full list of author information is available at the end of the article

Background

Hospital acquired infections in the Intensive Care Unit (ICU) result in patient morbidity and mortality [1]. Environmental contamination in hospitals wards and ICUs is a recognized problem for infection prevention and control [2–7], as the environment may facilitate transmission of several important health care-associated pathogens, including gram-negative bacilli (GNB) [8]. As part of the traditional hospital hand hygiene strategy and patient care, sinks are present in virtually all hospital wards and patient rooms. While sinks in the proximity of patients are advocated as a best practice of ICU design [9], involvement of these sinks in hospital-associated infections have been reported as early as the 1970s [10–14]. Recent publications have highlighted the role of sinks as a source of outbreaks and transmission of multidrug-resistant gram-negative bacilli (MDR-GNB) in intensive care units, including paediatric and neonatal ICUs [15–28]. Interventions to reduce transmission of MDR-GNB from sinks in outbreak settings have been explored [29–31], while the effect of sinks on overall infection and colonization rates has not been studied.

As multi-drug resistance (MDR) in GNB is an increasing problem in the management of hospitalized patients [32–34], we investigated the effect of the removal of sinks from the ICU patient rooms combined with 'water-free' patient care on ICU-acquired GNB colonization rates in patients admitted to the ICU.

Methods

Background and study design

In early 2014 an outbreak with extended-spectrum β-lactamase (ESBL)-producing *Enterobacter cloacae* was identified in our ICU that could be related to contaminated sinks. When the decision to remove the sinks and to implement the 'water-free' patient care method was taken, it was prospectively decided to evaluate its effect after 12 months. We conducted a pre/post quasi-experimental study to evaluate the effect of sink removal and introduction of 'water-free' patient care on colonization with GNB in patients admitted to the ICU for at least 48 h during a 12-month pre-intervention (May 2013–April 2014), the months of intervention (May 2014–August 2014) and a 12-month post-intervention period (September 2014–August 2015).

Study setting

This study was conducted in a large tertiary care medical center in the Netherlands with 953 beds. The ICU consists of five subunits, with a total 34 operational single patient rooms. Patients admitted to the ICU that need mechanical ventilation and are anticipated to stay >24 h receive selective digestive tract decontamination (SDD), which consists of 4 days of intravenous cefotaxime and topical application of tobramycin, colistin, and amphotericin B in the oropharynx and stomach [35]. No alterations were made to the SDD protocol during the study period. An essential part of SDD strategy is twice a week routine screening for colonization with gram-negative bacilli and yeasts from rectal, sputum and throat swabs.

The intervention

Between May and August 2014, all sinks were removed from all ICU patient rooms and a 'water-free' method of patient care was introduced, meaning that all patient care related activities that take place in the patient room and that would normally involve the use of tap water were adapted to a 'water-free' alternative, see Table 1.

Patient selection and medical ethical aspects

All patients of 18 years and older who were admitted to the ICU for at least 48 h were included in this study. The study was reviewed and approved (File number CMO: 2015–1764) by the ethics committee of the Radboud university medical centre and was carried out in accordance with the applicable rules concerning biomedical research using patient information. Patient data were collected and analyzed anonymously.

Data collection

Data were collected in a standardized manner according to standard definitions and were subject to data quality checks [36]. Demographic information including sex and age, referring specialty and location before ICU admission, type of admission, comorbidity, Acute Physiology and Chronic Health Evaluation (APACHE) score, days on mechanical ventilation, and ICU length of stay, were

Table 1 'Water-free' patient care activities

Patient care-related action	New method with 'water-free' working
Gloves and gowns	Universal gloving and gowning (pre- and post-intervention period)
Hand washing after visual contamination	'Quick & Clean', (Alpheios B.V., Heerlen, The Netherlands) wipes to remove extensive contamination from hands. Followed by disinfection with alcohol-based hand rub
Medication preparation	Dissolving of medication in bottled water (SPA reine, Spa, Belgium)
Drinks	Bottled water (SPA reine, Spa, Belgium)
Canula care	Disposable materials
Hair washing	Rinse-free shampoo cap (Comfort Personal cleansing products, USA)
Washing	Moistened disposable wash gloves, (D-care,Houten, The Netherlands)
Dental care	Bottled (SPA reine, Spa, Belgium)
Shaving	Electric shaving, or with warm bottled water (SPA reine, Spa, Belgium)

collected. We collected culture results (from routine SDD screenings) from the medical microbiology laboratory database. Culture results from cultures taken <48 h of admission, including all repeat findings, were excluded from further analyses. When a patient was readmitted to the ICU during the study period, culture results identical to the first ICU admission were excluded.

Outcomes and definitions

The primary outcome of this study was the GNB colonization rate, calculated as the number of primary positive microbiological results per 1000 ICU admission days, during the pre- and post-intervention periods. The colonization rates of patients with yeasts were used as a 'negative control', as yeasts do not thrive in sinks and the ICU sinks at all times had been free of yeast colonization.

Statistical analysis

'To compare the patient characteristics between pre-intervention and post-intervention period, we described continuous data as mean ± standard deviation and groups were compared using a Student-t-test, or as median (25th and 75th percentile) and compared using a Mann-Whitney U test, depending on the distribution. Dichotomous or categorical data were described as number with percentage and subgroups were compared using a Chi-squared test. The pre- and post-intervention GNB and yeast colonization rates were calculated per 1000 admission days. The colonization rate ratios were (with 95% confidence interval (CI)) calculated to quantify the effect of the intervention on these rates. For calculating the subsequent colonization rates related to ICU- length of stay (LOS), only admissions of ≥3, ≥5, ≥7, ≥10 or ≥14 days were used for the denominator (number of admission days).

Segmented regression analysis of interrupted time series data was conducted to estimate the effect of the intervention on the monthly GNB and yeast colonization rates, both immediately and over time and to identify whether there was a baseline or a post-intervention monthly trend in colonization rate [37]. An autoregressive integrated moving average (ARIMA) model was used. The model was adjusted for negative first order autocorrelation by including an autocorrelation parameter in the segmented regression model [37]. To determine if colonization was likely to be ICU-acquired and to relate it to exposure duration, time-dependent (ICU-LOS) effects were investigated. In this ARIMA model, β_0 estimates the baseline level of the monthly colonization rate at time zero; β_1 estimates the pre-intervention or baseline linear trend of the monthly colonization rate; β_2 estimates the level change in the monthly colonization rate immediately after the intervention (i.e. step change or change in level: immediate effect of the intervention); and β_3 estimates the

post-intervention change in linear trend of the monthly colonization rate. Predicted rates are calculated based on model parameters. The rates during the intervention months (May 2014 – August 2014) were excluded from this analysis.

First, the full regression model was specified for the GNB and the yeast colonization, meaning that the following estimates were given: β_0, β_1, β_2, and β_3. After stepwise elimination of non-significant terms, the most parsimonious model contained only the intercept (β_0) and the significant level change (β_2) in the monthly colonization rate. This segmented regression analysis was performed on all GNB identified ≥2 days after ICU admission, and subsequently repeated for GNB first identified ≥3, ≥5, ≥7, ≥10 or ≥14 days after ICU admission, respectively.

If the segmented regression analysis would show that there was no monthly trend in GNB colonization either before or after the intervention, overall GNB colonization rates were calculated and compared between pre- and post-intervention and were defined as the number of GNB (or MDR-GNB) per 1000 ICU admission days. The rates during the intervention months (May 2014 – August 2014) were excluded from this analysis. Colonization rate ratios (and 95% confidence intervals) were calculated to quantify the effect of the intervention on the outcome and rates were compared using a Chi-squared test. This analysis was repeated for GNB identified ≥3, ≥5, ≥7, ≥10 or ≥14 days after ICU admission, respectively.

Statistical analysis was performed using IBM SPSS Statistics version 22 and STATA/SE version 11.0. A two-sided p-value <0.05 was considered to indicate statistical significance.

Results

An increased number of *Enterobacter cloacae* ESBL positive isolates was detected and communicated to the ICU in May 2014. In total 11 isolates pre and one isolate post-intervention were identified. By molecular typing we were able to show that 5 isolates were related pre-intervention. Sinks in the ICU were tested positive for *Enterobacter cloacae* ESBL prior to removal. The outbreak developed despite routine use of extensive infection prevention measures including the use of protective clothing and gloves with all patient contacts. It was decided to remove the sinks from all ICU patient rooms in order to eradicate the source of MDR-GNB in the direct patient environment.

1644 patients were admitted to the ICU in the 12 months prior to the removal of sinks from the ICU patient rooms, of which 1496 patients had a ICU-LOS ≥2 days (total 9153 admission days). In the 12 months after the removal of sinks, 1618 patients were admitted to the ICU, of which 1444 were in the ICU for ≥2 days (total 9044 admission days). 145 (9.7%) in the pre-intervention period and 137 (9.5%) post-intervention were re-admissions ($P = 0.85$). See Fig. 1.

The baseline demographic characteristics of the patients at ICU admission are described in Table 2. Apart from a statistically significant difference between pre- and post-intervention patients for chronic respiratory insufficiency as a comorbidity, no other relevant differences in demographics were observed. The median ICU-length of stay was 3 days (IQR 2–6 days) pre-intervention, and 3 days (IQR 2–6 days) post-intervention ($p = 0.90$). In the pre- and post-intervention periods, 31.2% and 30.5% ($P = 0.66$) had an ICU-LOS ≥5 days, and 15.6% and 16.1% ($P = 0.71$) had an ICU-LOS ≥ 10 days, respectively. Over a third of the ICU admissions (38.3% pre-intervention; 34.9% post-intervention; $P = 0.06$) had a type of registered comorbidity at admission. A statistically significant difference between pre- and post-intervention patients (7.8% vs 4.9%, respectively; $P = 0.002$) was observed for chronic respiratory insufficiency.

Interrupted time series analysis

The results of the segmented regression analysis are shown in Additional file 1: Table S1. There was a statistically significant immediate effect of the removal of sinks on the monthly colonization rate of GNB, but not on the colonization rate of yeasts, with statistically significant $\beta 2$ level changes for all GNB colonization outcomes for the different ICU LOS ($P = 0.037$ for ICU LOS ≥48 h, $P = 0.005$ for ICU LOS ≥3 days; $P = 0.001$ for ICU LOS ≥5 days; $P < 0.001$ for ICU LOS ≥7 days; $P = 0.005$ for ICU LOS ≥10 days; $P = 0.011$ for ICU LOS ≥14 days) . There was no pre-intervention drift in monthly GNB rates and this was also the case in the ICU-LOS-dependent analyses. Graphs with the observed and predicted colonization rates are shown in Fig. 2. The data for the interrupted time series analysis for yeast colonization are shown in Additional file 2: Figure S4.

In the most parsimonious model, the pre-intervention trend (β_1) and post-intervention trend-change (β_3) were omitted, resulting in a statistically significant immediate effect of the intervention on the GNB colonization rates.

Overall GNB colonization rates

The overall GNB colonization rates were 26.3 and 21.6 GNB/1000 ICU admission days (rate ratio 0.82; 95%CI 0.67–0.99; $P = 0.02$) for pre- and post-intervention groups, respectively. The difference between the groups became more pronounced over time: GNB colonization rates that were first identified in cultures taken ≥3 days (22.5 vs. 15.2; RR 0.68; 95%CI 0.53–0.86; $P < 0.001$), cultures taken ≥5 days (15.0 vs. 9.4; RR 0.63; 95%CI 0.45–0.87;

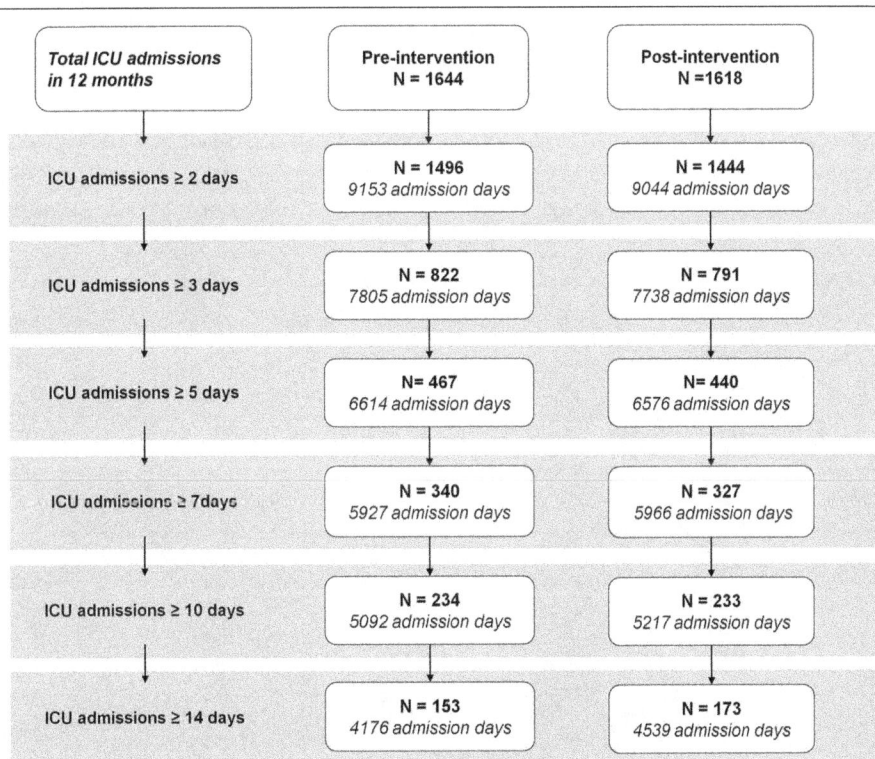

Fig. 1 Flow chart ICU admissions. Legend: Flowchart of the number of patients with an ICU-length of stay of ≥2 days, ≥3 days, ≥5 days, ≥7 days, ≥10 days and ≥14 days, and the subsequent number of admission days

Table 2 Characteristics of ICU admissions of ≥2 days before and after sink removal

	Pre intervention		Post intervention		
	n	%	n	%	P-value
ICU admissions with LOS of ≥48 h	N = 1496		N = 1444		
First or re-admission					
Primary admissions	1351	90.3%	1307	90.5%	0.85
Re-admissions	145	9.7%	137	9.5%	
Age, median (IQR)	62	[50–70]	63	[52–71]	0.07
Male sex, n (%)	890	59.5%	856	59.4%	0.94
BMI, mean (SD)	26.1	5.3	26.3	5.2	0.31
ICU mortality, n (%)	174	11.6%	146	10.1%	0.19
Hospital mortality, n (%)	225	15.0%	207	14.3%	0.59
ICU Lenght of stay (LOS), median days (IQR)	3	[2–6]	3	[2–6]	0.90
ICU LOS, n (%)					
2 days	674	45.1%	653	45.2%	0.38
3–4 days	355	23.7%	351	24.3%	
5–6 days	127	8.5%	113	7.8%	
7–9 days	106	7.1%	94	6.5%	
10–13 days	81	5.4%	60	4.2%	
≥ 14 days	153	10.2%	173	12.0%	
Apache score, mean (SD)	18.7	7.2	18.2	7.2	0.27
Days on respirator, median (IQR)	2	[0–4]	1	[0–4]	0.38
Comorbidity at ICU admission, n 'yes' (%)					
Any comorbidity	573	38.3%	504	34.9%	0.06
Cardiovascular insufficiency	93	6.2%	70	4.8%	0.11
Respiratory insufficiency	116	7.8%	71	4.9%	0.002
Diabetes	180	12.0%	168	11.6%	0.74
Chronic renal insufficiency	97	6.5%	83	5.7%	0.41
Neoplasm	130	8.7%	112	7.8%	0.36
Immune-insufficiency	166	11.1%	166	11.5%	0.93
Medical specialty, n (%)					
Surgery	330	22.1%	361	25.0%	0.04
Neurosurgery	239	16.0%	200	13.9%	
Thoracic surgery	234	15.6%	245	17.0%	
Pulmonary disease	125	8.4%	139	9.6%	
Internal medicine	64	4.3%	72	5.0%	
Other	504	33.7%	427	29.6%	
Admission type, n (%)					
Medical	732	48.9%	712	49.3%	0.06
Elective	528	35.3%	464	32.1%	
Emergency	236	15.8%	268	18.6%	
Admission source, n (%)					
Emergency	372	24.9%	344	23.8%	0.27
Clinical department	292	19.5%	302	20.9%	
Other IC unit	93	6.2%	69	4.8%	
Other	739	49.4%	729	50.5%	

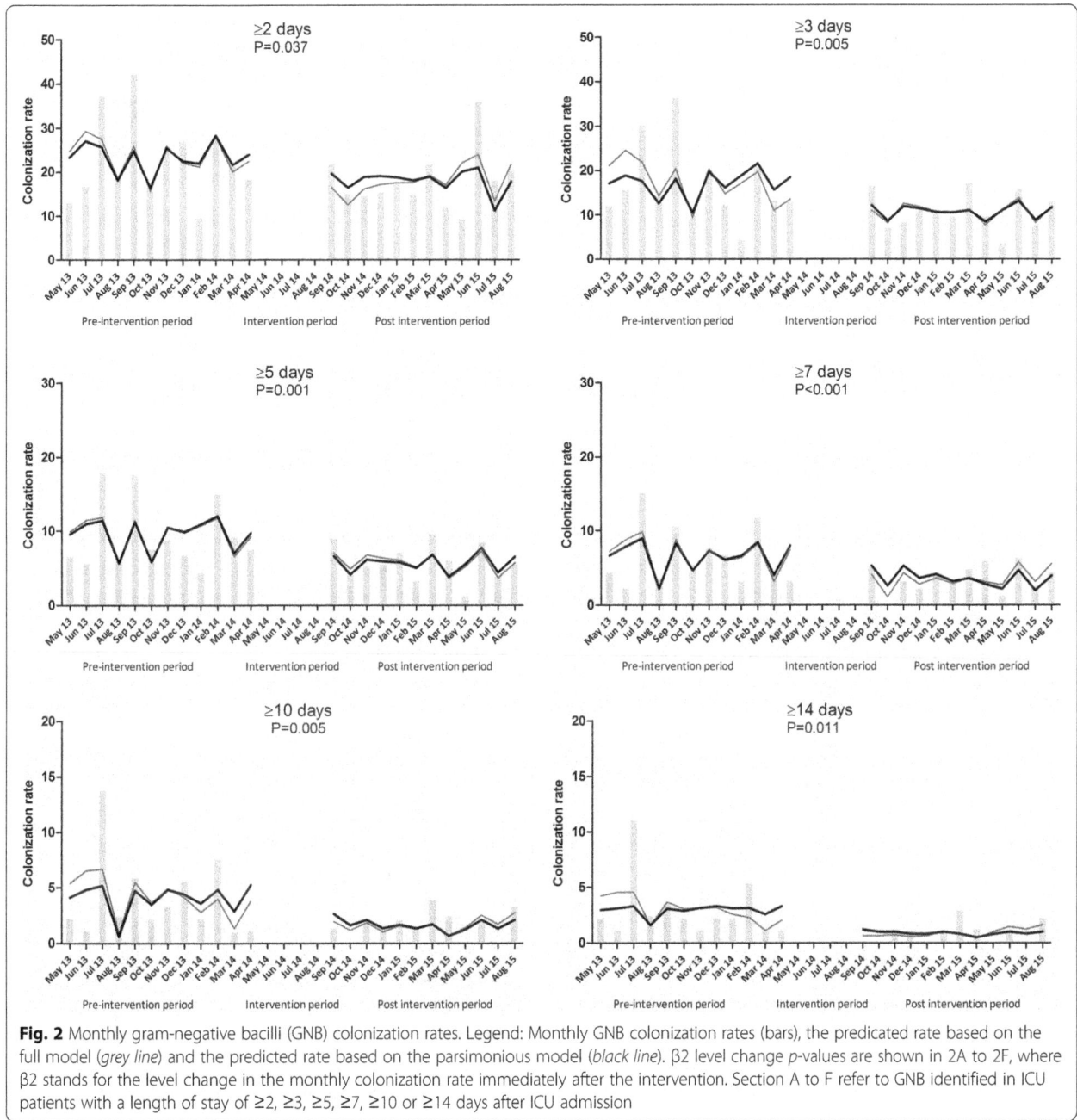

Fig. 2 Monthly gram-negative bacilli (GNB) colonization rates. Legend: Monthly GNB colonization rates (bars), the predicated rate based on the full model (*grey line*) and the predicted rate based on the parsimonious model (*black line*). β2 level change *p*-values are shown in 2A to 2F, where β2 stands for the level change in the monthly colonization rate immediately after the intervention. Section A to F refer to GNB identified in ICU patients with a length of stay of ≥2, ≥3, ≥5, ≥7, ≥10 or ≥14 days after ICU admission

P = 0.002), cultures taken ≥7 days (11.5 vs. 6.4; RR 0.56; 95%CI 0.36–0.84; P = 0.002), cultures taken ≥10 days (8.1 vs. 3.3; RR 0.40; 95%CI 0.22–0.73; P < 0.001) and cultures taken ≥14 days after ICU admission (7.2 vs. 2.0; RR 0.28; 95%CI 0.12–0.60; P < 0.001). As also illustrated by Fig. 3, the effect of the intervention in the GNB colonization rate increases with increasing LOS on patients at the ICU.

The (MDR-)GNB that were found on all time points are summarized in Additional file 3: Table S2.

Discussion

We have shown that the removal of sinks in patient rooms and implementation of water-free patient care is associated with a significant reduction of patient colonization with GNB and this effect was most pronounced in patients with a longer ICU length of stay.

The effect of the intervention on GNB colonization rates became even more apparent when pathogens that were first identified after longer durations of ICU stay were compared between the pre-intervention and post-

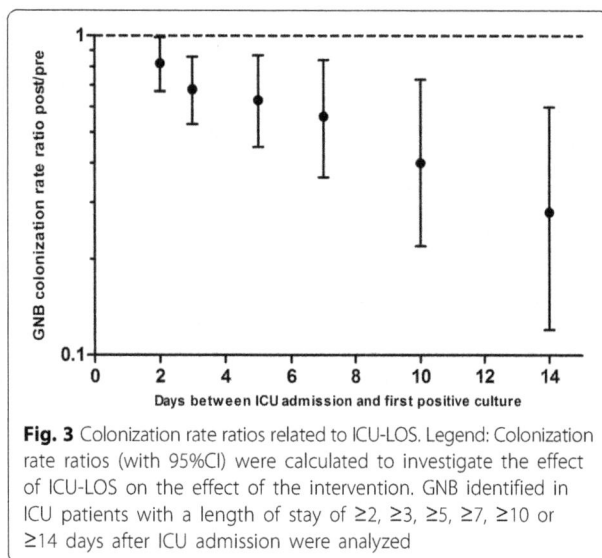

Fig. 3 Colonization rate ratios related to ICU-LOS. Legend: Colonization rate ratios (with 95%CI) were calculated to investigate the effect of ICU-LOS on the effect of the intervention. GNB identified in ICU patients with a length of stay of ≥2, ≥3, ≥5, ≥7, ≥10 or ≥14 days after ICU admission were analyzed

intervention period. Apart from the fact that with increased ICU-LOS the likelihood increases that these pathogens were acquired at the ICU, it appears plausible that a longer stay in an ICU increases the exposure to potential pathogens in the direct patient surroundings including those originated from the sinks.

The lower number GNB in the post-intervention period cannot be explained by an overall decrease in observed pathogens, as there was no effect of the intervention on yeast colonization rates. Yeast do not thrive in sinks or siphons and therefore we used them as a negative control. Furthermore, the overall number of cultures processed in the pre- and post-intervention study period were similar meaning that there was no reduction in the total number of screening cultures taken that could explain our findings.

In this study, we focused on colonization rates, and not infections. Even though infections caused by GNB would have been a more relevant clinical outcome than colonization, demonstrating the effect of an intervention on clinical infection rate would require a sample size that is not feasible. Previous work on the effects of SDD on infections with gram-negative bacilli showed that the cumulative incidence of ICU-acquired bacteremia in the SDD study group was 0.9%. To demonstrate a 30% reduction related to this intervention, approximately 26,000 patients would need to be included. Nevertheless, as colonization precedes infection, it is plausible that the intervention will have an impact on bloodstream infections with GNB.

Limitations of the study
Several limitations of this study need to be addressed. First and most importantly, this is an open label, non-randomized single-centre study. Naturally, the

implementation procedures importantly limited the feasibility of using other study designs. Despite of the design limitations, in the absence of alternative explanations, we believe that it is conceivable that the removal of sinks and implementation of water-free patient care resulted in a significant reduction of GNB colonization. There was no pre-existing downward drift in colonization rate, no changes were made during the study period in the hand hygiene protocol, protocol of standard or transmission-based precautions and the protocols of cleaning and disinfection. No chlorhexidine gluconate bathing is performed in our ICU. The quality of cleaning and disinfection remained constant and antibiotic guidelines did not alter during the study. The only difference between the pre- and post-intervention periods were the differences in some of the baseline demographic characteristics, e.g., patients in the pre-intervention period more often suffered chronic respiratory insufficiency compared to post-intervention admissions. However, as the vast majority (87%) of GNB colonization was identified in patients without chronic respiratory insufficiency, it appears unlikely that this difference could account for the observed effects. Importantly, no relevant changes in procedures, staffing levels, technical infrastructure, or other major changes that could influence patient management took place during the conduct of the study. No alternative confounders could be identified that could have influenced the outcome of the study. Second, our intervention was performed in a relatively "low GNB endemic setting" due to the use of SDD [35]. It is difficult to predict how the findings of this study can be generalized to a broader setting including non-SDD hospitals. On ICU's with a higher GNB colonization rate compared to our setting, it appears plausible that the effects could be more pronounced. Removing sinks from patient rooms could be a very effective intervention with a high impact for ICUs in low-resource settings, where nosocomial infections with GNB are very common [38]. Some may argue that the removal of the sinks could interfere with the prevention of nosocomial transmission of *Clostridium difficile*, as spores are resistant to alcohol-based handrub. In our hospital the incidence of *Clostridium difficile* infections is very low. Over the last 2.5 years 4 patients were diagnosed with *Clostridium difficile* in the ICU. Centers for Disease Control and Prevention advises to wear gloves when caring for patients with *C. difficile*-associated diarrhea. After gloves are removed, hands should be washed with a non-antimicrobial or an antimicrobial soap and water or disinfected with an alcohol-based handrub [39]. Our ICU setting with use of gloves in all patient contacts is in line with these recommendations. In our ICU, we have purchased a mobile hand washing sink that can be used as a back-up in case of a serious *Clostridium* infection outbreak.

In view of our results we should reconsider the necessity of sinks and other 'wet' areas in the patient rooms. Under time constraints, healthcare workers compliance with infection prevention and control measures is often reduced, specifically in the case of hand hygiene, infection prevention protocols and waste management protocols. Reconstructing the hospital infrastructure in a way that behavior of healthcare workers is more directed towards good clinical practice is a step in the direction of sustainable infection control.

Conclusions

This study shows that removal of the sinks from all patient rooms and the introduction of 'water-free' patient care is associated with a statistically significant lower number of ICU patients that become colonized with GNB, including MDR-GNB, especially among patients with a longer length of stay at the ICU. To our knowledge, this is the first study that indicates that sinks in patient rooms not only play a role in outbreak situations, but also in sporadic transmission of GNB from sinks to patients.

Acknowledgements
We acknowledge the significant work and dedication of Manon Tingen-Wieland (Infection control nurse) and Sanne Blonk, Monique Bonn, Jelle Driessen, Els van de Klok, Geerke van Kuijk, Mira de Lange, Ellen van der Mee, Sara Voet, (all ICU nurses) for their contributions to the implementation of the new 'water-free' procedures. Sjef van der Velde (Dept of Intensive Care) and Twan Klaassen (Dept of Medical Microbiology) are acknowledged for their valuable contribution to the ICT and data management.

Funding
No funding of this project was reported.

Authors' contributions
JH and AT had full access to all the data in the study and takes responsibility for the integrity of the data and the accuracy of the data analysis. Study concept and design: JH AT, PS, HvdH. Acquisition, analysis, or interpretation of data: JH, AT, PS, HvdH. Drafting of the manuscript: JH, AT, PS. Critical revision of the manuscript for important intellectual content: JH, AT, HW, AV, EK, PS, PPs, HvdH. Statistical analysis: AT, RA. Administrative, technical, or material support: MB. Study supervision: JH, AT, HvdH. All authors read and approved the final manuscript.

Competing interests
The authors declare that they have no competing interests.

Consent for publication
Not applicable.

Author details
¹Department of Medical Microbiology, Radboud university medical center, Geert Grooteplein 10, Postbus 9101, 6500, HB, Nijmegen, The Netherlands. ²Department of Medical Microbiology and Infectious Diseases, Canisius-Wilhelmina Hospital, Nijmegen, The Netherlands. ³Department of Primary and Community Care, Radboud university medical center, Nijmegen, The Netherlands. ⁴Department of Medical Microbiology, Laurentius hospital, Roermond, The Netherlands. ⁵Department of Intensive Care, Radboud university medical center, Nijmegen, The Netherlands.

References
1. Writing Group for the C-ICUI, the Brazilian Research in Intensive Care N, Cavalcanti AB, et al. Effect of a quality improvement intervention with daily round checklists, goal setting, and clinician prompting on mortality of critically ill patients: a randomized clinical trial. JAMA. 2016;315(14):1480–90.
2. Boyce JM. Environmental contamination makes an important contribution to hospital infection. J Hosp Infect. 2007;65(Suppl 2):50–4.
3. Carling PC, Parry MF, Bruno-Murtha LA, Dick B. Improving environmental hygiene in 27 intensive care units to decrease multidrug-resistant bacterial transmission. Crit Care Med. 2010;38(4):1054–9.
4. Carling PC, Von Beheren S, Kim P, Woods C, Healthcare Environmental Hygiene Study G. Intensive care unit environmental cleaning: an evaluation in sixteen hospitals using a novel assessment tool. J Hosp Infect. 2008;68(1):39–44.
5. Dancer SJ. The role of environmental cleaning in the control of hospital-acquired infection. J Hosp Infect. 2009;73(4):378–85.
6. Hopman J, Nillesen M, de Both E, et al. Mechanical vs manual cleaning of hospital beds: a prospective intervention study. J Hosp Infect. 2015;
7. Maltezou HC, Fusco FM, Schilling S, et al. Infection control practices in facilities for highly infectious diseases across Europe. J Hosp Infect. 2012;81(3):184–91.
8. Dancer SJ. Controlling hospital-acquired infection: focus on the role of the environment and new technologies for decontamination. Clin Microbiol Rev. 2014;27(4):665–90.
9. Rashid M. A decade of adult intensive care unit design: a study of the physical design features of the best-practice examples. Crit Care Nurs Q. 2006;29(4):282–311.
10. Ayliffe GA, Babb JR, Collins BJ, Lowbury EJ, Newsom SW. Pseudomonas aeruginosa in hospital sinks. Lancet. 1974;2(7880):578–81.
11. du Moulin GC. Airway colonization by Flavobacterium in an intensive care unit. J Clin Microbiol. 1979;10(2):155–60.
12. Edmonds P, Suskind RR, Macmillan BG, Holder IA. Epidemiology of Pseudomonas aeruginosa in a burns hospital: surveillance by a combined typing system. Appl Microbiol. 1972;24(2):219–25.
13. Levin MH, Olson B, Nathan C, Kabins SA, Weinstein RA. Pseudomonas in the sinks in an intensive care unit: relation to patients. J Clin Pathol. 1984;37(4):424–7.
14. Teres D. Pseudomonas in sinks, not taps. Lancet. 1973;1(7810):1001.
15. Boehmer TK, Bamberg WM, Ghosh TS, et al. Health care-associated outbreak of Salmonella Tennessee in a neonatal intensive care unit. Am J Infect Control. 2009;37(1):49–55.
16. Guyot A, Turton JF, Garner D. Outbreak of Stenotrophomonas maltophilia on an intensive care unit. J Hosp Infect. 2013;85(4):303–7.
17. Hong KB, Oh HS, Song JS, et al. Investigation and control of an outbreak of imipenem-resistant Acinetobacter baumannii Infection in a Pediatric Intensive Care Unit. Pediatr Infect Dis J. 2012;31(7):685–90.
18. Kotsanas D, Wijesooriya WR, Korman TM, et al. "Down the drain": carbapenem-resistant bacteria in intensive care unit patients and handwashing sinks. Med J Aust. 2013;198(5):267–9.
19. La Forgia C, Franke J, Hacek DM, Thomson RB Jr, Robicsek A, Peterson LR. Management of a multidrug-resistant Acinetobacter baumannii outbreak in an intensive care unit using novel environmental disinfection: a 38-month report. Am J Infect Control. 2010;38(4):259–63.
20. Leitner E, Zarfel G, Luxner J, et al. Contaminated handwashing sinks as the source of a clonal outbreak of KPC-2-producing Klebsiella oxytoca on a hematology ward. Antimicrob Agents Chemother. 2015;59(1):714–6.
21. Longtin Y, Troillet N, Touveneau S, et al. Pseudomonas aeruginosa outbreak in a pediatric intensive care unit linked to a humanitarian organization residential center. Pediatr Infect Dis J. 2010;29(3):233–7.
22. Lowe C, Willey B, O'Shaughnessy A, et al. Outbreak of extended-spectrum beta-lactamase-producing Klebsiella oxytoca infections associated with contaminated handwashing sinks(1). Emerg Infect Dis. 2012;18(8):1242–7.
23. Podnos YD, Cinat ME, Wilson SE, Cooke J, Gornick W, Thrupp LD. Eradication of multi-drug resistant Acinetobacter from an intensive care unit. Surg Infect. 2001;2(4):297–301.
24. Roux D, Aubier B, Cochard H, Quentin R, van der Mee-Marquet N. Centre HAIPGotRdHd. Contaminated sinks in intensive care units: an underestimated source of extended-spectrum beta-lactamase-producing Enterobacteriaceae in the patient environment. J Hosp Infect. 2013;85(2):106–11.

25. Tofteland S, Naseer U, Lislevand JH, Sundsfjord A, Samuelsen O. A long-term low-frequency hospital outbreak of KPC-producing *Klebsiella pneumoniae* involving Intergenus plasmid diffusion and a persisting environmental reservoir. PLoS One. 2013;8(3):e59015.

26. Verweij PE, Meis JF, Christmann V, et al. Nosocomial outbreak of colonization and infection with Stenotrophomonas maltophilia in preterm infants associated with contaminated tap water. Epidemiol Infect. 1998;120(3):251–6.

27. Wang SH, Sheng WH, Chang YY, et al. Healthcare-associated outbreak due to pan-drug resistant Acinetobacter baumannii in a surgical intensive care unit. J Hosp Infect. 2003;53(2):97–102.

28. Wendel AF, Kolbe-Busch S, Ressina S, et al. Detection and termination of an extended low-frequency hospital outbreak of GIM-1-producing Pseudomonas aeruginosa ST111 in Germany. Am J Infect Control. 2015;

29. Fusch C, Pogorzelski D, Main C, Meyer CL, El Helou S, Mertz D. Self-disinfecting sink drains reduce the Pseudomonas aeruginosa bioburden in a neonatal intensive care unit. Acta paediatrica. 2015;104(8)344–9.

30. Knoester M, de Boer MG, Maarleveld JJ, et al. An integrated approach to control a prolonged outbreak of multidrug-resistant Pseudomonas aeruginosa in an intensive care unit. Clin Microbiol infect. 2014;20(4):O207–15.

31. Wolf I, Bergervoet PW, Sebens FW, van den Oever HL, Savelkoul PH, van der Zwet WC. The sink as a correctable source of extended-spectrum beta-lactamase contamination for patients in the intensive care unit. J Hosp Infect. 2014;87(2):126–30.

32. Liu YY, Wang Y, Walsh TR, et al. Emergence of plasmid-mediated colistin resistance mechanism MCR-1 in animals and human beings in China: a microbiological and molecular biological study. Lancet Infect Dis. 2016;16(2):161–8.

33. Walsh TR, Weeks J, Livermore DM, Toleman MA. Dissemination of NDM-1 positive bacteria in the New Delhi environment and its implications for human health: an environmental point prevalence study. Lancet Infect Dis. 2011;11(5):355–62.

34. Neuhauser MM, Weinstein RA, Rydman R, Danziger LH, Karam G, Quinn JP. Antibiotic resistance among gram-negative bacilli in US intensive care units: implications for fluoroquinolone use. JAMA. 2003;289(7):885–8.

35. de Smet AM, Kluytmans JA, Cooper BS, et al. Decontamination of the digestive tract and oropharynx in ICU patients. N Engl J Med. 2009;360(1):20–31.

36. Arts D, de Keizer N, Scheffer GJ, de Jonge E. Quality of data collected for severity of illness scores in the Dutch National Intensive Care Evaluation (NICE) registry. Intensive Care Med. 2002;28(5):656–9.

37. Wagner AK, Soumerai SB, Zhang F, Ross-Degnan D. Segmented regression analysis of interrupted time series studies in medication use research. J Clin Pharm Ther. 2002;27(4):299–309.

38. Allegranzi B, Bagheri Nejad S, Combescure C, et al. Burden of endemic health-care-associated infection in developing countries: systematic review and meta-analysis. Lancet. 2011;377(9761):228–41.

39. Boyce J, Pittet D. Guideline for Hand Hygiene in Health-Care Settings. MMWR. Recommendations and reports : Morbidity and mortality weekly report. Recommendations and reports / Centers for Disease Control. 2002 October 25, 2002 / 51(RR16);1–44.

4

Implementation of central line-associated bloodstream infection prevention bundles in a surgical intensive care unit using peer tutoring

Sang-Won Park[1,2*], Suhui Ko[1], Hye-sun An[1], Ji Hwan Bang[1,2] and Woo-Young Chung[2,3]

Abstract

Background: Central line-associated bloodstream infections (CLABSIs) can be prevented through well-coordinated, multifaceted programs. However, implementation of CLABSI prevention programs requires individualized strategies for different institutional situations, and the best strategy in resource-limited settings is uncertain. Peer tutoring may be an efficient and effective method that is applicable in such settings.

Methods: A prospective intervention was performed to reduce CLABSIs in a surgical intensive care unit (SICU) at a tertiary hospital. The core interventions consisted of implementation of insertion and maintenance bundles for CLABSI prevention. The overall interventions were guided and coordinated by active educational programs using peer tutoring. The CLABSI rates were compared for 9 months pre-intervention, 6 months during the intervention and 9 months post-intervention. The CLABSI rate was further observed for three years after the intervention.

Results: The rate of CLABSIs per 1000 catheter-days decreased from 6.9 infections in the pre-intervention period to 2.4 and 1.8 in the intervention (6 m; $P = 0.102$) and post-intervention (9 m; $P = 0.036$) periods, respectively. A regression model showed a significantly decreasing trend in the infection rate from the pre-intervention period ($P < 0.001$), with incidence-rate ratios of 0.348 (95% confidence interval [CI], 0.98–1.23) in the intervention period and 0.257 (95% CI, 0.07–0.91) in the post-intervention period. However, after the 9-month post-intervention period, the yearly CLABSI rates reverted to 3.0–5.4 infections per 1000 catheter-days over 3 years.

Conclusions: Implementation of CLABSI prevention bundles using peer tutoring in a resource-limited setting was useful and effectively reduced CLABSIs. However, maintaining the reduced CLABSI rate will require further strategies.

Keywords: Central line-associated bloodstream infection, Intensive care unit, Education, Intervention, Learning by teaching, Peer tutoring

Background

Central line-associated bloodstream infection (CLABSI) is one of serious healthcare-associated infections that cause increased medical costs, morbidity and mortality; however, CLABSIs have been prevented in many developed and developing countries using multifaceted approaches [1–5]. Several guidelines for the prevention of CLABSIs are available, but the core contents of the evidence-based recommendations are shared in common [6, 7]. Although the objectives of the CLABSI prevention guidelines are evident and simple, the implementation of these guidelines in clinical practices requires many factors to be well-coordinated. Heterogeneity in compliance or performance with the guidelines exists worldwide, and interventions have not always been successful [8]. The importance of infection control in healthcare settings for patient safety and quality of care cannot be emphasized enough, but the available resources including expert personnel, reimbursement systems and

* Correspondence: hswon1@snu.ac.kr
[1]Infection Control Office, Boramae Medical Center, Seoul, Republic of Korea
[2]Department of Internal Medicine, Boramae Medical Center, Seoul National University College of Medicine, 20 Boramae-ro 5-Gil, Dongjak-gu, Seoul 07061, Republic of Korea
Full list of author information is available at the end of the article

managerial support are not always sufficient to deal with many active issues in most healthcare facilities. Different strategies for different regional or institutional situations are needed for the successful implementation of CLABSI prevention guidelines.

The education of and feedback from healthcare workers are core components of implementing an intervention program. The education component should be organized in a manner that allows the healthcare workers to collaborate, learn from, and support each other. We used 'learning by teaching method'-based education to implement CLABSI prevention bundles in a surgical intensive care unit (SICU) with a high CLABSI rate. This peer tutoring approach was intended to motivate the healthcare workers to actively participate in their own workplace problems and to develop a safety culture in the unit through the sharing of a common understanding.

Methods

Setting and subjects

This study was conducted in a surgical intensive care unit at a 767-bed tertiary hospital. The SICU had 15 beds, and most of the beds were occupied by patients from the neurosurgery and thoracic surgery departments. The patient to nurse ratio was 3:1. The SICU did not have a full-time intensivist responsible for overall clinical care but instead had a medical director whose main responsibility was administrative. All patients admitted to the SICU during the study period were included. The infection control office at the hospital comprised one infectious diseases physician who concurrently served as the director and one full-time and one part-time nurse.

Study design and data collection

The primary goals of the intervention were to reduce CLABSIs in a SICU and to maintain the reduced rate. The secondary goals were to improve the perception of core knowledge related to CLABSI prevention and to retain compliance with the use of insertion and maintenance bundles. This study consisted of three periods, a pre-intervention period of 9 months (August 2011 to April 2012), an intervention period of 6 months (May 2012 to October 2012), and a post-intervention period of 9 months (November 2012 to July 2013). In addition, long-term follow-up of CLABSIs was performed for 3 years after 2013, and the infection control office intervened minimally during this period as specified in the 'Intervention Program' section below. The insertion bundle included hand hygiene, maximal barrier precautions, chlorhexidine skin antisepsis, and optimal catheter site selection with the subclavian vein identified as the preferred site for insertion that were explained in detail in previous reports [1, 9, 10]. The maintenance

bundle included hand hygiene, catheter site dressing, hub care, and daily review of central line necessity [1, 9, 10]. For catheter site dressing, either sterile gauze or transparent semipermeable dressing was used and replaced every 2 days and 1 week respectively if not otherwise indicated. The site was disinfected with 2% chlorhexidine tincture. Before accessing catheter hubs, 70% alcohol was used for cleansing to reduce contamination.

Hand hygiene performance in the SICU was monitored weekly by an infection control nurse using the World Health Organization hand hygiene guide as a part of hospital-wide surveillance [11]. As the monitoring has a role of both measuring the performance and educating the healthcare workers on the spot, feedback about the hand hygiene performance was given to the health care workers immediately on the spot and monthly to each department. We only irregularly audit the hand hygiene performance by pre-trained unrelated external personnel to estimate the magnitude of Hawthorne effect for reference only. The perception of core knowledge was assessed for all nurses in the SICU. The survey consisted 20 questions total and was performed three times during the intervention period of 6 months. Residents or physicians in charge inserted catheter. The nurse in charge of each patient assisted the procedure and before the insertion, the nurse explained the checklist of insertion bundle and checked the adherence. The default of bundle was pointed out by the nurse in the middle of procedure and the persistence of default was recorded in the checklist. However, the nurse did not have the authority to stop the procedure.

CLABSIs were defined as laboratory-confirmed bloodstream infections in which a central line was in place for >2 calendar days on the date of event, and the line was in place on the date of the event or the day before [12]. To capture data for infections acquired during hospitalization only, the designation of CLABSI was considered valid only if the positive blood culture and clinical signs/symptoms of infection occurred at least 48 h after admission. The infection control office monitored the CLABSI events as well as compliance with use of the central line bundles. The number of pairs of blood cultures per 1000 patient-days was calculated during the study period to monitor the appropriate ordering practices of blood cultures [13].

Intervention program

Regular team meetings between the infection control office and the SICU were held to implement and coordinate the CLABSI prevention bundles. The SICU team included the director of the unit, the head nurse and all of the working nurses. The infection control office designed the overall CLABSI prevention bundles and working programs and adjusted them based on the feedback received at the regular meetings.

Implementation of the insertion and maintenance bundles was initiated through education, which provided working knowledge of the bundles, as well as individual and group feedback related to bundle use adherence. The educational sessions were conducted for all of the nurses in the SICU and were taught using the 'learning by teaching' or peer tutoring method in which the nurses themselves prepared and delivered the lecture contents (Fig. 1). After an initial introductory overview of the CLABSI bundles by the infection control office, these 30-min weekly educational sessions were held for 6 months (May 2012 – Oct 2012). The content of the lecture given by each nurse consisted of a repetitive summary of the core contents of the CLABSI bundles followed by a detailed review of one section of the published guidelines for the prevention of intravascular catheter-related infections, which was allocated to each lecturer [10]; a self-assessment of the current departmental problems in view of the reviewed content; and suggestions for possible solutions to these problems. The educational sessions were designed such that all of the SICU nurses served as lecturer, and the nurses had the opportunity to actively study and discuss the CLABSI-related problems. The framework of the lecture was suggested by the infection control office. The review sections included the guideline references to share their scientific basis. All of the participants were encouraged to discuss their problems or suggestions during every session. To educate doctors and encourage their cooperative compliance with the prevention bundles, separate monthly meetings were held between the infection control office and representative doctors from every clinical department that used the SICU because there was no intensivist or physician dedicated to patient care in the SICU.

Indirect education for all of the doctors in clinical departments was performed through these representative doctors using presentation materials created by the infection control office. Regular group feedback and instant individual feedback were given pertaining to the performance of the CLABSI prevention checklists. The checklists used in the insertion and maintenance bundles were incorporated into the electronic medical record (EMR) system during the interventional period, and then automatic data collection in the infection control office and a short message alert service for the removal of central catheters were implemented. An all-in-one cart that had all of the necessary items for central line insertion was prepared.

After the intervention period, systematically fixed programs continued. There was weekly hand hygiene monitoring. The performance of checklists in the insertion and maintenance bundles of CLABSI prevention checked by the nurses in the SICU was monitored through EMR by the infection office, and the feedback for violation was provided to individual healthcare workers daily and clinical departments monthly. However, active educational meetings were not held any more. There was no systematic educational program about CLABSI bundle for new nurses of SICU, but they were expected to learn from their colleagues and fixed work pattern like daily checklists embedded in the EMR system. For new residents or physicians, educational material illustrated in a PowerPoint file was provided monthly through their e-mail. Active audit for the individual component of checklists on the spot was not performed.

Statistical analysis

Comparisons of the CLABSI incidence rates during and after the intervention period with that of the baseline were analyzed by Poisson regression and are presented

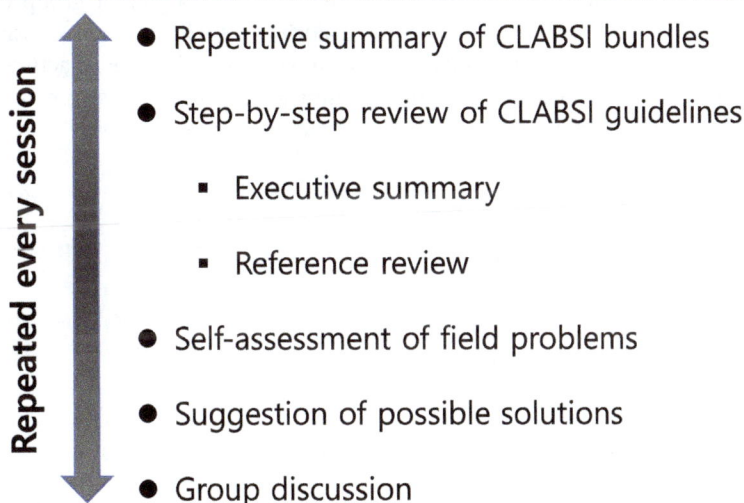

Fig. 1 Contents of the peer tutoring educational session for nurses in the surgical intensive care unit

with 95% confidence intervals (CIs). All statistical tests were two-tailed, and P values <0.05 were considered significant (SPSS 22.0; SPSS Inc., Chicago, IL, USA).

Results

The rate of CLABSIs per 1000 catheter-days decreased from 6.9 infections in the pre-intervention period to 2.4 and 1.8 in the intervention (6 m; P = 0.102) and post-intervention (9 m; P = 0.036) periods, respectively (Table 1 and Fig. 2). The regression model showed a significantly decreasing trend in the infection rate from the pre-intervention period (P < 0.001) with incidence-rate ratios of 0.348 (95% confidence interval [CI], 0.98–1.23) in the intervention period and 0.257 (95% CI, 0.07–0.91) in the post-intervention period. However, after the 9 months post-intervention period, the yearly CLABSI rates reverted to 3.0–5.4 per 1000 catheter-days (Table 1).

Adherence to each component in the insertion bundle reached 100% in the 5th month. Adherence to each component in the maintenance bundle reached 100% in the 2nd month. The absolute amount of central line use increased gradually but central line utilization ratio taking patient-days into account has been steadily decreasing since the initial rise during intervention period from 0.58 to 0.48 (Table 1). The places of central line insertion during intervention (6 m) and post-intervention (9 m) periods were operating room (58.6%), interventional radiology (20.8%), SICU (16.4%), emergency room (3.5%) and general ward (0.7%). The awareness of core knowledge about CLABSI prevention practices during the interventional period of 6 months increased, with scores of 15.8 (1st month), 17.1 (3rd month), and 18.9 (6th month) points out of a total of 20 points for the 20-question assessment. The performance of hand hygiene which was monitored weekly were 93.4% (range, 92–96), 89.7% (range, 79–97) and 90.9% (range, 83–96) during the pre-intervention, intervention and post-intervention periods, respectively.

Twenty pathogens were responsible for the CLABSIs during the 3 study periods, which totaled 24 months (Table 2). In the pre-interventional period, the predominant causative organisms were *Enterococcus* species (20%), *Acinetobacter baumannii* (20%), and coagulase-negative staphylococci (10%); one case each (5%) of *Staphylococcus aureus*, viridans streptococci, *Pseudomonas aeruginosa* and *Stenotrophomonas maltophilia* also occurred. In the intervention and post-intervention periods, *Candida* was the most common pathogen (4/6, 66.7%) of the 6 total causative agents, though the total number of infections was small. The *Candida* cases were not related to neutropenia. The mean pairs of blood cultures per 1000 patient-days during study periods were 201 (pre-intervention), 190 (intervention), and 196 (post-intervention).

Discussion

Our intervention to reduce CLABSIs by implementing CLABSI prevention bundles using peer tutoring was effective during the interventional period of 6 months and a post-interventional period of approximately 1 year. However, without continuous active interactions and dominating internal governance, the virtuous reduction of CLABSIs was not sustained. Our educational method had several advantages. Each healthcare worker had the opportunity to voice her/his own work-related problems, to hear from other colleagues, to understand the principles behind their routine activities and to receive responses to their problems. These factors minimized resistance to the introduction of a new job pattern. The purpose of the educational sessions was to motivate the healthcare workers, to provide them with expert knowledge for practical use and to improve knowledge retention over longer time periods. Determining the most effective educational method has been an area of utmost interest for a long time. Generally, active participatory education is more effective than passive learning. 'Learning by teaching' or peer tutoring is one of the active participatory educational methods in which the core idea is to have a pair or group of students teaching the majority of topics to their classmates in a way that encourages their classmates' active participation and communication in the best possible way [14]. 'Learning Pyramids' have shown that learners can retain

Table 1 Central line utilization ratios and central line-associated blood stream infections in a surgical intensive care unit over 5 years

Period	Central line-days	Patient-days	Central line utilization ratio	[a]CLABSI events	[b]CLABSI rate
Pre-intervention, 9 m	1734	3273	0.53	12	6.9
Intervention, 6 m	1245	2147	0.58	3	2.4
After intervention,					
9 m	1684	3207	0.53	3	1.8
1st year (12 m)	1994	3920	0.51	9	4.5
2nd year (12 m)	2030	4137	0.49	6	3.0
3rd year (12 m)	2222	4657	0.48	12	5.4

[a]*CLABSI* central line-associated bloodstream infection
[b]*CLABSI rate* CLABSI events per 1000 central line-days

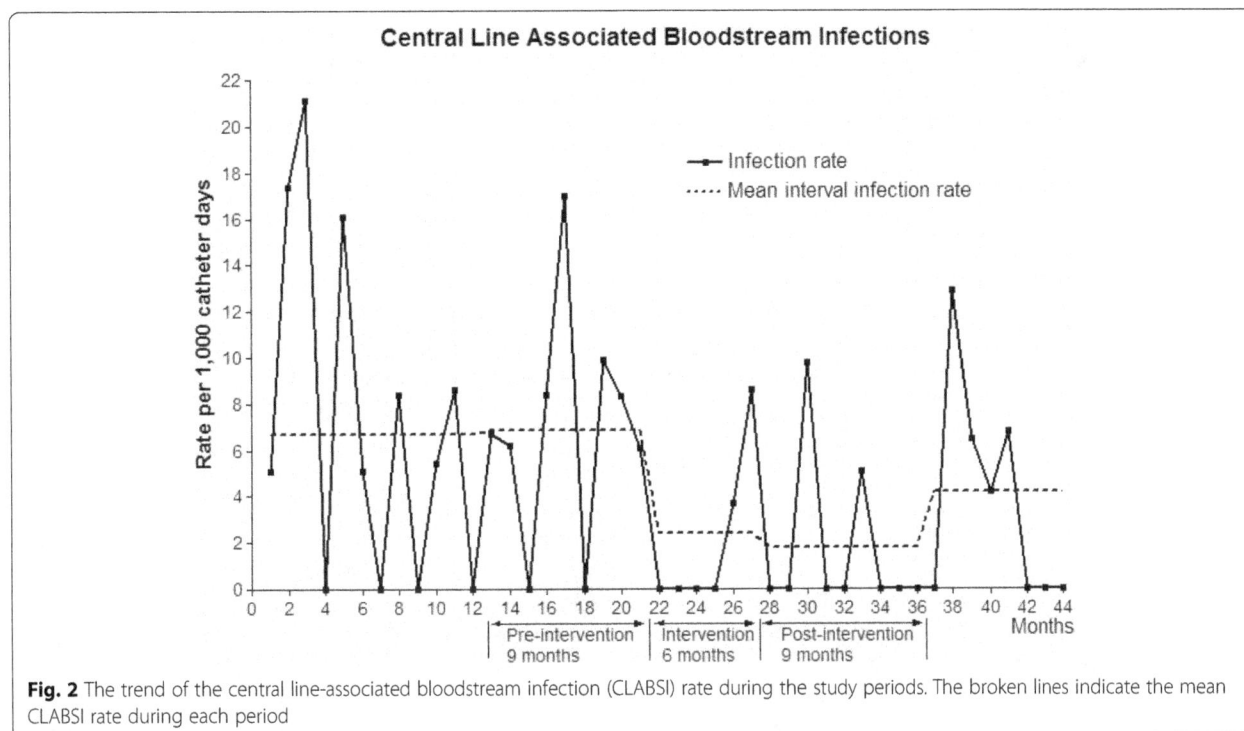

Fig. 2 The trend of the central line-associated bloodstream infection (CLABSI) rate during the study periods. The broken lines indicate the mean CLABSI rate during each period

approximately 90% of the content of a subject matter when they teach the material to someone else.

The commitment of the infection control staffs to co-ordinate the overall program and the presence of governing leadership in the unit to maintain a level of practice quality were basic components of the intervention.

Table 2 Microorganisms responsible for the central line-associated bloodstream infections during the three study periods

Organisms	Pre-intervention (9 m, n = 12)	During intervention (6 m, n = 3)	Post-intervention (9 m, n = 3)
Gram-positive bacteria			
Staphylococcus aureusv	1[a]	.	.
Coagulase-negative staphylococci	2[a]	.	1
viridans streptococci	1	.	.
Enterococcus species	4	.	.
Corynebacterium species		1	
Gram-negative bacteria			
Acinetobactera baumannii	4[a]	.	.
Pseudomonas aeruginosa	1	.	.
Stenotrophomonas maltophilia	1	.	.
Fungi			
Candida albicans	.	2	1
Candida parapsilosis	.	.	1

[a]Two cases were polymicrobial with A. baumannii + S. aureus and A. baumannii + coagulase-negative staphylococci, respectively

Regardless of the strong positive aspects of our educational approach, the intervention failed to sustain a reduced CLABSI rate beyond 9 months post-intervention. Several complex factors seem to be responsible for this lack of sustainability. High job turnover in the unit coupled with the lack of a continuing education system for new nurses and doctors after the intervention period likely weakened the effectiveness of the prevention protocols. The turnover rates of nurses in the SICU were 24.9% and 59.5% due to resignation, leave of absence and rotation during intervention (6 m) and post-intervention (9 m) periods. Thereafter, the rate was 39.1% - 46.8% annually for 3 years. Interns or residents had a rotational program every 1 or 2 months among 3 affiliated family hospitals. The patient-to-nurse ratio of 1:3 was much higher than the previously reported rate of 1:2 which was a risk factor for CLABSIs [15]. Moreover, there was no dedicated intensivist in the SICU who could have led and maintained the program at the hospital.

Successful large-scale interventions with sustained reductions in CLABSIs have been reported worldwide [2, 3, 5, 16, 17]. In South Korea, there have been a few single center or small-scale trials to reduce CLABSIs [18–21]. The only recent multicenter interventional study involving 58 ICUs in 26 hospitals funded by the Korea Centers for Disease Control and Prevention resulted in a CLABSI rate of 2.23 infections per 1000 catheter-days, which did not significantly improve the pre-interventional rate of 2.09 infections per 1000 catheter-days [22]. There have been no reports about sustaining a reduced CLABSI rate in South Korea. The distribution of CLABSI pathogens in the pre-interventional period was similar to recent Korean National Healthcare-associated Infections Surveillance System (KONIS) data from 166 ICUs, which showed *A. baumannii* (14.6%) as second most common pathogen of CLABSI in 2013 [23]. The high number of *A. baumannii* infections in our study might reflect high *A. baumannii* infection/colonization in the SICU. Regarding relatively higher frequency of candida infection during the intervention and the immediate post-intervention periods, there were no changes of antibiotics prophylaxis or strategies of treatment of surgical site infection. The only systematic change was a use of 2% chlorhexidine tincture for skin disinfection before catheter insertion and catheter site dressing instead of 10% povidone-iodine as a CLABSI bundle component. Whether the chlorhexidine had weaker effect on candida that on other bacterial pathogens requires further data due to the small absolute number of candida infections in our study, but previous studies about CLABSI have not supported the role of chlorhexidine in candida infections.

There are diverse institutional situations and cultures that deal with infection control programs and patient safety issues. Although standard CLABSI prevention guidelines are well-known, their translation into clinical practice needs to be individualized according to regional or institutional feasibility. Our educational method was efficient in the initial implementation of the program and effectively reduced the CLABSI rate for a short time period of approximately one year. To maintain the reduced rate, a multifaceted integrative approach must be continued [15]. Intra-departmental or intra-unit effort hardly maintained the effects of the program over a longer time period. Our approach may not be effective in certain situations, but it deserves to be considered by institutions implementing a CLABSI prevention program for the first time, especially in resource-limited settings.

Our study has some limitations. First, as this was a single-center study, the effectiveness of our approach may not be generalizable. However, one institutional success may provide a good model for generalization, as has been shown previously [1, 24]. Second, we did not perform a comparative study to prove the effectiveness of the peer tutoring method. However, from a practical point of view, it was a useful tool to guide the program as it received the cooperation of the participants and improved the understanding between healthcare workers. Third, the indirect educational approach implemented for doctors in the SICU might have weakened the effect of the intervention. As residents from each clinical department who were mainly involved in the insertion procedure in the SICU rotated at 1 or 2 months interval among 3 family hospitals, integrative successive group education and follow-up assessment were impractical.

And maintenance bundles were mainly related to the nurses. So, we decided to educate indirectly the doctors through preceptors in each department who had regular meetings with infection control office. The doctors had individual feedbacks on the spot in the SICU for their performance. Fourth, the performance of insertion bundle might be incomplete. Operating room was the most frequent place of central line insertion, but fully adopted the insertion bundle only after intervention period. They had been using a similar protocol except for skin disinfection with 10% povidone-iodine and a small sized drape. Emergency room (3.5%) and general ward (0.7%) had no insertion bundle though the number was small.

Conclusions

A peer tutoring educational method was useful for the implementation of CLABSI prevention bundles in a SICU and effectively reduced infection rates for a short time period of approximately 1 year. This approach is applicable for hospitals with limited resources that are trying to initiate prevention bundles. However, to maintain the reduced CLABSI rates, resources support and multifaceted cooperative approaches may be essential.

Abbreviations

CIs: Confidence intervals; CLABSI: Central line-associated bloodstream infection; EMR: Electronic medical record; SICU: Surgical intensive care unit

Acknowledgements

Not applicable.

Funding

This work was supported by a clinical research grant-in-aid from the Seoul Metropolitan Government - Seoul National University (SMG-SNU) Boramae Medical Center (03–2012-3).

Authors' contributions

SWP, SHK, and WYC designed the study. SWP, SHK, HAS, JHB and WYC performed the intervention as well as collected and analyzed the data. SWP and SHK wrote the manuscript. All of the authors read and approved the final manuscript.

Consent for publication

Not applicable.

Competing interests

The authors declare that they have no competing interests.

Author details

[1]Infection Control Office, Boramae Medical Center, Seoul, Republic of Korea. [2]Department of Internal Medicine, Boramae Medical Center, Seoul National University College of Medicine, 20 Boramae-ro 5-Gil, Dongjak-gu, Seoul 07061, Republic of Korea. [3]Intensive Care Units, Boramae Medical Center, Seoul, Republic of Korea.

References

1. Pronovost P, Needham D, Berenholtz S, Sinopoli D, Chu H, Cosgrove S, Sexton B, Hyzy R, Welsh R, Roth G, et al. An intervention to decrease catheter-related bloodstream infections in the ICU. N Engl J Med. 2006;355:2725–32.

2. Bion J, Richardson A, Hibbert P, Beer J, Abrusci T, McCutcheon M, Cassidy J, Eddleston J, Gunning K, Bellingan G, et al. 'Matching Michigan': a 2-year stepped interventional programme to minimise central venous catheter-blood stream infections in intensive care units in England. BMJ Qual Saf. 2013;22:110–23.

3. Berenholtz SM, Lubomski LH, Weeks K, Goeschel CA, Marsteller JA, Pham JC, Sawyer MD, Thompson DA, Winters BD, Cosgrove SE, et al. Eliminating central line-associated bloodstream infections: a national patient safety imperative. Infect Control Hosp Epidemiol. 2014;35:56–62.

4. Yaseen M, Al-Hameed F, Osman K, Al-Janadi M, Al-Shamrani M, Al-Saedi A, Al-Thaqafi A. A project to reduce the rate of central line associated bloodstream infection in ICU patients to a target of zero. BMJ Qual Improv Rep. 2016. https://doi.org/10.1136/bmjquality.u212545.w4986.

5. Marsteller JA, Sexton JB, Hsu YJ, Hsiao CJ, Holzmueller CG, Pronovost PJ, Thompson DA. A multicenter, phased, cluster-randomized controlled trial to reduce central line-associated bloodstream infections in intensive care units. Crit Care Med. 2012;40:2933–9.

6. Latif A, Halim MS, Pronovost PJ. Eliminating infections in the ICU: CLABSI. Curr Infect Dis Rep. 2015;17:491.

7. Ling ML, Apisarnthanarak A, Jaggi N, Harrington G, Morikane K, Thu le TA, Ching P, Villanueva V, Zong Z, Jeong JS, Lee CM. APSIC guide for prevention of central line associated bloodstream infections (CLABSI). Antimicrob Resist Infect Control. 2016;5:16.

8. Valencia C, Hammami N, Agodi A, Lepape A, Herrejon EP, Blot S, Vincent JL, Lambert ML. Poor adherence to guidelines for preventing central line-associated bloodstream infections (CLABSI): results of a worldwide survey. Antimicrob Resist Infect Control. 2016;5:49.

9. Marschall J, Mermel LA, Classen D, Arias KM, Podgorny K, Anderson DJ, Burstin H, Calfee DP, Coffin SE, Dubberke ER, et al. Strategies to prevent central line-associated bloodstream infections in acute care hospitals. Infect Control Hosp Epidemiol. 2008;29(Suppl 1):S22–30.

10. O'Grady NP, Alexander M, Burns LA, Dellinger EP, Garland J, Heard SO, Lipsett PA, Masur H, Mermel LA, Pearson ML, et al. Guidelines for the prevention of intravascular catheter-related infections. Clin Infect Dis. 2011;52:e162–93.

11. World Health Organization. WHO Guidelines on hand hygiene in health care. http://apps.who.int/iris/bitstream/10665/44102/1/9789241597906_eng.pdf. 2009. Accessed 1 Aug 2017.

12. Centers for Disease Control and Prevention. Bloodstream infection event (central line-associated bloodstream infection and non-central line-associated bloodstream infection). http://www.cdc.gov/nhsn/pdfs/pscmanual/4psc_clabscurrent.pdf. 2017. Accessed 1 Aug 2017.

13. Baron EJ, Weinstein MP, Dunne WM Jr, Yagupsky P, Welch DF, Wilson DM. Cumitech 1C: Blood cultures IV. Washington DC: ASM Press; 2005.

14. Grzega J, Schöner M. The didactic model LdL (Lernen durch Lehren) as a way of preparing students for communication in a knowledge society. J Educ Teach. 2008;34:167–75.

15. Fridkin SK, Pear SM, Williamson TH, Galgiani JN, Jarvis WR. The role of understaffing in central venous catheter-associated bloodstream infections. Infect Control Hosp Epidemiol. 1996;17:150–8.

16. Palomar M, Alvarez-Lerma F, Riera A, Diaz MT, Torres F, Agra Y, Larizgoitia I, Goeschel CA, Pronovost PJ, Bacteremia Zero Working G. Impact of a national multimodal intervention to prevent catheter-related bloodstream infection in the ICU: the Spanish experience. Crit Care Med. 2013;41:2364–72.

17. Pronovost PJ, Watson SR, Goeschel CA, Hyzy RC, Berenholtz SM. Sustaining reductions in central line-associated bloodstream infections in Michigan intensive care units: a 10-year analysis. Am J Med Qual. 2016;31:197–202.

18. Kim OS, Kim SM. Prevention of central venous catheter-related infections. Korean J Nosocomial Infect Control. 1999;4:35–40.

19. Yoo S, Ha M, Choi D, Pai H. Effectiveness of surveillance of central catheter-related bloodstream infection in an ICU in Korea. Infect Control Hosp Epidemiol. 2001;22:433–6.

20. Lee DH, Jung KY, Choi YH. Use of maximal sterile barrier precautions and/or antimicrobial-coated catheters to reduce the risk of central venous catheter-related bloodstream infection. Infect Control Hosp Epidemiol. 2008;29:947–50.

21. Yoo S, Jung SI, Kim GS, Lim DS, Sohn JW, Kim JY, Kim JE, Jang YS, Jung S, Pai H. Interventions to prevent catheter-associated blood-stream infections: A multicenter study in Korea. Infect Chemother. 2010;42:216–22.

22. Yoon YK, Lee SE, Seo BS, Kim HJ, Kim JH, Yang KS, Kim MJ, Sohn JW. Current status of personnel and infrastructure resources for infection prevention and control programs in the Republic of Korea: A national survey. Am J Infect Control. 2016;44:e189–93.

23. Choi JY, Kwak YG, Yoo H, Lee SO, Kim HB, Han SH, Choi HJ, Kim HY, Kim SR, Kim TH, et al. Trends in the distribution and antimicrobial susceptibility of causative pathogens of device-associated infection in Korean intensive care units from 2006 to 2013: results from the Korean Nosocomial Infections Surveillance System (KONIS). J Hosp Infect. 2016;92:363–71.

24. Berenholtz SM, Pronovost PJ, Lipsett PA, Hobson D, Earsing K, Farley JE, Milanovich S, Garrett-Mayer E, Winters BD, Rubin HR, et al. Eliminating catheter-related bloodstream infections in the intensive care unit. Crit Care Med. 2004;32:2014–20.

5

Management and investigation of a *Serratia marcescens* outbreak in a neonatal unit in Switzerland – the role of hand hygiene and whole genome sequencing

Walter Zingg[1*], Isabelle Soulake[1], Damien Baud[2], Benedikt Huttner[1,3], Riccardo Pfister[4], Gesuele Renzi[5], Didier Pittet[1], Jacques Schrenzel[2,5] and Patrice Francois[2,5]

Abstract

Background: Many outbreaks due to *Serratia marcescens* among neonates have been described in the literature but little is known about the role of whole genome sequencing in outbreak analysis and management.

Methods: Between February and March 2013, 2 neonates and 2 infants previously hospitalised in the neonatal unit of a tertiary care centre in Switzerland, were found to be colonised with *S. marcescens*. An investigation was launched with extensive environmental sampling and neonatal screening in four consecutive point prevalence surveys between April and May 2013. All identified isolates were first investigated by fingerprinting and later by whole genome sequencing. Audits of best practices were performed and a hand hygiene promotion programme was implemented.

Results: Twenty neonates were colonised with *S. marcescens*. No invasive infection due to *S. marcescens* occurred. All 231 environmental samples were negative. Hand hygiene compliance improved from 51% in April 2013 to 79% in May 2013 and remained high thereafter. No *S. marcescens* was identified in point prevalence surveys in June and October 2013. All strains were identical in the fingerprinting analysis and closely related according to whole genome sequencing.

Conclusions: Improving best practices and particularly hand hygiene proved effective in terminating the outbreak. Whole genome sequencing is a helpful tool for genotyping because it allows both sufficient discrimination of strains and comparison to other outbreaks through the use of an emerging international database.

Keywords: Neonates, Neonatal intensive care unit, *Serratia Marcescens*, Outbreak, Hand hygiene, Isolation, Infection control, Whole genome sequencing, Cross-transmission, Healthcare-associated infection

Background

Serratia marcescens has long been recognized as an important pathogen in neonatal intensive care units (NICUs). It is the third most common pathogen identified in published NICU outbreaks [1], and it has been found to account for 15% of all culture-positive nosocomial infections in this setting [2]. The large number of outbreak reports underestimates the true occurrence of *S. marcescens* in neonatology units and NICUs. According to the results of the mandatory surveillance of healthcare-associated infections (HAIs) in very low birth weight infants in Germany from 2006 to 2011, at least one to two *Serratia* outbreaks per year are expected for Germany alone [3].

S. marcescens causes a wide range of clinical manifestations in neonates, from asymptomatic colonization to infections such as urinary tract infections, pneumonia, sepsis or meningitis [4, 5]. Risk factors for *Serratia* spp. acquisition by neonates are related to

* Correspondence: walter.zingg@hcuge.ch

Presented in part at the 2nd International Conference on Prevention and Infection Control, Geneva, Switzerland, 2015; and the "15th Rencontres Internationales Francophones des Infirmier(e)s en Hygiène et Prévention de l'Infection", Lille, France, 2016.

[1]Infection Control Program and WHO Collaborating Center for Patient Safety, University of Geneva Hospitals, 4 Rue Gabrielle Perret-Gentil, 1211, 14 Geneva, Switzerland

Full list of author information is available at the end of the article

immaturity, prolonged hospital stay, antibiotic use, and mechanical ventilation [4, 6].

The objective of this outbreak report was to summarize the investigation and successful management of a *S. marcescens* outbreak in neonates and to investigate the contribution of using whole genome sequencing. This report follows the ORION (Outbreak Reports and Intervention Studies Of Nosocomial infection) statement [7].

Methods

Setting

The University of Geneva Hospitals (HUG), are a 1'800-bed primary and tertiary care center with about 47,000 admissions accounting for 660,000 patient-days per year. At the time of the outbreak it offered 17 places in the NICU, and 12 places in the geographically separate pediatric intensive care unit (PICU), where neonates are cared for when mechanical ventilation is needed. Neonates who are clinically stable but need prolonged stay for non-medical reasons are transferred to the unit for child development (UCD).

Outbreak

The outbreak started in February 2013 and ended in June 2013 (Fig. 1). Between February and March 2013, two neonates in the NICU and 2 infants in the UCD were found with *S. marcescens* (2 vascular catheters, 2 eye swabs, and 1 urine sample). Given the organizational ties and the patient flow between NICU, PICU, and UCD, an investigation was launched by a first point prevalence survey in the three units (Fig. 2) on 23 April 2013. Eight out of 41 screened children were identified as cases in this survey, one in the PICU, 3 in the UCD and 4 in the NICU. All new cases were neonates with a present or past history of stay in the NICU. Based on these findings, we focused further activity on the NICU with extensive environmental sampling and neonatal screening during 4 consecutive prevalence surveys.

Outbreak management

Audits of best practices in the use of surface disinfectants, ointments and cosmetic products were performed, as well as weekly direct hand hygiene

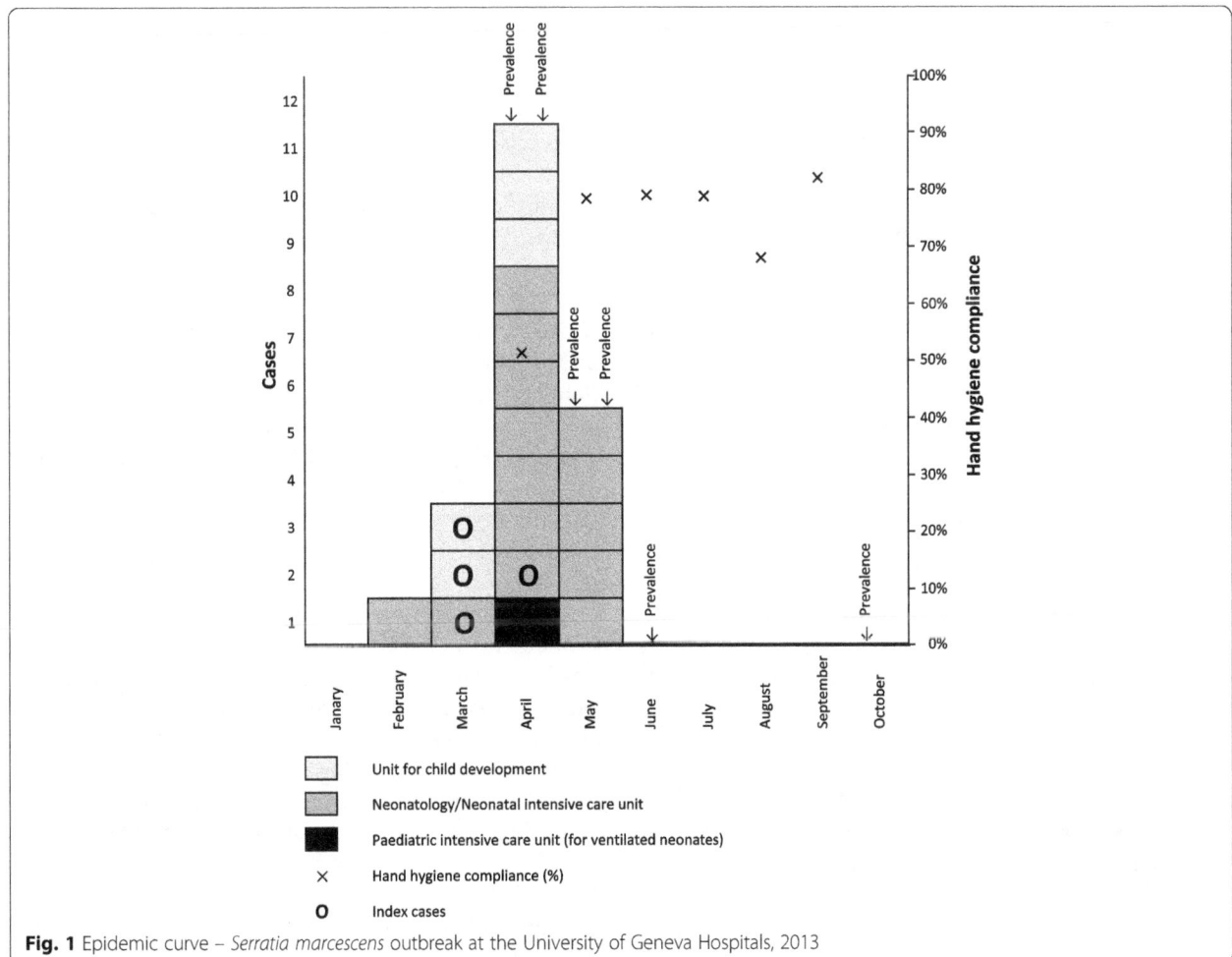

Fig. 1 Epidemic curve – *Serratia marcescens* outbreak at the University of Geneva Hospitals, 2013

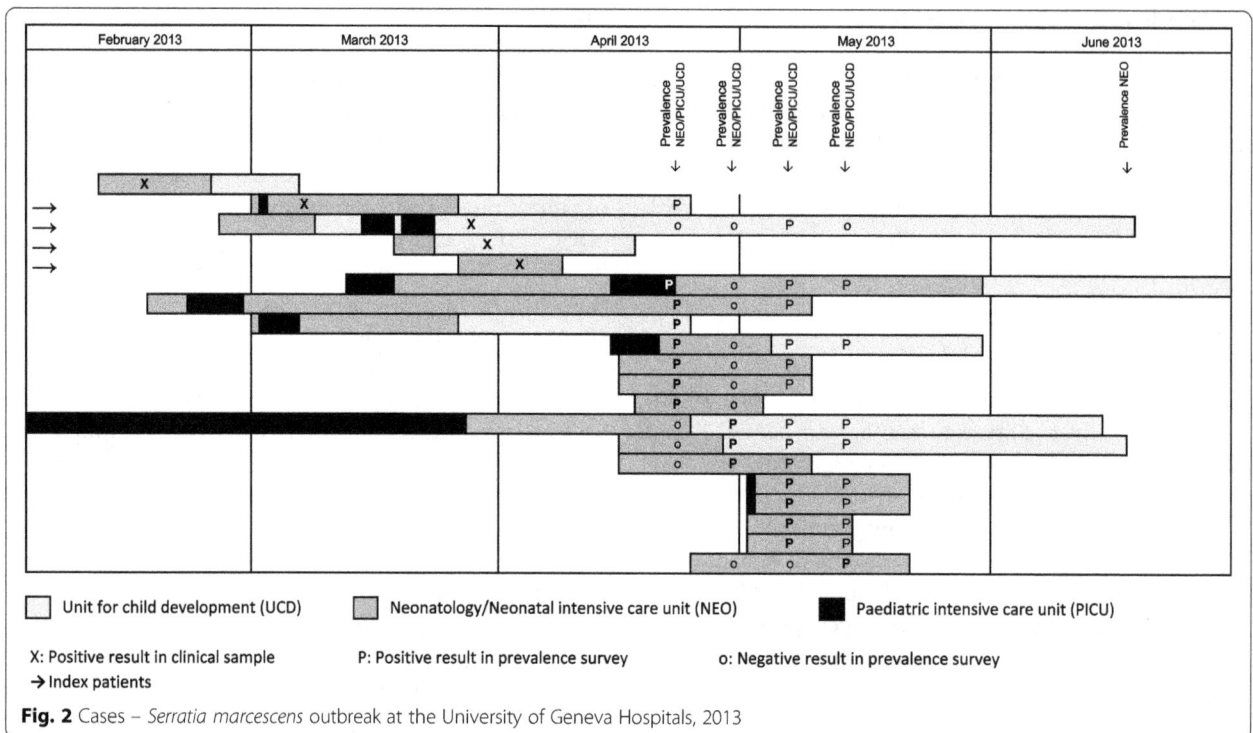

Fig. 2 Cases – *Serratia marcescens* outbreak at the University of Geneva Hospitals, 2013

observations (439 opportunities in total). An intensive hand hygiene promotion programme was offered to the staff working in the NICU: daily presence in the NICU, education and training, and weekly hand hygiene audits with individual feedback.

Microbiological investigation/genotyping

In 2013, the genomes of the *S. marcescens* isolates obtained in the prevalence surveys were tested by a commercial fingerprinting assay (DiversiLab®, Biomerieux, France). In 2016, the genomes *S. marcescens* isolates were fully sequenced using an Illumina HiSeq 2500 sequencer as previously described [8].

Results

A total of 232 neonatal screenings (117 stool samples, 115 nasal swabs) [9] were performed. In addition to the 4 index cases and the 8 cases identified in the first prevalence survey, an additional three, four and one cases were identified in the second, third and fourth prevalence surveys in April and May, respectively (Fig. 2). The proportions of positive rectal and nasal swabs were 11.1% (13/117) and 6.1% (7/115), respectively. Five infants had a positive result for both rectal and nasal swabs. All cases were preterm-, and seven were very-low-birth weight infants. No new *S. marcescens* cases were identified until October 2016, including two further prevalence surveys, which were performed in June and October. There was no invasive infection due to *S. marcescens*, neither during the outbreak nor until end of

December 2013. A total of 231 environmental samplings were performed (Table 1). All tested products, materials and surfaces were negative for *S. marcescens*. Hand hygiene compliance improved from 51% in April 2013 to 79% in May 2013 following the promotion programme. Compliance remained above 65% in the following months (Fig. 1).

Fingerprinting of 24 isolates from 16 neonates showed identical strains (Fig. 3). Whole genome sequencing was carried out on the set of 24 *S. marcescens* strains (Sm01-Sm24) belonging to the outbreak. The sequencing on an Illumina HiSeq produced on average a total of 13 million 150 bp reads per sample, exhibiting very high theoretical coverage values (between 300 and 900 fold). Assembly was achieved using SPAdes 3.9.0 software, after read quality trimming and filtering was applied to the raw reads. The assembly produced very similar results for each strain from the outbreak, resulting in an average genome size of 5′080′124 bp with a standard deviation of 1097 bp. This shows extreme similarity between the strains of the outbreak. Moreover, pairwise comparisons using MUMmer software were performed between each couple of strains and showed similarity above 99.999% [10]. Figure 4 shows an unrooted tree displaying all the isolates from the outbreak (Sm01-24), and one representative strain isolated in Germany during a SM outbreak in 2016 (SMB2099) [11].

Discussion

This report suggests that focusing on and improving hand hygiene is effective in terminating a *S. marcescens*

Table 1 Products, materials and surfaces tested for microbiological growth – *Serratia marcescens* outbreak at the University of Geneva Hospitals, 2013

Products, materials and surfaces	N (%)
Hand and skin disinfectants	66 (28.6)
Hypochlorite solution 225 ppm to disinfect pacifiers and nipple shields	25 (10.8)
Ointments and body lotions	25 (10.8)
Computer keyboards	20 (8.7)
Medicated and non-medicated soaps	20 (8.7)
Bowls for body care	17 (7.4)
Water from incubators	11 (4.8)
Tap water	10 (4.3)
Tubs	9 (3.9)
Sinks	9 (3.9)
Water from CPAP[a] tubes	6 (2.6)
Other materials or surfaces	13 (5.6)
Total	231 (100)

There was no growth for *S. marcescens* on any of the tested products, materials or surfaces
[a]*CPAP* continuous positive airway pressure

outbreak among neonates. Whole genome sequencing is a useful tool for outbreak investigation because it is more discriminative than standard fingerprinting tests and allows benchmarking with other outbreaks thanks to a growing gene bank.

The source of *S. marcescens* outbreaks in NICUs is rarely identified. A review summarizing 48 NICU outbreaks reported an identified source in only 40% (19/48), the most frequent being a colonized or infected index patient (8/48), followed by equipment for patient care (6/48), an (unspecified) environment (4/48), and food (1/48) [12]. Colonized or infected patients are thought to represent the most important reservoir of *S. marcescens* outbreaks in NICUs [4, 13]. In the currently described situation, the investigation revealed two additional NICU cases prior to the outbreak. A mother of one of them hadan amnion infection syndrome due to *S. marcescens* three months before the start of the outbreak, and thus, may have been the most likely source [12]. In the literature, healthcare workers were never identified as a source, but few studies investigated this specifically [14]. Like in our study, extensive environmental screening rarely yielded positive results in the

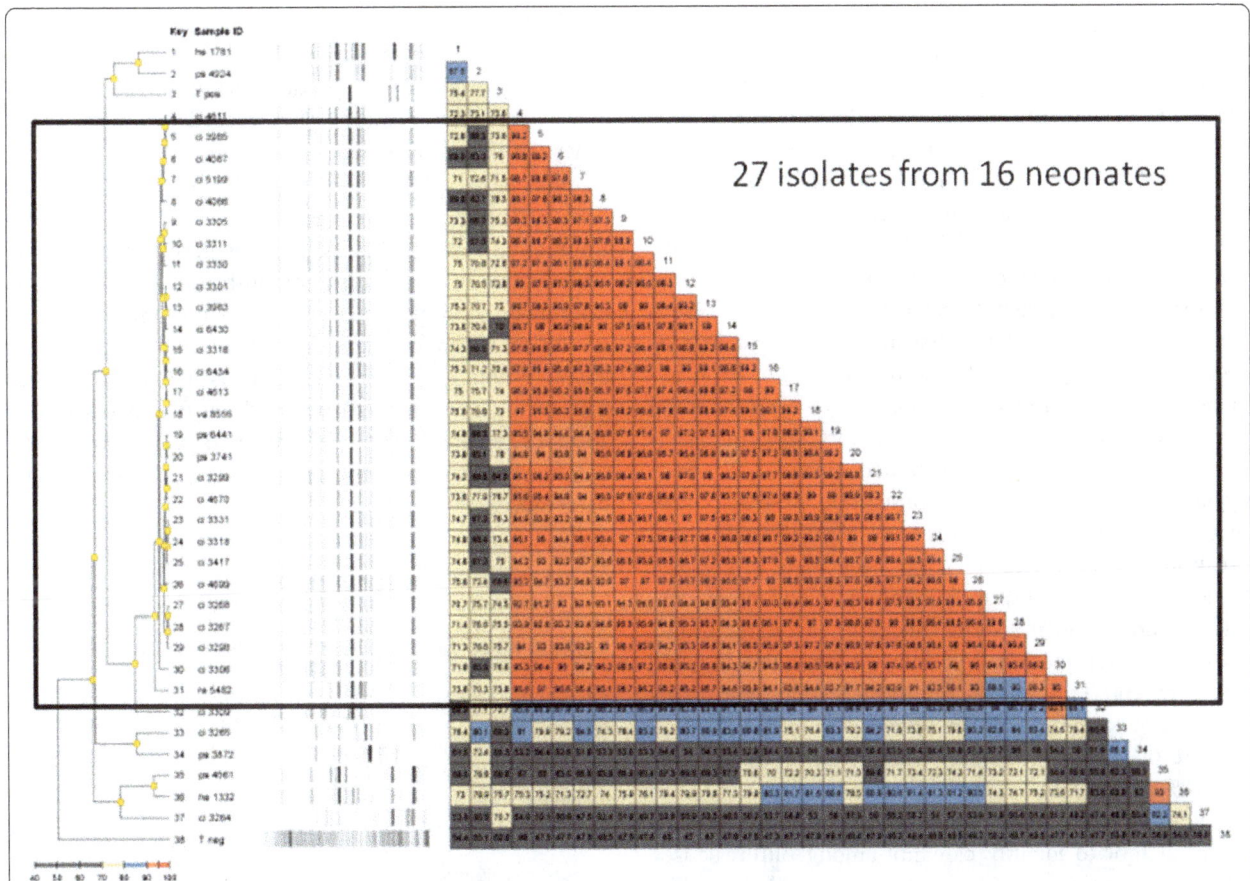

27 isolates from 16 neonates

Fig. 3 Fingerprinting of *S. marcescens* strains using the DiversiLab® kit – *Serratia marcescens* outbreak at the University of Geneva Hospitals, 2013

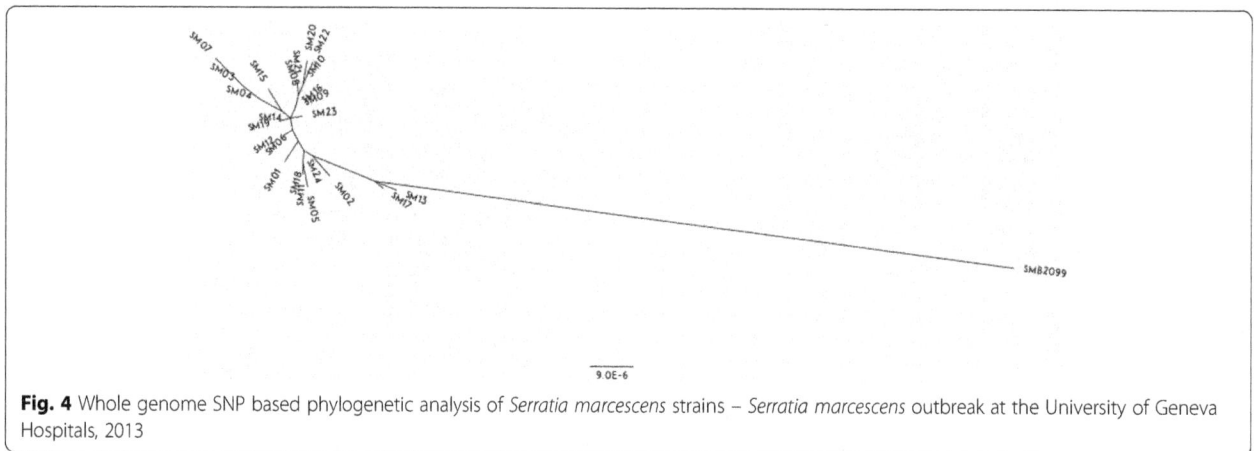

Fig. 4 Whole genome SNP based phylogenetic analysis of *Serratia marcescens* strains – *Serratia marcescens* outbreak at the University of Geneva Hospitals, 2013

reported outbreaks, suggesting that environmental contamination may play a limited role.

The clinical implication of colonization with *S. marcescens* in neonates and its implication in outbreaks is not always clear. A number of studies reported that *S. marcescens* is rather commonly isolated in stool of preterm neonates within the first weeks of life [6, 15, 16]. However, the pathogen was not isolated consistently in preterm neonates either [17], and *S. marcescens* has not been isolated in healthy term babies [18]. Thus, while the finding of *S. marcescens* in neonatal stool can be considered a regular event in NICUs, the pathogen per se is not part of the normal early gut flora of healthy newborns in the community. Once the intestines of a neonate are colonized with *S. marcescens* from the (pathologic) outside, they can become the "source" of an outbreak. This makes control of *Serratia* outbreaks very difficult, and underlines the importance of hands in the transmission of the pathogen and the possible successful management of an outbreak.

Already in 1981, contaminated hand-washing brushes were reported to be implicated in a *S. marcescens* outbreak, indirectly pointing to the pivotal role of hand hygiene in the spread of the pathogen [19]. Contaminated soaps were identified in another report [20]. Interventions to control outbreaks included always both hand hygiene and environmental control [9, 21–28]. Given that all environmental samples were negative in our outbreak investigation and work had been done in the past to dedicate equipment, drugs, ointments and other cosmetic products to individual neonates (avoiding multivials) [29], our intervention focused on hand hygiene improvement. This was all the more justified because a decrease of hand hygiene compliance had been identified as part of the investigation; hand hygiene compliance was 72% in the year before the outbreak.

Whole genome sequencing technology emerged as a powerful tool to identify clonality among outbreak isolates. The genome of a *S. marcescens* strain that sparked an outbreak among infants in Germany was reported

very recently [11, 12]. Comparison with our index case revealed a moderate difference around 200 SNPs. Other isolates identified from our institution and not related to the outbreak were sequenced and the number of SNPs was higher than 100'000 (data not shown).

There are limitations in our outbreak investigation. First, environmental sampling was large but we did not consistently use neutralizing agents for testing the different cosmetic products, resulting in potential underreporting. However, cosmetic products were strictly confined to the neonates and no multivials were in use. A positive finding of a product with a case would not have been prove of the product being the source. Second, we did not produce formal records from the audits other than hand hygiene.

Conclusions
Improving best practice and particularly hand hygiene are effective in terminating the outbreak. This highlights the role of hand hygiene in the cause but also in the successful management of *S. marcescens* outbreaks in neonates. Whole genome sequencing is a helpful tool for genotyping because it allows both sufficient discrimination of strains within the outbreak and comparison to other outbreaks through an emerging international database.

Abbreviations
HAI: Healthcare-associated infection; HUG: University of Geneva hospitals; NICU: Neonatal intensive care unit; ORION: Outbreak reports and intervention studies of nosocomial infection; PICU: Pediatric intensive care unit; SNP: Single nucleotide polymorphism; UCD: Unit for child development

Acknowledgments
We would like to thank Delphine Scalia-Perreard, Claude Ginet, and Sylvie Touveneau for the outbreak investigation.

Funding
No external funding.

Authors' contributions
BH, IS, and WZ organised and performed the investigation and management of the outbreak. DB, GR and PF performed the microbiological investigation

and whole genome sequencing. WZ, DB, and PF did the data analysis. WZ wrote the first draft of the manuscript. WZ, IS, DB, BH, RP, GR, DP, JS, and PF reviewed and contributed to subsequent drafts. All authors approved the final version for publication.

Consent for publication
Not applicable.

Competing interests
The authors declare that they have no competing interests.

Author details
[1]Infection Control Program and WHO Collaborating Center for Patient Safety, |University of Geneva Hospitals, 4 Rue Gabrielle Perret-Gentil, 1211, 14 Geneva, Switzerland. [2]Genomic Research Laboratory, Division of Infectious Diseases, University of Geneva Hospitals, Geneva, Switzerland. [3]Division of Infectious Diseases, University of Geneva Hospitals and Faculty of Medicine, Geneva, Switzerland. [4]Neonatal Intensive Care Unit, Department of Paediatrics, University of Geneva Hospitals, Geneva, Switzerland. [5]Bacteriology Laboratory, Department of Genetics and Laboratory Medicine, University of Geneva Hospitals, Geneva, Switzerland.

References
1. Gastmeier P, Loui A, Stamm-Balderjahn S, Hansen S, Zuschneid I, Sohr D, Behnke M, Obladen M, Vonberg RP, Ruden H. Outbreaks in neonatal intensive care units - they are not like others. Am J Infect Control. 2007;35(3):172–6.
2. Raymond J, Aujard Y. Nosocomial infections in pediatric patients: a European, multicenter prospective study. European study group. Infect Control Hosp Epidemiol. 2000;21(4):260–3.
3. Schwab F, Geffers C, Piening B, Haller S, Eckmanns T, Gastmeier P. How many outbreaks of nosocomial infections occur in German neonatal intensive care units annually? Infection. 2014;42(1):73–8.
4. Voelz A, Muller A, Gillen J, Le C, Dresbach T, Engelhart S, Exner M, Bates CJ, Simon A. Outbreaks of Serratia Marcescens in neonatal and pediatric intensive care units: clinical aspects, risk factors and management. Int J Hyg Environ Health. 2010;213(2):79–87.
5. David MD, Weller TM, Lambert P, Fraise AP. An outbreak of Serratia Marcescens on the neonatal unit: a tale of two clones. J Hosp Infect. 2006; 63(1):27–33.
6. Moles L, Gomez M, Heilig H, Bustos G, Fuentes S, de Vos W, Fernandez L, Rodriguez JM, Jimenez E. Bacterial diversity in meconium of preterm neonates and evolution of their fecal microbiota during the first month of life. PLoS One. 2013;8(6):e66986.
7. Stone SP, Cooper BS, Kibbler CC, Cookson BD, Roberts JA, Medley GF, Duckworth G, Lai R, Ebrahim S, Brown EM, et al. The ORION statement: guidelines for transparent reporting of outbreak reports and intervention studies of nosocomial infection. Lancet Infect Dis. 2007;7(4):282–8.
8. Von Dach E, Diene SM, Fankhauser C, Schrenzel J, Harbarth S, Francois P. Comparative genomics of community-associated Methicillin-resistant Staphylococcus Aureus shows the emergence of clone ST8-USA300 in Geneva, Switzerland. J Infect Dis. 2016;213(9):1370–9.
9. Steppberger K, Walter S, Claros MC, Spencker FB, Kiess W, Rodloff AC, Vogtmann C. Nosocomial neonatal outbreak of Serratia Marcescens–analysis of pathogens by pulsed field gel electrophoresis and polymerase chain reaction. Infection. 2002;30(5):277–81.
10. Kurtz S, Phillippy A, Delcher AL, Smoot M, Shumway M, Antonescu C, Salzberg SL. Versatile and open software for comparing large genomes. Genome Biol. 2004;5(2):R12.
11. Serratia marcescens SMB2099 complete genome; GenBank: HG738868.1. https://www.ncbi.nlm.nih.gov/nuccore/HG738868.1. Accessed 1 Dec 2017.
12. Gastmeier P. Serratia Marcescens: an outbreak experience. Front Microbiol. 2014;5:81.
13. Duggan TG, Leng RA, Hancock BM, Cursons RT. Serratia Marcescens in a newborn unit–microbiological features. Pathology. 1984;16(2):189–91.
14. Assadian O, Berger A, Aspock C, Mustafa S, Kohlhauser C, Hirschl AM. Nosocomial outbreak of Serratia Marcescens in a neonatal intensive care unit. Infect Control Hosp Epidemiol. 2002;23(8):457–61.
15. Moles L, Gomez M, Jimenez E, Fernandez L, Bustos G, Chaves F, Canton R, Rodriguez JM, Del Campo R. Preterm infant gut colonization in the neonatal ICU and complete restoration 2 years later. Clin Microbiol Infect. 2015;21(10): e931–10. 936
16. Drell T, Lutsar I, Stsepetova J, Parm U, Metsvaht T, Ilmoja ML, Simm J, Sepp E. The development of gut microbiota in critically ill extremely low birth weight infants assessed with 16S rRNA gene based sequencing. Gut Microbes. 2014;5(3):304–12.
17. Aujoulat F, Roudiere L, Picaud JC, Jacquot A, Filleron A, Neveu D, Baum TP, Marchandin H, Jumas-Bilak E. Temporal dynamics of the very premature infant gut dominant microbiota. BMC Microbiol. 2014;14:325.
18. Palmer C, Bik EM, DiGiulio DB, Relman DA, Brown PO. Development of the human infant intestinal microbiota. PLoS Biol. 2007;5(7):e177.
19. Anagnostakis D, Fitsialos J, Koutsia C, Messaritakis J, Matsaniotis N. A nursery outbreak of Serratia Marcescens infection. Evidence of a single source of contamination. Am J Dis Child. 1981;135(5):413–4.
20. Archibald LK, Corl A, Shah B, Schulte M, Arduino MJ, Aguero S, Fisher DJ, Stechenberg BW, Banerjee SN, Jarvis WR. Serratia Marcescens outbreak associated with extrinsic contamination of 1% chlorxylenol soap. Infect Control Hosp Epidemiol. 1997;18(10):704–9.
21. Al Jarousha AM, El Qouqa IA, El Jadba AH, Al Afifi AS. An outbreak of Serratia Marcescens septicaemia in neonatal intensive care unit in Gaza City Palestine. J Hosp Infect. 2008;70(2):119–26.
22. Bates CJ, Pearse R. Use of hydrogen peroxide vapour for environmental control during a Serratia outbreak in a neonatal intensive care unit. J Hosp Infect. 2005;61(4):364–6.
23. Braver DJ, Hauser GJ, Berns L, Siegman-Igra Y, Muhlbauer B. Control of a Serratia Marcescens outbreak in a maternity hospital. J Hosp Infect. 1987; 10(2):129–37.
24. Buffet-Bataillon S, Rabier V, Betremieux P, Beuchee A, Bauer M, Pladys P, Le Gall E, Cormier M, Jolivet-Gougeon A. Outbreak of Serratia Marcescens in a neonatal intensive care unit: contaminated unmedicated liquid soap and risk factors. J Hosp Infect. 2009;72(1):17–22.
25. Casolari C, Pecorari M, Fabio G, Cattani S, Venturelli C, Piccinini L, Tamassia MG, Gennari W, Sabbatini AM, Leporati G, et al. A simultaneous outbreak of Serratia Marcescens and Klebsiella Pneumoniae in a neonatal intensive care unit. J Hosp Infect. 2005;61(4):312–20.
26. Gillespie EE, Bradford J, Brett J, Kotsanas D. Serratia Marcescens bacteremia - an indicator for outbreak management and heightened surveillance. J Perinat Med. 2007;35(3):227–31.
27. Jang TN, Fung CP, Yang TL, Shen SH, Huang CS, Lee SH. Use of pulsed-field gel electrophoresis to investigate an outbreak of Serratia Marcescens infection in a neonatal intensive care unit. J Hosp Infect. 2001;48(1):13–9.
28. Sarvikivi E, Lyytikainen O, Salmenlinna S, Vuopio-Varkila J, Luukkainen P, Tarkka E, Saxen H. Clustering of Serratia Marcescens infections in a neonatal intensive care unit. Infect Control Hosp Epidemiol. 2004;25(9):723–9.
29. Pessoa-Silva CL, Hugonnet S, Pfister R, Touveneau S, Dharan S, Posfay-Barbe K, Pittet D. Reduction of health care associated infection risk in neonates by successful hand hygiene promotion. Pediatrics. 2007;120(2):e382–90.

6

Barriers and facilitators to infection control at a hospital in northern India

Anna K. Barker[1] (iD), Kelli Brown[1], Dawd Siraj[2], Muneeb Ahsan[3], Sharmila Sengupta[4] and Nasia Safdar[2,5*]

Abstract

Background: Hospital acquired infections occur at higher rates in low- and middle-income countries, like India, than in high-income countries. Effective implementation of infection control practices is crucial to reducing the transmission of hospital acquired infections at hospitals worldwide. Yet, no comprehensive assessments of the barriers to sustained, successful implementation of hospital interventions have been performed in Indian healthcare settings to date. The Systems Engineering Initiative for Patient Safety (SEIPS) model examines problems through the lens of interactions between people and systems. It is a natural fit for investigating the behavioral and systematic components of infection control practices.

Methods: We conducted a qualitative study to assess the facilitators and barriers to infection control practices at a 1250 bed tertiary care hospital in Haryana, northern India. Twenty semi-structured interviews of nurses and physicians, selected by convenience sampling, were conducted in English using an interview guide based on the SEIPS model. All interview data was subsequently transcribed and coded for themes.

Results: Person, task, and organizational level factors were the primary barriers and facilitators to infection control at this hospital. Major barriers included a high rate of nursing staff turnover, time spent training new staff, limitations in language competency, and heavy clinical workloads. A well developed infection control team and an institutional climate that prioritizes infection control were major facilitators.

Conclusions: Institutional support is critical to the effective implementation of infection control practices. Prioritizing resources to recruit and retain trained, experienced nursing staff is also essential.

Keywords: Infection control, Global health, Qualitative methodology, Human factors, India

Background

Healthcare associated infections (HAIs) affect millions of patients every year and are the most common complication of healthcare delivery globally [1]. They complicate clinical care, increase length of hospital stays, and are particularly debilitating for patients and healthcare facilities with limited income and resources [2–4].

While HAIs are a considerable problem in high-income countries, low- and middle-income counties are disproportionately burdened by these infections [5, 6]. In India, a majority of healthcare settings lack robust infection

control infrastructure and no nationwide HAI surveillance system exists [7]. Low- and middle-income countries also tend to have higher rates of antimicrobial resistance [5]. A recent multi-center study conducted at twelve Indian intensive care units found an overall rate of 9.06 HAIs per 1000 intensive care days, which is close to the global average in high income countries [8]. However, there is considerable variability in infection rates at institutions across the country. Several single site studies have reported considerably higher HAI rates, with levels reaching between 25 and 40 infections per 1000 patient days [9–11].

Effective implementation of infection control practices is crucial to controlling the transmission of HAIs in settings with high infection rates. A recent meta-analysis found that over ninety-five percent intervention

* Correspondence: ns2@medicine.wisc.edu
[2]Department of Medicine, University of Wisconsin-Madison, School of Medicine and Public Health, Madison, WI, USA
[5]William S. Middleton Memorial Veterans Affairs Hospital, Madison, WI, USA
Full list of author information is available at the end of the article

compliance is required to reduce central line-associated bloodstream infections [12]. While the necessary rate of compliance is not known for other infections, all infection control interventions are complex, multifaceted, and challenging to sustain [13]. In order for infection prevention measures to be successful, barriers to effective implementation must be identified and overcome [14]. Likewise, facilitators to intervention implementation must also be identified and championed.

The Systems Engineering Initiative for Patient Safety (SEIPS) is one of the leading conceptual frameworks in human factors engineering research [15]. This model examines problems through the lens of complex interactions between people and systems, which includes organizations, technology and tools, the environment, tasks, and people (Fig. 1). It has been utilized as the guiding framework for patient safety analyses in over fifty studies, ranging from primary care clinics to intensive care units (ICUs [16]). The SEIPS model improves upon earlier patient safety frameworks by evaluating both the causes and control of medical errors [15]. Thus, it is a natural fit for investigating the behavioral and systematic components of infection control practices. SEIPS has previously been used to identify barriers and facilitators to infection prevention practices for *Clostridium difficile* infection [17], ventilator associated pneumonia [18], and HAIs in the ICU [19].

Despite the high rate of HAIs in India, no study of the comprehensive barriers and facilitators to infection control has been conducted at an Indian hospital, to our knowledge. Thus, we conducted a qualitative study of infection control practices at a tertiary care hospital in Haryana, northern India, based on the SEIPS conceptual framework.

Methods

We conducted a qualitative study of facilitators and barriers to infection control at a private tertiary care hospital in Haryana, India. Semi-structured interviews were conducted in June and July 2015.

Study population

Ten physicians and ten nurses were recruited at a 1250-bed tertiary care private hospital in Haryana, India. The hospital includes ten ICUs for a total of 350 ICU beds. Participants were selected by convenience sampling and represented a wide range of clinical departments and career levels. They were recruited in the hospital employee cafeteria, on clinical wards, and by word of mouth. To ensure a range of clinical expertise, some participants from less common sectors, for example infectious disease nursing and ICU leadership, were approached directly. All hospital employees directly involved in patient care were eligible for enrollment. Student trainees and non-English speakers were excluded, although no potential participants met exclusion criteria.

Interviews

We conducted twenty semi-structured interviews to assess facilitators and barriers to a hospital infection control program. English language competency is a requirement for employment as a healthcare worker at the study hospital, thus, all interviews were conducted in English. Interviews took place at the hospital, in a room adjacent to the participant's work environment. The initial interview guide was developed based on the SEIPS model (Fig. 1) and was refined during the study based on participant responses (Additional file 1). Interview questions assessed the hospital's infection control

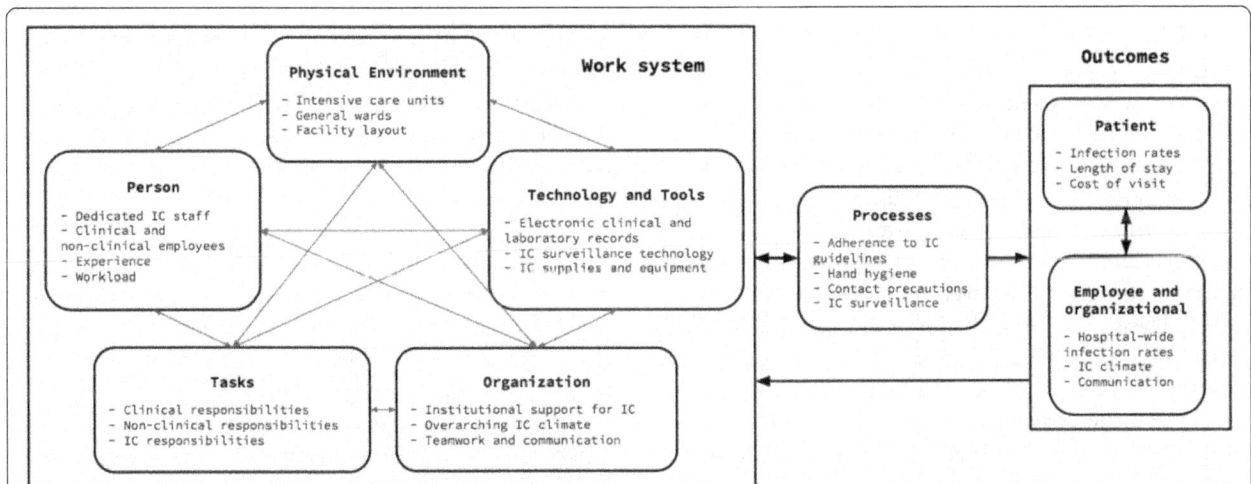

Fig. 1 SEIPS model of infection control in an Indian hospital. Adaptation of the SEIPS model by Carayon, et al. to infection control in an Indian hospital [15]. The work system includes five factors: tools and technology, organization, environment, person, and tasks. These affect related processes and outcomes. IC: infection control

policies, focusing on how people, physical environments, tasks, organizations, and tools are barriers and facilitators to the success of ongoing interventions. Most interviews lasted between ten and twenty minutes. All were audio recorded and transcribed for qualitative analysis.

Analysis

Preliminary data analyses were conducted concurrently with study procedures to direct iterative revisions of the interview guide and determine theoretical saturation. Reworking the interview guide allowed the focus of the interview content to shift overtime, so that new information was gleaned even among later participants. After interviewing the twentieth participant, we decided that the responses to interview questions were becoming highly repetitive and that no new data were likely to appear. Thus, a twenty participant sample size was finalized based on theoretical saturation. Interview transcripts were subsequently analyzed using NVivo software (Version 11.3, QSR International), with responses coded for themes based on the SEIPS framework [15]. NVivo is a qualitative software that aids data analysis by organizing the key themes that are identified by researchers in large quantities of open-ended text. Data were independently coded in NVivo by two investigators (AB and KB) who then jointly reviewed the analyses.

Ethics approval

The institutional review board of the participating institution approved this study and the Health Sciences Institutional Review Board at the University of Wisconsin-Madison granted this study exemption from review. All participants provided oral consent before any data were collected.

Results

Participants' characteristics

Participants were comprised of ten nurses (80% female) and ten doctors (30% female), selected from a wide range of clinical departments including internal medicine, neurology, anesthesia, infectious disease, and three ICUs (cardiac, pediatric, and medicine). Three nurses were recruited from the hospital's infection control department. Participants were enrolled from a range of career levels including junior and senior consulting physicians, residents, head nurses, and general nursing staff.

Tools and technology

Hospital staff overwhelmingly reported that an adequate supply of contact precautions equipment was readily available for use (Table 1). On the general wards, gowns, gloves, and masks were stored outside of the rooms of patients placed under contact precautions. Gloves,

masks, and shoe covers, for dust control, were available within and outside of the ICUs, with gowns available inside the rooms of patients under contact precautions. Although mask use was only required when interacting with patients under droplet or airborne precautions, healthcare workers often put on a mask before entering the ICU. They wore masks intermittently in the ICU and switched them after visiting patients under infection control precautions. Despite their availability, participants reported that both healthcare workers and visitors struggled with mask compliance for patients under droplet or airborne precautions, in large part because of issues surrounding comfort. *"We have to remind visitors all the time [to wear the mask...] The mask is very difficult, especially when they are in the room. If they are sitting there all the time, the mask makes them very hot."* -Internal medicine resident; *"Staff know the importance of personal protective equipment, but they do not always wear the mask. [...] They report that when they wear the mask for a long time, they feel like they are suffocating."* -Infection control head nurse.

Although the hospital's health record was not fully electronic, an electronic microbial database served as the primary resource for treating physicians to access final laboratory results. Critical results were communicated from the microbiologist to the physician by phone and documented. Infection control nurses also utilized the electronic database for tracking patients, accessing microbiology results, and ensuring that correct contact precautions signage was promptly hung and precautions implemented.

Organization

Physicians identified nursing staff turnover as the single greatest barrier to infection control. This was also identified as a barrier by the infection control nurses, but not general nursing staff. Several participants reported high turnover rates, with nurses leaving primarily to take higher paying positions abroad. This was complicated by the fact that many new nurses entered directly from nursing school, without any prior work experience. *"We have a huge turnover of nurses in our hospital. We lose around one-third of our intensive care staff every six months to the west or the Middle East."* -ICU, senior physician. While physicians knew that investing in the training of new nurses was crucial to patient care, it was also acknowledged to be time consuming and rarely resulted in long-term benefits for the healthcare team.

Participants also identified the limited Hindi language capabilities of incoming nurses as a considerable barrier to effective infection control. This was cited as a concern by general and infection control nurses, but no physicians. Hindi was the primary language used between healthcare workers when discussing clinical care. It is

Table 1 Barriers and facilitators to infection control, categorized by components of the Systems Engineering Initiative for Patient Safety (SEIPS)

Tools and Technology	Organization	Environment	Person	Tasks
Barriers				
Clinician and visitors find mask uncomfortable	High nursing turnover	Shoe covers required in ICUs because of dust	New nurse hires often lack clinical experience	Heavy patient workload
No comprehensive electronic health record	Limited initial Hindi language capabilities	Ongoing construction within hospital	Frustration with the frequency of IC training	Perceived understaffing
Facilitators				
Ample IC supplies	Institutional climate that prioritizes IC	Centrally located sinks, hand gel at bedside	IC team well integrated into clinical care	Staff knowledgeable about IC practices
Electronic database for laboratory results	Funding and support for dedicated IC team	Sufficient beds to prevent overcrowding	Large environmental cleaning staff (600)	IC nurses help new hires complete IC tasks

IC infection control, *ICU* intensive care unit

predominately spoken in northern India, but a majority of the nursing schools nationwide are located in the south. Thus, many nurses join the hospital with limited Hindi speaking abilities and initially struggle to communicate with patients and other staff. *"There is a language barrier because a majority of nurses are from South India, but here (in Haryana), they use Hindi. [...] In two or three months the nurses will pick up the language. Before, when I lived in southern India, I did not know Hindi. Now I do."* -Staff nurse.

Because most infection control training takes place in the first few months of employment, this is particularly hindered by limited language proficiency. *"The nurses from Kerala [a southern state of India] do not know much Hindi or English, so sometimes we wonder how we should teach them to make them understand. [...] There are so many things that are very difficult to teach them."* Infection control staff nurse. To help new nurses learn Hindi, head nurses often communicated with them in broken Hindi, even if they shared the same local language from the south.

Despite these barriers, the organization was committed to infection control and has facilitated it through the creation and staffing of a large infection control team. This includes sixteen nurses dedicated full-time to infection control activities. The hospital has also designated several physicians as leaders in ongoing infection control and antibiotic stewardship initiatives. These actions have created an institutional climate that prioritizes and values infection control. *"Other institutions talk about infection control, but nobody emphasizes it like they are doing now. I have realized that this [hospital-acquired infections] is a major reason why my patients are staying in the hospital longer."*-Anesthesia, physician.

Environment

The hospital's physical environment was structured and maintained to facilitate infection control. Each general ward had a centrally located sink with running water

and alcohol based hand rub at the patients' bedside. Rooms contained between one and six beds and patients under contact precautions were either placed into single rooms or cohorted. Overcrowding was not a problem and every patient was given their own bed. Each ICU had several sinks and a hand rub bottle for each patient.

Environmental cleaning was prioritized by the hospital, which employs more than six hundred cleaning staff on site. Housekeeping staff were recognized by study participants as key stakeholders in infection prevention. Anecdotally, they had the best hand hygiene compliance rates in the hospital and participants were adamant that environmental cleaning was comprehensive and timely. Staff decontaminated patient rooms three times a day, with common areas cleaned even more frequently. *"Every two to three hours [housekeeping] will come."*-Cardiac ICU, senior staff nurse.

Person

Sixteen nurses were dedicated to front-line implementation of hospital infection control policies. Each worked on specific units rounding with physicians, conducting daily hand hygiene and environmental cleaning audits, and providing new nurses with infection control training at the patient's bedside. Because of the high rate of nursing turnover, these trainings occurred on a daily basis. *"I am very strict and will say to them [the nurses] again and again, don't do this or don't do that. I instruct them, because I do not want my staff transmitting infections from one patient to another."* - Infection control staff nurse.

Infection control nurses were also responsible for ensuring that nursing staff completed infection control checklists for high risk patients at each shift. Most nurse and physician participants were receptive to the work of the infection control nurses. *"If the nurse sees that someone is not doing it [hand hygiene], she will point it out, whether it is a doctor or a nurse. She's like a police woman. [...] We always do whatever she says, because even we forget that infection is such a problem in the ICUs. We have to take advice from her. We do not mind." -ICU, senior physician.* A few non-infection control nurses described frustration with the continual training and audits. *"If it is a new person then it is fine, because they need training. But if you've been here for awhile, it is not so good." -Staff nurse.*

Tasks

The typical nurse to patient ratio on the general wards was 1:6 and 1:1 or 1:2 in the ICU. Several non-infection control nurses expressed concern that they were understaffed and the daily workload was difficult to manage. *"We are not getting any time to sit, or even to stand. We have to run just like in the Olympics." -Pediatrics ICU, staff nurse.*

The perceived workload had direct implications for infection control practices. Both staff nurses and infection control nurses reported that staff nurses were less likely to practice infection control properly when they were busy. *"The knowledge is there, but some people are not implementing it [the practices...] If they are busy, sometimes they avoid it." -Infection control nurse.*

Discussion

In this interview-based, qualitative analysis of the barriers and facilitators to infection control implementation in an Indian hospital, we found that staff turnover, time spent training new staff, limitations in language competency, and workload were major barriers to effective infection control. A well developed infection control team and an institutional climate that prioritizes infection control were major facilitators. Most of these barriers and facilitators mapped to the tasks, person, and organizational components of SEIPS.

These findings have implications for hospital leadership, infection control departments, and clinicians. It is especially imperative in resource constrained environments to implement interventions that are the most likely to be impactful. With the recognition of major barriers related to staffing, support from the highest levels of leadership is needed to implement policies that incentivize healthcare worker retention and recruitment. Hospital leadership must also prioritize the allocation of resources to rapidly build language and infection control skills for incoming healthcare workers. We recommend that hospitals incorporate intensive language training focused on medically relevant vocabulary into initial staff onboarding programs.

Two interventional studies from India also report on the role of person and organizational level factors in improving the implementation of infection control interventions. The first, assessing airborne infection control practices in thirty-five Indian healthcare settings, found that an intervention bundle focused on capacity building and systems development at the organizational level substantially improved the implementation of infection control policies [20]. The second study introduced an organizational change process intervention known as appreciative inquiry to the maternity wards of three hospitals in Gujarat, India. Researchers found that the introduction of the appreciative inquiry program improved decision making and inter-personal relationships between healthcare workers, which in turn facilitated improved implementation and compliance of infection control practices [21]. Furthermore, a recent international survey of infection prevention practices in thirty countries found that limited trained staff, infrastructure, and supplies were major barriers to preventing multidrug resistant organism transmission [22].

In our study, responses regarding the SEIPS factors physical environment and tools and technology primarily discussed facilitators to infection control. Participants reported an ample supply of gowns, masks, and gloves, placed in highly visible locations. Barriers to compliance centered around complex behavioral issues, instead of a lack of supplies. In contrast, a lack of personal protective equipment has previously been identified as a barrier to infection control in other Indian hospitals [21, 23]. These findings must be contextualized for the study institutions. One limitation of our study is that it focuses on a single tertiary care hospital that is internationally accredited by Joint Commission International. As such, our findings are likely not generalizable to India's more resource limited healthcare settings.

Additional studies are needed from public government hospitals and other institution types. The Indian healthcare system is varied and complex with a high burden of antimicrobial resistance. Organized infection control programs are not routinely practiced, except in accredited healthcare organizations. Data regarding the barriers and facilitators from multiple types of healthcare settings are required to create a broader action plan of curbing antimicrobial resistance and healthcare associated infections.

Another limitation of the study is that we were not able to correlate self-reported practices with direct observations of infection control behavior. Future studies may identify additional barriers and facilitators of relevance by collecting such data via direct observation of hospital infection control practices.

Despite these limitations, we conducted, to our knowledge, the first SEIPS work system analysis of infection control practices at a hospital in India. Furthermore, our findings and methods provide institutions with an approach to identifying local barriers and facilitators to infection prevention that guide intervention implementation.

Adaptation and tailoring interventions to local contexts is crucial. Designing solutions without identifying and accounting for such underlying inter-related barriers may lead to unsuccessful interventions and is a potential reason why interventions that have been successful in one setting may fail in another.

Conclusions

A work systems evaluation is a valuable exercise for organizations to identify new and evolving areas for improvement. At our Indian study hospital, tasks, person, and organizational level factors were key to the success of infection control practices. Institutional support for infection control and prioritizing resources to recruit and retain trained, experienced nursing staff are critical to the effective implementation of infection control practices.

Abbreviations
HAI: Healthcare associated infections; ICU: Intensive care unit; SEIPS: Systems engineering initiative for patient safety

Acknowledgements
None.

Funding
The research presented was supported by the Indo-US Science and Technology Forum S. N. Bose Scholars Program and a Graduate Student Award from the Global Health Institute at the University of Wisconsin, Madison. AB received funding as a pre-doctoral trainee under NIH award TL1TR000429 administered by the Clinical and Translational Science Award site funded by NIH award UL1TR000427. Content is the responsibility of the authors and does not necessarily represent the views of the funding agencies. These funding bodies had no role in the design of the study, data collection, data analysis, interpretation of data, writing of the manuscript, or the decision to submit the article for publication.

Authors' contributions
AB drafted and critically edited the manuscript, and contributed to study conception, design, data acquisition, and data analysis. KV and MA contributed to data collection, data analysis, and critical manuscript editing. DS drafted the discussion and edited the manuscript. SS and NS contributed to the study design and critical manuscript editing. All authors read and approved the final version of this manuscript.

Competing interests
The authors declare that they have no competing interests.

Consent for publication
Not applicable.

Author details
[1]Department of Population Health Sciences, University of Wisconsin-Madison, School of Medicine and Public Health, Madison, WI, USA. [2]Department of Medicine, University of Wisconsin-Madison, School of Medicine and Public Health, Madison, WI, USA. [3]Medanta Institute of Eduation and Research, Medanta the Medicity Hospital, Gurgaon, Haryana, India. [4]Department of Clinical Microbiology & Infection Control, Medanta the Medicity Hospital, Gurgaon, Haryana, India. [5]William S. Middleton Memorial Veterans Affairs Hospital, Madison, WI, USA.

References

1. World Health Organization. Patient Safety: Health care-associated infections [Internet]. WHO. 2014 [cited 2016 Dec 1]. Available from: http://www.who.int/gpsc/country_work/gpsc_ccisc_fact_sheet_en.pdf.
2. Dubberke ER, Olsen MA. Burden of Clostridium difficile on the healthcare system. Clin Infect Dis. 2012;55(Suppl 2):S88–92.
3. Lloyd-Smith P, Younger J, Lloyd-Smith E, Green H, Leung V, Romney MG. Economic analysis of vancomycin-resistant enterococci at a Canadian hospital: assessing attributable cost and length of stay. J Hosp Infect. 2013;85:54–9.
4. Perencevich EN, Stone PW, Wright SB, Carmeli Y, Fisman DN, Cosgrove SE, et al. Raising standards while watching the bottom line: making a business case for infection control. Infect Control Hosp Epidemiol. 2007;28:1121–33.
5. Allegranzi B, Bagheri Nejad S, Combescure C, Graafmans W, Attar H, Donaldson L, et al. Burden of endemic health-care-associated infection in developing countries: systematic review and meta-analysis. Lancet. 2011; 377:228–41.
6. World Health Organization. The Burden of Health Care-Associated Infection Worldwide [Internet]. WHO. [cited 2016 Dec 3]. Available from: http://www.who.int/gpsc/country_work/summary_20100430_en.pdf.
7. World Health Organization. Antimicrobial resistance: Global report on surveillance [Internet]. 2014. Available from: http://apps.who.int/iris/bitstream/10665/112642/1/9789241564748_eng.pdf.
8. Mehta A, Rosenthal VD, Mehta Y, Chakravarthy M, Todi SK, Sen N, et al. Device-associated nosocomial infection rates in intensive care units of seven Indian cities. Findings of the International Nosocomial Infection Control Consortium (INICC). J Hosp Infect. 2007;67:168–74.
9. Kamat U, Ferreira A, Savio R, Motghare D. Antimicrobial resistance among nosocomial isolates in a teaching hospital in Goa. Indian J Community Med. 2008;33:89–92.
10. Taneja N, Emmanuel R, Chari PS, Sharma M. A prospective study of hospital-acquired infections in burn patients at a tertiary care referral centre in North India. Burns. 2004;30:665–9.
11. Habibi S, Wig N, Agarwal S, Sharma S, Lodha R, Pandey R, et al. Epidemiology of nosocomial infections in medicine intensive care unit at a tertiary care hospital in northern India. Trop Doct. 2008;38:233–5.
12. Furuya EY, Dick A, Perencevich EN, Pogorzelska M, Goldmann D, Stone PW. Central line bundle implementation in US intensive care units and impact on bloodstream infections. PLoS One. 2011;6:e15452.
13. Whitby M, McLaws M-L, Slater K, Tong E, Johnson B. Three successful interventions in health care workers that improve compliance with hand hygiene: Is sustained replication possible? Am J Infect Control. 2008;36:349–55.
14. Anderson J, Gosbee LL, Bessesen M, Williams L. Using human factors engineering to improve the effectiveness of infection prevention and control. Crit Care Med. 2010;38:S269–281.
15. Carayon P, Hundt AS, Karsh B, Gurses AP, Alvarado CJ, Smith M, et al. Work system design for patient safety: the SEIPS model. Qual Saf Health Care. 2006;15:i50–8.
16. Holden RJ, Carayon P, Gurses AP, Hoonakker P, Hundt AS, Ozok AA, et al. SEIPS 2.0: A human factors framework for studying and improving the work of healthcare professionals and patients. Ergonomics. 2013;56:1669–86.
17. Yanke E, Zellmer C, Van Hoof S, Moriarty H, Carayon P, Safdar N. Understanding the current state of infection prevention to prevent clostridium difficile infection: a human factors and systems engineering approach. Am J Infect Control. 2015;43:241–7.
18. Safdar N, Musuuza JS, Xie A, Hundt AS, Hall M, Wood K, et al. Management of ventilator-associated pneumonia in intensive care units: a mixed methods study assessing barriers and facilitators to guideline adherence. BMC Infect Dis. 2016;16:349.
19. Caya T, Musuuza J, Yanke E, Schmitz M, Anderson B, Carayon P, et al. Using a systems engineering initiative for patient safety to evaluate a hospital-wide daily chlorhexidine bathing intervention. J Nurs Care Qual. 2015;30:337–44.
20. Parmar MM, Sachdeva KS, Rade K, Ghedia M, Bansal A, Nagaraja SB, et al. Airborne infection control in India: baseline assessment of health facilities. Indian J Tuberc. 2015;62:211–7.
21. Sharma B, Ramani KV, Mavalankar D, Kanguru L, Hussein J. Using "appreciative inquiry" in India to improve infection control practices in maternity care: a qualitative study. Glob Health Action. 2015;8:26693.

7

Molecular characteristics and successful management of a respiratory syncytial virus outbreak among pediatric patients with hemato-oncological disease

Claas Baier[1][*][†] (iD), Sibylle Haid[2†], Andreas Beilken[3], Astrid Behnert[3], Martin Wetzke[4], Richard J. P. Brown[2], Corinna Schmitt[5], Ella Ebadi[1], Gesine Hansen[4], Thomas F. Schulz[5], Thomas Pietschmann[2†] and Franz-Christoph Bange[1†]

Abstract

Background: Respiratory syncytial virus (RSV) is responsible for upper and lower respiratory tract infection in adults and children. Especially immunocompromised patients are at high risk for a severe course of infection, and mortality is increased. Moreover RSV can spread in healthcare settings and can cause outbreaks. Herein we demonstrate the successful control and characteristics of a RSV outbreak that included 8 patients in our Department of Pediatric Hematology and Oncology.

Methods: We performed an epidemiologic investigation and a molecular analysis of the outbreak strains. Moreover we present the outbreak control bundle and our concept for RSV screening in the winter season.

Results: RSV A and B strains caused the outbreak. RSV B strains affected 3 patients, 2 of whom were co-infected with RSV A. Exactly this RSV A strain was detected in another 5 patients. Our multimodal infection control bundle including prophylactic RSV screening was able to rapidly stop the outbreak.

Conclusion: An infection control bundle in RSV outbreaks should address all potential transmission pathways. In pediatric settings the restriction of social activities might have a temporal negative impact on quality of life but helps to limit transmission opportunities. Molecular analysis allows better understanding of RSV outbreaks and, if done in a timely manner, might be helpful for guidance of infection control measures.

Keywords: RSV, Respiratory syncytial virus, Outbreak, Infection control, Molecular typing, Pediatric patients, Hematology and oncology, Cancer patients

Background

Respiratory syncytial virus (RSV) of the family *Pneumoviridae* is a single stranded RNA-virus with two antigenic different subtypes (A and B). It causes upper and lower respiratory tract infection (URTI and LRTI) in children and adults in a seasonal pattern [1–4]. The median incubation period is 4.4 days [5], ranging from 2 to 8 days. Human to human transmission takes place via droplets as well as direct and indirect contact (e.g. contaminated surfaces or hands of medical staff). Patients with hemato-oncological disease are at risk for severe RSV-caused infection - especially in the context of hematopoietic stem cell transplantation (HSCT) [6, 7]. In the literature varying RSV-related case fatality rates are reported in children with cancer to range from 5% to 33% [8–10].

Respiratory tract infection (RTI) due to RSV is typically community/household-acquired. RSV is a member of the so called community-acquired respiratory viruses such as influenza virus. Nevertheless, hospital (nosocomial) acquisition is possible as well and transmission

* Correspondence: baier.claas@mh-hannover.de
[†]Equal contributors
[1]Institute for Medical Microbiology and Hospital Epidemiology, Hannover Medical School, Carl-Neuberg-Straße 1, 30625 Hannover, Germany
Full list of author information is available at the end of the article

may occur by other infected patients, staff or visitors [11, 12]. RSV outbreaks in inpatient pediatric oncologic care facilities and in adult hematology and oncology units have been described [9, 12–16]. An understanding of transmission pathways helps to guide adequate outbreak control measures and to implement prophylactic measures. Finally, RSV-caused respiratory tract infections are a differential diagnosis worth considering in neutropenic cancer patients with fever [17, 18].

Therapeutic options for patients in hematopoietic stem cell transplantation and with intensive cancer therapy, who are severely infected by RSV, include the use of systemic or aerosolized ribavirin and polyclonal intravenous immunoglobulins (IVIG)[19, 20]. The RSV-specific monoclonal antibody Palivizumab has been used for treatment and for passive immunization (prophylaxis) in high risk pediatric patient groups [19–21].

Here we describe the successful management and characteristics of a RSV outbreak in a single non-HSCT pediatric hematology and oncology ward including 8 patients in March and April 2016. Moreover, we show the results of the molecular strain analysis.

Methods
Outbreak Case definition
An outbreak case is a patient with a positive RSV laboratory testing in samples from the upper or lower respiratory tract and a definite or possible nosocomial onset. A definite nosocomial case was defined as a positive RSV laboratory testing on day 5 or later of the hospital stay. A possible nosocomial case was defined as a positive RSV laboratory testing on day 2 to 4 of hospital stay. Patients who were admitted to the ward with a new positive RSV laboratory testing, and had been on the ward within 8 days prior to admission were also considered a possible nosocomial case. All patients that were accommodated in the same room with cases were considered contacts.

Processing of patient specimens
A combined nose/throat swab was taken for routine viral diagnostics. Material from the lower respiratory tract was suitable as well.

Samples taken for diagnostic purposes were processed at the Institute of Virology using real-time RT-PCR or direct fluorescent antibody (DFA) staining. RNA was extracted from the specimens using a QiaAmp Viral RNA Mini Kit in a QIAcube according to the manufacturer's instruction (Qiagen, Hilden, Germany). cDNA synthesis, amplification and detection of nucleic acid were performed in an Applied Biosystems® 7500 Real-Time PCR System (Life Technologies, Carlsbad, California) by a commercially available one-step real-time RT-PCR kit (RSV/hMPV r-gene® PCR Kit, bioMérieux, Nürtingen,

Germany) according to the manufacturer's instructions. For DFA staining a ready to use FITC (fluorescein isothiocyanate) -labeled monoclonal RSV antibody (LIGHT DIAGNOSTICS, Merck, Darmstadt, Germany) was used according to a protocol described before [22]. PCR and DFA did not differentiate between RSV A and B. One diagnostic specimen was tested using a point-of-care test (POCT) system (Sofia, Quidel, Kornwestheim, Germany), which is available in the pediatric emergency room.

Strain typing
Nasopharyngeal aspirates from 6 outbreak patients (case 1, 2, 3, 5, 6, and 7) were taken only for strain typing purposes on one occasion (March18[th]), which were exclusively processed at the Institute for Experimental Virology, Twincore - Centre for Experimental and Clinical Infection Research. In addition, selected archived (frozen) samples taken for diagnostic purposes from outbreak patients (case 2, 3, 4, 5, 7, 8) were provided by the Institute of Virology and processed at the Institute for Experimental Virology, Twincore - Centre for Experimental and Clinical Infection Research.

Linearized acrylamide (Ambion, Thermo Fisher Scientific; 35 µg/ml final concentration) was added to the sample and total RNA was extracted from 140 µl of aspirate according to the manufacturer's description (QiaAmp Viral RNA Mini Kit, Qiagen, Hilden, Germany). cDNA synthesis was performed using the Superscript III kit from Invitrogen (Invitrogen, Darmstadt, Germany) and random hexamer primers. Next, a nested PCR was performed first amplifying the RSV-G and F protein coding region and in a second round amplifying the G protein gene. PCR products were sent for Sanger sequencing (GATC, Konstanz, Germany) and the sequences were analyzed using MEGA software and the Highlighter analysis tool [23].

Results
Outbreak Setting
The outbreak occurred in the Clinic for Pediatric Hematology and Oncology which is a tertiary referral center for children from 0-18 years with hematologic and solid neoplasia. The affected ward harbors 5 single- and 5 two-bed rooms. Each single room has an anteroom and a high-efficiency particulate air filtration with the air flow directed to the hallway. The same floor houses the outpatient clinic and a recreation room for the hemato-oncological pediatric patients. Exchange from patients between the ward and the outpatient clinic

occurs regularly. Moreover two recreation rooms for social activities are part of the ward. Most patients receive antineoplastic therapy during their stay. A substantial number of patients have a neutrophil count below 500 cells / µl. The ward is serviced by permanent health care workers (HCWs) and house-keeping staff. External personnel (such as medical consultants or physiotherapists) enter the ward when necessary. Autologous and allogenic HSCT are performed on a separate ward with 6 single rooms. Parents are allowed to stay overnight with their children.

Standard infection control measures on the ward

Patients with a positive RSV test are electronically marked in the hospital alert system. Besides single room accommodation, contact and droplet precautions (surgical mask, gown, gloves) are used at any time by visitors and HCWs when entering the room of a RSV positive patient. Affected patients are encouraged to stay in their room and are trained in hygienic hand washing to minimize spread via contact. When leaving the room becomes necessary (e.g. for examination), patients wear a surgical mask. These measures also apply for patients with typical respiratory symptoms (e.g. cough or sneezing) before a pathogen is identified. Measures are usually suspended when there are two negative RSV PCR-based test results at a minimum 2-day interval and therefore patients are not anymore considered infectious. HCWs with symptoms of URTI are suspended from direct patient care and wear a surgical mask while on the ward. Visitors with symptoms of acute RTI are not permitted to enter the ward. Strict hand hygiene following WHO guidelines is implemented. Targeted RSV diagnostics are performed in case of suspected viral RTI. Positive testing for respiratory viruses is regularly reported for epidemiologic and infection control reasons to the infection control staff.

Cases

In March a total of 8 patients (cases 1 to 8) were tested RSV-positive in respiratory samples. Patient characteristics are shown in Table 1. 6 patients fulfilled criteria for nosocomial acquisition. The remaining 2 patients had a possible nosocomial acquisition, as they had been on the ward within 8 days prior to admission. Epidemic curve and an outbreak timeline with the diagnostic results can be seen in Figs 1 and 2.

Case 1 was neutropenic and developed severe LRTI with a RSV positive bronchoalveolar lavage and a requirement for oxygen. Case 2 also suffered from LRTI, which was less severe. Cases 3 to 8 had respiratory symptoms of an URTI such as cough, sneeze and a positive RSV testing in secretions from the upper respiratory tract. Case 6 was co-infected with influenza A virus .

4 patients received oral Ribavirin therapy (case 1, 2, 5, 8) and 5 patients (case 1 to 5) temporarily required supportive oxygen administration via nasal cannula. IVIG or Palivizumab was not administered. No direct RSV-associated mortality was observed. In addition, all patients were empirically treated by antibiotics presuming bacterial co- respectively superinfection according to in-house standards (Table 1).

Viral persistence (viral shedding) is defined as the time period from first positive diagnostic test to sustained negativity. Duration of viral persistence was minimally 4 days (case 7) and maximally at least 63 days (case 1) – see also Table 1.

Outbreak control measures

Active outbreak management was started after detection of 3 new RSV infected patients in calendar week 10 (see Fig. 1). An outbreak control team consisting of the infection control unit and the physicians in charge was established. The head of the Clinic for Pediatric Hematology and Oncology, the medical director of our institution, and the public health authority were informed. In addition to the existing standard infection control measures described above, interventional measures were introduced. All HCWs (including permanent staff members and external personnel), visitors and outpatients were required to wear a surgical mask at any time (patient care and non-patient care activities) when on the ward and in the outpatient clinic (preemptive barrier precaution). Moreover, roommates of patients tested positive for RSV in their clinical course were moved to single rooms for 8 days (typical maximum incubation period; so called quarantine). They were repeatedly tested for RSV using PCR. All newly admitted patients were tested for RSV (admission screening). Twice weekly PCR RSV prevalence screening for *all* patients on ward was established (prevalence screening). If possible, elective patient admissions were delayed to reduce patient-to-nurse ratio. Moreover, only parents were allowed as visitors. All social activities for the patients and relatives were suspended. During outbreak, all two bed-rooms were occupied by one patient only, meaning single room isolation for *all* patients on the ward. Repeated training sessions for staff were provided by the infection control team. They addressed RSV transmission pathways and underlined the importance of droplet precautions (e.g. masks and cough etiquette for HCWs and visitors) as well as hand hygiene.

Intervention measures were fully implemented on 22nd of March. The last nosocomial case occurred on 29th of March (case 8). However, the patient had been discharged from the ward on 22nd of March, and readmitted on 29th of March (Fig. 2). Thus, after intervention measures had been in place no further nosocomial RSV

Table 1 Patients' characteristics

Case	Nosocomial (Yes/No)	Age[a] (years)	Sex (M/F)	Underlying Disease	RSV infection	WBC[b] (per microliter)	RSV Treatment, Duration (days)	Additional antibiotic treatment	Oxygen (Yes/No)	RSV-related outcome	Virus shedding (days)
1	yes	16	M	Acute myeloid leukemia (recurrent)	LRTI	0	oral Ribavirin, 64	Yes	Yes	Remission	At least 63
2	yes	15	M	Severe aplastic anemia	LRTI	800	oral Ribavirin, 10	Yes	Yes	Remission	7
3	Yes	16	M	Acute lymphoid leukemia	URTI	1200	-	Yes	Yes (at night)	Remission	At least 6
4[c]	Yes	9	M	Post-transplant Burkitt's leukemia	URTI	300	-	Yes	Yes	Remission	17[d]
5	Yes	1	F	Neuroblastoma	URTI	9500	intravenous Ribavirin, 8	Yes	Yes	Remission	44
6	Possible	3	F	Ewing Sarcoma	URTI	500	-	Yes	Yes	Remission	5
7	Yes	10	F	Acute lymphoid leukemia	URTI	700	-	Yes	No	Remission	4
8	Possible	14	F	Acute lymphoid leukemia	URTI	290	oral Ribavirin, 8	Yes	No	Remission	13

[a]At time of virus detection
[b]At time (+/- 2 days) of virus detection
[c]Onset of disease after discharge (treatment in home town hospital)
[d]There had been no in-house tests between first positive and first negative testing

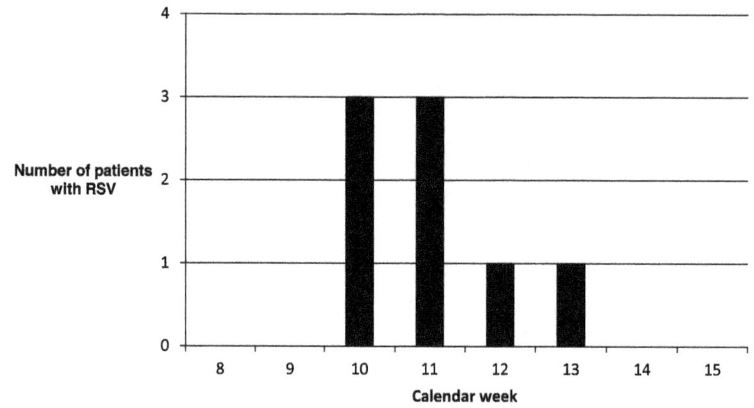

Fig. 1 Epidemic curve for the RSV outbreak

cases occurred. At the beginning of May the last positive patients were discharged respectively sustainably tested negative and all outbreak control measures were suspended.

Molecular analysis

For phylogenetic analysis of the RSV genome we focused on the viral glycoprotein G of RSV as this gene is highly variable and shows the highest sequence variance between the RSV subgroups A and B (53% amino acid sequence identity [24]). From the total of 8 patients, five of them were infected with a RSV A strain (Case 1, 3, 4, 5, 6), one was tested positive for RSV B (case 8) and two patients were infected with RSV A and B (case 2 and 7) dependent on the time point of sampling. Despite the coexistence of genetically definite genotypic strains with many nucleotide exchanges especially in the C-terminal variable region of RSV-G [25–27], we detected the very same nucleotide sequence for the coding region of the RSV-G protein for all patients infected with RSV A (Fig. 3a). Only one single nucleotide exchange was detected in the intergenic region of the virus infecting patient C3 and only at one time point of sampling (Fig. 3a; C3_13_3). In the specimen taken 5 days later (C3_18_3), this variation was no longer detectable. Among the three patients infected with RSV B, we observed 4 nucleotide differences in the coding region

of the G protein (Fig. 3b). Two additional variations were observed in the intergenic region of the G gene (Fig. 3b). The RSV B viruses infecting patients C2 and C7 were almost identical with merely three nucleotide differences between them. Notably, the chromatograms of the Sanger sequencing from these patients revealed sequence ambiguity at exactly these three positions: between G/A at position 907, between T/A at position 974 and G/A at residue 979. While in case C7, residues G, T and G were dominant, in patient C2, residues A, A, A predominated. This result suggested that these two patients were infected with an essentially identical viral quasispecies and that merely the relative number of viruses with G, T, G residues compared to viruses with A, A, A nucleotides at these positions varied between these two patients. In contrast, patient C8 carried a RSV B virus with an unambiguous sequence at these three positions G, T, G (Fig. 3d). Moreover, it displayed three additional polymorphisms in the G protein coding region relative to the virus infecting patients C2 and C7, thus supporting the conclusion that this patient was infected with a different RSV B virus. Noticeably, case 2 was tested RSV negative in two samples taken and processed for routine diagnostic on March 15th and 18th. RSV strain sequences available from other, non-outbreak pediatric patients (same season as the outbreak) were used for comparison. These strains show a predominantly polyclonal pattern for RSV A (Fig. 3c).

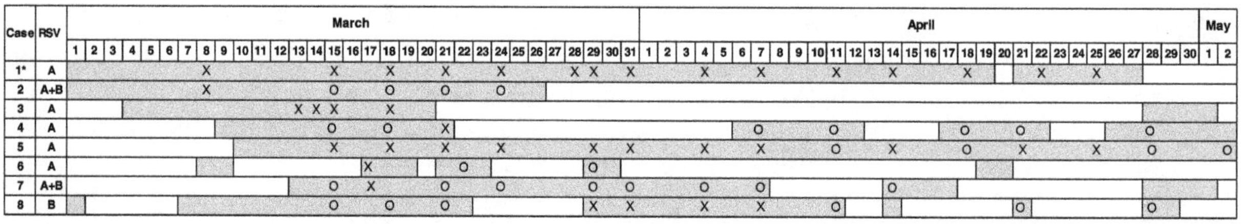

Fig. 2 Outbreak timeline. Grey bars indicate the patient's stay on the ward. 'X' indicates positive routine diagnostic RSV testing (DFA, PCR, POCT). 'O' indicates a negative routine diagnostic RSV testing. *Case 1 was readmitted on May 6th and had another positive testing on May 9th (not shown)

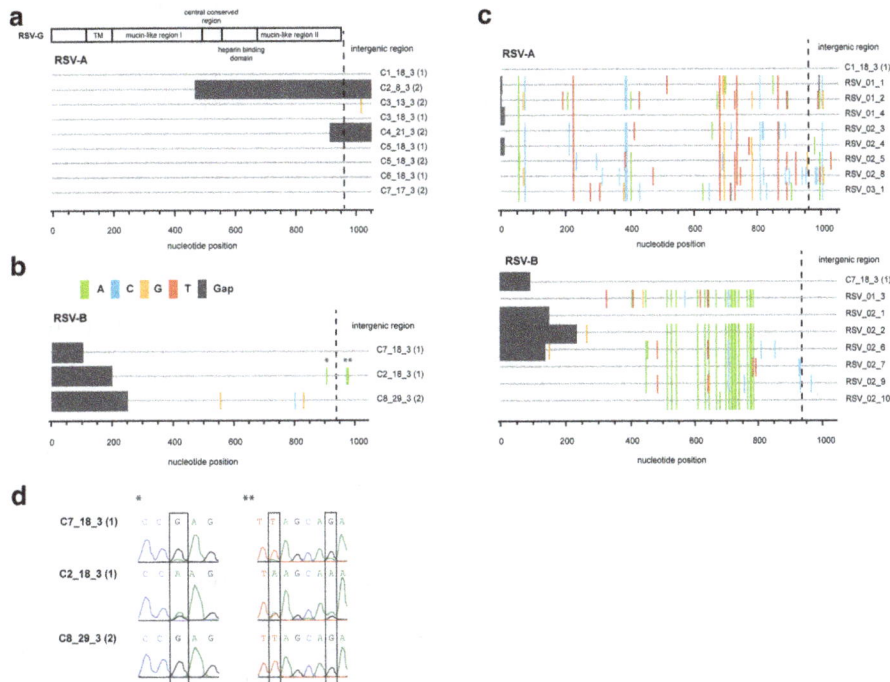

Fig. 3 Highlighter plot depicting nucleotide mismatches comparing the sequence of the strain obtained from patient C1 to all other RSV A strains, and the sequence of the strain obtained from patient C7 to all other RSV B strains. **a** RSV A and (**b**) RSV B glycoprotein sequences were aligned using MEGA and depicted as highlighter plot using the highlighter analysis tool [23]. Nucleotide exchanges compared to a reference sequence (C1_18_3 (1) for RSV A and C7_18_3 (1) for RSV B) are depicted in color. Absence of sequence information is depicted as grey bar. A schematic of the RSV G protein with the different domains is depicted on top [modified from [39]]. (1) indicates samples taken exclusively for strain typing at the 18th of March and (2) indicates samples collected for routine viral diagnostics. **c** RSV-G sequence alignment from other pediatric, non-outbreak patients compared to the references C1 and C7, respectively. **d** Sequencing chromatograms for RSV B cases. The depicted area is highlighted by * and ** in Figure 3B. Overlying sequence information from different quasispecies detected in the samples are highlighted in a box

Interestingly, one patient (RSV_02_1) was infected with the very same RSV B strain as cases 2 and 7 (Fig. 3c, lower part), whereas there were clear sequence differences for the other RSV B strains isolated from non-outbreak pediatric patients.

Discussion

For our Clinic of Pediatric Hematology and Oncology this was the first actively managed RSV-outbreak. In the previous two winter seasons in total only 3 RSV-positive patients were detected on the affected ward.

We studied the epidemiologic and molecular background of this outbreak.

Considering bed and room occupancy on the ward during the outbreak, direct patient to patient transmission (e.g. via droplets or contaminated surfaces) in cases 1 and 2 as well as 3 and 4 seemed epidemiologically possible as each pair was accommodated in the same room before samples were tested positive for RSV. Cases 5 and 7 acquired RSV at day 6 and 5 of their stay on the ward, respectively, suggesting nosocomial RSV acquisition. These two patients did not share rooms with other infected patients but were on ward during the outbreak.

Cases 6 and 8 were tested positive for RSV on admission. Nosocomial acquisition was considered possible, as case 6 and 8 had been discharged 8 and 7 days, respectively, from the affected ward prior to re-admission. During this previous stay patients with symptoms of RTI and a positive RSV test were already on the ward. Nonetheless, community-onset still was an option for case 6 and 8.

Based on this epidemiologic background, our main hypothesis was that direct and indirect patient to patient transmission (the latter for example via the HCWs' hands) caused the outbreak. However, at this point transmission by an infected visitor or HCWs acting as a point source could not be excluded. Moreover, taking all epidemiological data into account, a random introduction of several different community-acquired strains seemed unlikely to us. We suspected ongoing transmission of a single RSV variant and sequencing was used retrospectively to test this hypothesis (see below).

The standard, pre-outbreak infection control measures regarding RSV were mainly in line with previously made recommendations for hospitalized patients with hemato-oncologic disease[19, 28]. The additionally implemented measures, in particular single room accommodation for contact patients (quarantine), suspension of all social activities, and surgical masks for all HCWs and visitors at any time, addressed the postulated RSV transmission pathways during this outbreak. These postulated pathways were direct patient to patient transmission (e.g. roommate to roommate), but also transmission via HCWs and visitors.

Direct patient to patient transmission as the most probable route of infection has been shown by Lehners et al. in a large RSV outbreak in a German hematology and transplant unit [11]. Jensen et al. described direct patient to patient transmission, mixed with introduction of strains from outside, in an outbreak affecting immunocompromised adults [29]. We therefore focused on patient to patient transmission early during the outbreak by strict isolation precautions for RSV infected patients and contacts. Isolation for infected patients was also a key measure in a multimodal control bundle described by Inkster et al. [15]. Contact patients were isolated for 8 days and repeatedly tested in order to disrupt infection chains as described in literature [11]. This so called quarantine concerned 2 patients in our outbreak. One of them (case 4) was eventually tested RSV-positive at day 8 of quarantine while being negative at day 2 and 5. This underlines the value of the measure. Finally, we re-emphasized in training sessions the need for preemptive isolation of patients with respiratory symptoms. As all these measures required more isolation capacity on the ward, we restricted elective admissions and located all patients in single rooms.

As another measure we reduced direct patient to patient contacts on the ward by suspending community events, as active social behavior can be a risk factor for nosocomial RSV acquisition [30]. Even so this noticeably restricted the social life for the patients and their families during the outbreak, we enforced this measure. We further restricted social contacts by temporally limiting visits of infants to the ward, as (especially young) infants are known to be the main reservoir for RSV and as our outbreak was approximately concurrent (slightly delayed) to the RSV community peak. Only parents were allowed to the ward, which is in line with an intervention done by Kelley et al. [12]. A restrictive visiting policy is as well described by Singh et al. in a pediatric RSV outbreak [14].

The use of surgical masks for everyone on the ward is an important measure to prevent droplet associated nosocomial RSV transmissions. This is even more rational as RSV may be transmitted via symptomless or oligosymptomatic persons (e.g. HCWs or visitors) and the infectious period can in fact already begin 1 to 2 days before actual onset of symptoms. A literature review by French et al. concluded that personal protective equipment might be advantageous for reducing nosocomial RSV transmission [31]. Kelly et al. showed that five HCWs showing only mild symptoms were involved in a RSV outbreak on an adult stem cell transplant unit [12]. This underlines the necessity that HCWs with respiratory symptoms should not participate in direct patient care activities, at least in a high risk patient care setting. We re-emphasized this issue in training sessions for the HCWs. Although staff screening is described in literature [15], we were able to terminate this outbreak without staff screening. A cohort of HCWs to take care of solely RSV-positive patients as reported before [9] had also not been established but would have been another option in case of an ongoing outbreak.

Temporal survival of respiratory viruses in general [32] and specifically RSV [33] on inanimate surfaces is described, thus contact transmission via the hands of staff was conceivable for nosocomial acquisition. This is especially of importance as cough etiquette and compliance to basic hygienic principles may be reduced for obvious reasons in pediatric patients, so a higher environmental RSV burden is probable. Nonetheless we did not implement changes in the well established cleaning and disinfection procedures on the ward.

We detected prolonged RSV persistence (virus shedding), which has been reported in patients with hematological disorders [34]. This finding needs to be considered for efficient outbreak control and favors the practice of repeated testing in immunocompromised patients as we did. Likewise, this is important as pediatric hemato-oncologic patients are often readmitted several times for cancer treatment cycles or fever in neutropenia. When symptoms are no longer present or mild but viruses are still being shed, RSV may be re-introduced to the ward. Thus, for termination of isolation precautions during the outbreak, we required negative results as reported before [35]. In fact, two subsequent negative results at a minimum 2-day interval were necessary. The usefulness of this requirement is supported by the longitudinal course of the samples from patient 5 which were obtained in April and May. This patient produced positive specimens on two occasions, after one specimen had been tested negative (see Fig. 2).

Active RSV-surveillance by screening on admission and twice weekly for all patients on the ward insured rapid detection of RSV-positive patients. This is in line with successful infection control measures reported in literature [9, 12]. We presume that a prophylactic admission and prevalence RSV screening for all patients in the winter season might be helpful as a preventive measure in high risk populations. Therefore, one consequence of this outbreak was the implementation of an active RSV surveillance (admission and prevalence screening once weekly) in our Clinic for Pediatric Hematology and Oncology during the RSV season. The beginning and ending of this seasonal screening period is determined by in-house and regional/national RSV epidemiology [36]. Moreover, pre-RSV-season audits involving clinicians, infection control staff and the Institute of Virology take place to ensure timely beginning of screening procedures and adherence to the existing infection control practices.

Molecular characterization of RSV strains, for instance by whole genome sequencing [37] or characterization of RSV G-Protein [16, 38], has been used to investigate nosocomial RSV outbreaks. We were able to collect and examine selected outbreak strains by G-Protein gene sequencing. We found that cases 1 to 7 were infected with an RSV A virus with identical G protein coding region. In case of patient C3 one nucleotide difference in the intergenic region of the G gene was observed in one of two samples collected five days apart (Fig. 3a. It is possible that this change was due to natural drift of the infecting virus over time or that this polymorphism is indicative of the presence of two slightly different viruses replicating in parallel and dominating on the one and the other day of sampling, respectively.

Moreover we found that case 8 had a RSV-B infection and that cases 2 and 7 were co-infected by RSV A and RSV B viruses. While sequence analysis of the earlier samples of case 2 and 7 revealed infection by the RSV A virus, the sequence analysis of the later specimen showed infection by an RSV B virus. With the available specimen, we were unable to distinguish if these two patients had a prolonged co-infection between these viruses or if they were sequentially infected by RSV A and RSV B. These findings became available only after the outbreak ended, as routine virological testing during the outbreak did not include molecular differentiation of RSV A and B. In retrospect, these results indicated the decision not to cohort RSV-patients during the outbreak, as we probably might have cohorted RSV-patients with different subtypes. Detailed sequencing analysis suggests that cases 2 and 7 were infected by an almost identical RSV B virus population. We observed three nucleotide differences between these viruses; however, nucleotides of the viruses at these three positions were ambiguous in both cases (G,T,G versus A,A,A residues). Thus, both patients were likely infected by a highly similar RSV B quasispecies which was characterized by two different nucleotide signatures varying in abundance between patients. In contrast, the RSV B virus infecting patient C8 differed in two key criteria. First, it did not show any sequence ambiguity at the three above mentioned residues that was characteristic for the RSV B virus population observed in patients C2 and C7. Second, it displayed three additional polymorphisms in the coding region of the G protein. Taken together, this suggests that patient C8 was infected by another RSV B virus and that there was no transmission from patients C2 and C7 to patient C8.

Outbreak strains of the subtype RSV A were highly similar and different from polyclonal strains from other non-outbreak pediatric patients (Fig. 3c). We therefore conclude that a single RSV A strain was introduced to the ward and then spread within the ward. Interestingly, the RSV B isolate C7_18_3 (1) was identical to the community strain RSV_02_1, however further epidemiologic and clinical information are not accessible for the non-outbreak patient. Taken together, the nucleotide analysis suggests independent introductions of at least 2 different RSV B strains into the ward affecting patient C2, C7 and C8, and transmission of one RSV A strain on the ward between patients C1 to C7.

Looking exclusively at the molecular analysis, it is not possible to disclose the exact transmission pathway of RSV A. RSV A might have been introduced to the ward by an infected patient (index patient) on the ward (maybe case 1) and was then successively transmitted from patient to patient. Alternatively, a point source, such as a RSV-positive HCW, may have caused the outbreak. However, in correlation with the epidemiologic observations such as overlapping patient stays on the ward, stay of case 1 and 2, and case 3 and 4 in a double room, and social activity on the ward in the initial phase of the outbreak, we consider a direct and indirect patient to patient transmission most likely.

Conclusions

RSV poses a significant infectious threat to pediatric patients with an underlying oncologic disease. This outbreak and other outbreaks reported in literature demonstrate the potential of RSV to spread in a hospital. We strictly enforced our existing infection control practices and implemented temporally additional measures to terminate the outbreak. According to our experiences an outbreak control bundle for RSV should include (preemptive) barrier precautions (especially masks), prevalence and admission screenings for *all* patients, and strict isolation procedures for infected patients and contact patients. Quarantine for contacts should at least be for 8 days, the usual maximal incubation period of RSV. In pediatric settings the restriction of visitors (especially siblings) and social activities on the ward can be helpful to prevent transmission and RSV introduction from outside, but definitely limits social life quality. As shown in other outbreaks with viral and bacterial pathogens restriction of admissions still is a very effective measure as it enables single room accommodation for all or the majority of the patients. Moreover, a decrease of the patient to nurse ratio makes transmission more unlikely. In our case the molecular analysis was very helpful to verify the true outbreak character of the RSV cluster and revealed ongoing transmission of an unique RSV A strain on the ward, and an probable independent introduction of different RSV B strains into the ward.

Abbreviations
RSV: Respiratory syncytial virus; URTI: Upper respiratory tract infection; LRTI: Lower respiratory tract infection; HSCT: Hematopoietic stem cell transplantation; RTI: Respiratory tract infection; IVIG: Intravenous immunoglobulins; DFA: Direct fluorescent antibody staining; FITC: Fluorescein isothiocyanate; POCT: Point-of-care-testing; HCWs: Health care workers.

Acknowledgements
Not applicable.

Funding
This research did not receive any specific grant from funding agencies in the public, commercial, or not-for-profit sectors.

Authors' contributions
All authors contributed to the manuscript according to the ICMJE (International Committee of Medial Journal Editors) recommendations: All authors were involved in data acquisition, analysis and interpretation. SH, RB and TP carried out molecular analysis. CB, SH, TP and F-CB prepared the manuscript. CB organized the drafting process. AsB and AnB, CB and F-CB were involved in the active outbreak management. TS and CS carried routine RSV diagnostic. MW collected specimens for typing purposes. All authors critically revised the manuscript and account for accuracy and correctness. All authors have read and agreed to the final draft before submission.

Consent for publication
Not applicable (No individual details such as images or videos are included).

Competing interests
The authors declare that they have no competing interests.

Author details
[1]Institute for Medical Microbiology and Hospital Epidemiology, Hannover Medical School, Carl-Neuberg-Straße 1, 30625 Hannover, Germany. [2]Institute for Experimental Virology; Twincore- Centre for Experimental and Clinical Infection Research; a joint venture of Hannover Medical School (MHH) and Helmholtz Centre for Infection Research (HZI), Hannover, Germany. [3]Department of Paediatric Haematology and Oncology, Hannover Medical School (MHH), Hannover, Germany. [4]Department for Paediatric Pneumology, Allergy and Neonatology, Hannover Medical School (MHH), Hannover, Germany. [5]Institute of Virology, Hannover Medical School (MHH), Hannover, Germany.

References
1. Borchers AT, Chang C, Gershwin ME, Gershwin LJ. Respiratory syncytial virus - A comprehensive review. Clin Rev Allergy Immunol. 2013;45:331–79.
2. Ogra PL. Respiratory syncytial virus: the virus, the disease and the immune response. Paediatr Respir Rev. 2004;5(Suppl A):S119–26.
3. Bont L, Checchia PA, Fauroux B, Figueras-Aloy J, Manzoni P, Paes B, et al. Defining the Epidemiology and Burden of Severe Respiratory Syncytial Virus Infection Among Infants and Children in Western Countries. Infect Dis Ther. 2016;5:271–98.
4. Rodriguez R, Ramilo O. Respiratory syncytial virus: how, why and what to do. J Infect. 2014;68(Suppl 1):S115–8.
5. Lessler J, Reich NG, Brookmeyer R, Perl TM, Nelson KE, Cummings DA. Incubation periods of acute respiratory viral infections: a systematic review. Lancet Infect Dis. 2009;9:291–300.
6. Khanna N, Widmer AF, Decker M, Steffen I, Halter J, Heim D, et al. Respiratory Syncytial Virus Infection in Patients with Hematological Diseases: Single-Center Study and Review of the Literature. Clin Infect Dis. 2008;46: 402–12.
7. Avetisyan G, Mattsson J, Sparrelid E, Ljungman P. Respiratory syncytial virus infection in recipients of allogeneic stem-cell transplantation: a retrospective study of the incidence, clinical features, and outcome. Transplantation. 2009; 88:1222–6.
8. Hatanaka M, Miyamura T, Koh K, Taga T, Tawa A, Hasegawa D, et al. Respiratory syncytial virus infection in infants with acute leukemia: a retrospective survey of the Japanese Pediatric Leukemia/Lymphoma Study Group. Int J Hematol. 2015;102:697–701.
9. Shachor-Meyouhas Y, Zaidman I, Kra-Oz Z, Arad-Cohen N, Kassis I. Detection, control, and management of a respiratory syncytial virus outbreak in a pediatric hematology-oncology department. J Pediatr Hematol Oncol. 2013;35:124–8.
10. Chemaly RF, Ghantoji SS, Shah DP, Shah JN, El-Taoum KK, Champlin RE, et al. Respiratory syncytial virus infections in children with cancer. J Pediatr Hematol Oncol. 2014;36:e376–81.
11. Lehners N, Schnitzler P, Geis S, Puthenparambil J, Benz MA, Alber B, et al. Risk factors and containment of respiratory syncytial virus outbreak in a hematology and transplant unit. Bone Marrow Transplant. 2013;48:1548–53.
12. Kelly SG, Metzger K, Bolon MK, Silkaitis C, Mielnicki M, Cullen J, et al. Respiratory syncytial virus outbreak on an adult stem cell transplant unit. Am J Infect Control. 2016;44:1022–6.
13. Anak S, Atay D, Unuvar A, Garipardic M, Agaoglu L, Ozturk G, et al. Respiratory syncytial virus infection outbreak among pediatric patients with oncologic diseases and/or BMT. Pediatr Pulmonol. 2010;45:307–11.
14. Singh AK, Jain B, Verma AK, Kumar A, Dangi T, Dwivedi M, et al. Hospital outbreak of human respiratory syncytial virus (HRSV) illness in immunocompromised hospitalized children during summer. Clin Respir J. 2015;9:180–4.
15. Inkster T, Ferguson K, Edwardson A, Gunson R, Soutar R. Consecutive yearly outbreaks of respiratory syncytial virus in a haemato-oncology ward and efficacy of infection control measures. J Hosp Infect. 2017;96:353–9.
16. Nabeya D, Kinjo T, Parrott GL, Uehara A, Motooka D, Nakamura S, et al. The clinical and phylogenetic investigation for a nosocomial outbreak of respiratory syncytial virus infection in an adult hemato-oncology unit. J Med Virol. 2017;89:1364–72.
17. Torres JP, De la Maza V, Kors L, Villarroel M, Piemonte P, Izquierdo G, et al. Respiratory Viral Infections and Co-Infections in Children with Cancer, Fever and Neutropenia. Pediatr Infect Dis J. 2016;35:1.
18. Söderman M, Rhedin S, Tolfvenstam T, Rotzén-Östlund M, Albert J, Broliden K, et al. Frequent Respiratory Viral Infections in Children with Febrile Neutropenia - A Prospective Follow-Up Study. Schildgen O, editor. PLoS One. 2016;11:e0157398.
19. Hirsch HH, Martino R, Ward KN, Boeckh M, Einsele H, Ljungman P. Fourth European conference on infections in leukaemia (ECIL-4): Guidelines for diagnosis and treatment of human respiratory syncytial virus, parainfluenza virus, metapneumovirus, rhinovirus, and coronavirus. Clin Infect Dis. 2013;56: 258–66.
20. Waghmare A, Englund JA, Boeckh M. How I treat respiratory viral infections in the setting of intensive chemotherapy or hematopoietic cell transplantation. Blood. 2016;127:1–3.
21. American Academy of Pediatrics. Updated guidance for palivizumab prophylaxis among infants and young children at increased risk of hospitalization for respiratory syncytial virus infection. Pediatrics. 2014;134: 415–20.
22. Ganzenmueller T, Kluba J, Hilfrich B, Puppe W, Verhagen W, Heim A, et al. Comparison of the performance of direct fluorescent antibody staining, a point-of-care rapid antigen test and virus isolation with that of RT-PCR for the detection of novel 2009 influenza A (H1N1) virus in respiratory specimens. J Med Microbiol. 2010;59:713–7.
23. Keele BF, Giorgi EE, Salazar-Gonzalez JF, Decker JM, Pham KT, Salazar MG, et al. Identification and characterization of transmitted and early founder virus envelopes in primary HIV-1 infection. Proc Natl Acad Sci U S A. 2008;105:7552–7.
24. Johnson PR, Spriggs MK, Olmsted RA, Collins PL. The G glycoprotein of human respiratory syncytial viruses of subgroups A and B: extensive sequence divergence between antigenically related proteins. Proc Natl Acad Sci U S A. 1987;84:5625–9.
25. Cane PA, Pringle CR. Evolution of subgroup A respiratory syncytial virus: evidence for progressive accumulation of amino acid changes in the attachment protein. J Virol. 1995;69:2918–25.
26. Sullender WM, Mufson MA, Anderson LJ, Wertz GW. Genetic diversity of the attachment protein of subgroup B respiratory syncytial viruses. J Virol. 1991; 65:5425–34.
27. Cane PA, Matthews DA, Pringle CR. Identification of variable domains of the

attachment (G) protein of subgroup A respiratory syncytial viruses. J Gen Virol. 1991;72(Pt 9):2091–6.

28. Tomblyn M, Chiller T, Einsele H, Gress R, Sepkowitz K, Storek J, et al. Guidelines for Preventing Infectious Complications among Hematopoietic Cell Transplantation Recipients: A Global Perspective. Biol Blood Marrow Transplant. 2009;15:1143–238.

29. Jensen TO, Stelzer-Braid S, Willenborg C, Cheung C, Andresen D, Rawlinson W, et al. Outbreak of respiratory syncytial virus (RSV) infection in immunocompromised adults on a hematology ward. J Med Virol. 2016;88: 1827–31.

30. RSV Nosocomial Outbreak Investigation Team. Contributing and Terminating Factors of a Large RSV Outbreak in an Adult Hematology and Transplant Unit. PLoS Curr. 2014

31. French CE, Mckenzie BC, Coope C, Rajanaidu S, Paranthaman K, Pebody R, et al. Risk of nosocomial respiratory syncytial virus infection and effectiveness of control measures to prevent transmission events: A systematic review. Influenza Other Respi. Viruses. 2016;10:268–90.

32. Kramer A, Schwebke I, Kampf G. How long do nosocomial pathogens persist on inanimate surfaces? A systematic review. BMC Infect. Dis. 2006;6:130.

33. Hall CB, Douglas RG, Geiman JM. Possible transmission by fomites of respiratory syncytial virus. J Infect Dis. 1980;141:98–102.

34. Lehners N, Tabatabai J, Prifert C, Wedde M, Puthenparambil J, Weissbrich B, et al. Long-term shedding of influenza virus, parainfluenza virus, respiratory syncytial virus and nosocomial epidemiology in patients with hematological disorders. PLoS One. 2016;11:1–17.

35. von Lilienfeld-Toal M, Berger A, Christopeit M, Hentrich M, Heussel CP, Kalkreuth J, et al. Community acquired respiratory virus infections in cancer patients—Guideline on diagnosis and management by the Infectious Diseases Working Party of the German Society for haematology and Medical Oncology. Eur J Cancer. 2016;67:200–12.

36. Terletskaia-Ladwig E, Enders G, Schalasta G, Enders M. Defining the timing of respiratory syncytial virus (RSV) outbreaks: an epidemiological study. BMC Infect Dis. 2005;5:20.

37. Zhu Y, Zembower TR, Metzger KE, Lei Z, Green SJ, Qi C. Investigation of Respiratory Syncytial Virus Outbreak on an Adult Stem Cell Transplant Unit using Whole Genome Sequencing. J Clin Microbiol. 2017;55:2956–63.

38. Geis S, Prifert C, Weissbrich B, Lehners N, Egerer G, Eisenbach C, et al. Molecular characterization of a respiratory syncytial virus outbreak in a hematology unit in Heidelberg. Germany J Clin Microbiol. 2013;51:155–62.

39. McLellan JS, Ray WC, Peeples ME. Structure and function of respiratory syncytial virus surface glycoproteins. Anderson L, Graham B, editors. Curr. Top. Microbiol. Immunol. vol 372. 2013;372:83–104.

Cost-effectiveness of ceftolozane/tazobactam plus metronidazole versus piperacillin/tazobactam as initial empiric therapy for the treatment of complicated intra-abdominal infections based on pathogen distributions drawn from national surveillance data in the United States

Vimalanand S. Prabhu[1,7]* ⓘ, Joseph S. Solomkin[2], Goran Medic[3], Jason Foo[3], Rebekah H. Borse[1], Teresa Kauf[4], Benjamin Miller[5], Shuvayu S. Sen[1] and Anirban Basu[6]

Abstract

Background: The prevalence of antimicrobial resistance among gram-negative pathogens in complicated intra-abdominal infections (cIAIs) has increased. In the absence of timely information on the infecting pathogens and their susceptibilities, local or regional epidemiology may guide initial empirical therapy and reduce treatment failure, length of stay and mortality. The objective of this study was to assess the cost-effectiveness of ceftolozane/tazobactam + metronidazole compared with piperacillin/tazobactam in the treatment of hospitalized US patients with cIAI at risk of infection with resistant pathogens.

Methods: We used a decision-analytic Monte Carlo simulation model to compare the costs and quality-adjusted life years (QALYs) of persons infected with nosocomial gram-negative cIAI treated empirically with either ceftolozane/tazobactam + metronidazole or piperacillin/tazobactam. Pathogen isolates were randomly drawn from the Program to Assess Ceftolozane/Tazobactam Susceptibility (PACTS) database, a surveillance database of non-duplicate bacterial isolates collected from patients with cIAIs in medical centers in the USA from 2011 to 2013. Susceptibility to initial therapy was based on the measured susceptibilities reported in the PACTS database determined using standard broth micro-dilution methods as described by the Clinical and Laboratory Standards Institute (CLSI).

Results: Our model results, with baseline resistance levels from the PACTS database, indicated that ceftolozane/tazobactam + metronidazole dominated piperacillin/tazobactam, with lower costs ($44,226/patient vs. $44,811/patient respectively) and higher QALYs (12.85/patient vs. 12.70/patient, respectively). Ceftolozane/tazobactam + metronidazole remained the dominant choice in one-way and probabilistic sensitivity analyses.

(Continued on next page)

* Correspondence: vimalanand.prabhu@merck.com
[1]Merck & Co., Inc., Kenilworth, NJ, USA
[7]Center for Observational and Real World Evidence (CORE), Merck & Co., Inc., 2000 Galloping Hill Road, Kenilworth, NJ 07033, USA
Full list of author information is available at the end of the article

(Continued from previous page)

Conclusions: Based on surveillance data, ceftolozane/tazobactam is more likely to be an appropriate empiric therapy for cIAI in the US. Results from a decision-analytic simulation model indicate that use of ceftolozane/tazobactam + metronidazole would result in cost savings and improves QALYs, compared with piperacillin/tazobactam.

Keywords: Cost-effectiveness analysis, Ceftolozane, Piperacillin, Tazobactam, Intraabdominal infections, United States, Drug resistance

Background

Intra-abdominal infections (IAIs) represent a wide variety of pathological conditions caused by inflammation or perforation of the intra-abdominal organs. In the latter case, complicated IAIs (cIAIs) arise causing localized or diffuse peritonitis [1]. Gram-negative pathogens, including resistant pathogens are responsible for over 70% of cIAIs [2]. Patients at a higher risk of treatment failure due to a resistant infection include those with health care-associated infection or prior antibiotic exposure [3]. Studies have shown that 'high-risk' patients are more likely to experience a delay in the receipt of appropriate therapy, increased length of hospital stay, more frequent intensive care unit (ICU) admission, increased cost of care (including antibiotic costs) and increased mortality [4–8].

Treatment guidelines recommend initiation of antibiotic therapy as soon as a patient is diagnosed or suspected of an intra-abdominal infection [3]. Since culture and susceptibility results are not available at diagnosis, empiric antibiotic therapy is often considered. If the initial empiric therapy chosen has in vitro activity against the pathogen isolated it is termed initial appropriate antibiotic therapy (IAAT), whereas one without in vitro activity is termed initial inappropriate empiric therapy (IIAT).

Important considerations for choosing empiric therapy include consideration of the most likely pathogens at the site of infection, knowledge of any prior colonization, and finally, local resistance epidemiology [9–12]. Surgical Infection Society and Infectious Diseases Society of America (IDSA) joint guidelines for treatment of cIAI suggest routine culture and susceptibility studies if there is significant resistance (10–20% of isolates) of a common isolate to an antimicrobial regimen in widespread local use [3]. Improving the chances of IAAT is likely to improve clinical outcomes and impart economic benefits. A US study with cIAI patients identified the additional length of stay (LOS) for IIAT relative to IAAT as 4.6 days (11.6 days vs. 6.9 days total), with additional hospital costs per patient of $6368 ($16,520 vs. $10,152) and substantial excess mortality (9.5% vs. 1.3%) [13].

Given the acute nature of cIAI and the substantial clinical and economic benefits associated with IAAT, the antibacterial spectrum of the empiric antibiotic agent considered should cover the most relevant pathogens to increase the likelihood of IAAT. The economic benefits that could be obtained because of improved susceptibility and increased coverage of IAAT is an important consideration.

A case in point is the comparison of piperacillin/tazobactam and ceftolozane/tazobactam + metronidazole. Piperacillin/tazobactam is recommended for empiric therapy for the treatment of cIAI in various treatment guidelines [14, 15]. Ceftolozane/tazobactam is a novel cephalosporin/β-lactamase inhibitor combination with activity against multidrug resistant gram-negative pathogens, including extended-spectrum β-lactamase-producing *Enterobacteriaceae* and drug-resistant *P. aeruginosa* [16]. Metronidazole is an oral synthetic antiprotozoal and antibacterial agent which may be used for initial empiric treatment of complicated intra-abdominal infections alongside other agents including ceftolozane/tazobactam. In this study, we assess the cost-effectiveness of ceftolozane/tazobactam + metronidazole compared with piperacillin/tazobactam (considered standard of care) as empiric therapy in the treatment of hospitalized US patients with cIAI.

Methods

Model structure

We developed a decision-analytic microsimulation model to estimate the quality-adjusted life expectancy and cost of patients admitted to an inpatient facility, diagnosed with cIAI, and administered empiric antibiotic therapy. A graphical representation of the model structure with all treatment pathways is provided in Fig. 1. The methodology and model structure is similar to the one used to assess the cost-effectiveness of ceftolozane/tazobactam in complicated urinary tract infections [17].

Patients enter the microsimulation model at the time of cIAI diagnosis, which is assumed to be concurrent with initiation of empiric antimicrobial therapy. Each patient in the model receives empiric antibiotic treatment with ceftolozane/tazobactam + metronidazole in one arm and piperacillin/tazobactam in another. A specimen is isolated for culture after diagnosis to determine the pathogen and its in-vitro susceptibility to different antibiotic therapies.

Pathogen distribution and in-vitro susceptibility was based on that of a US isolate randomly selected from the Program to Assess Ceftolozane/Tazobactam Susceptibility (PACTS) surveillance dataset, an international

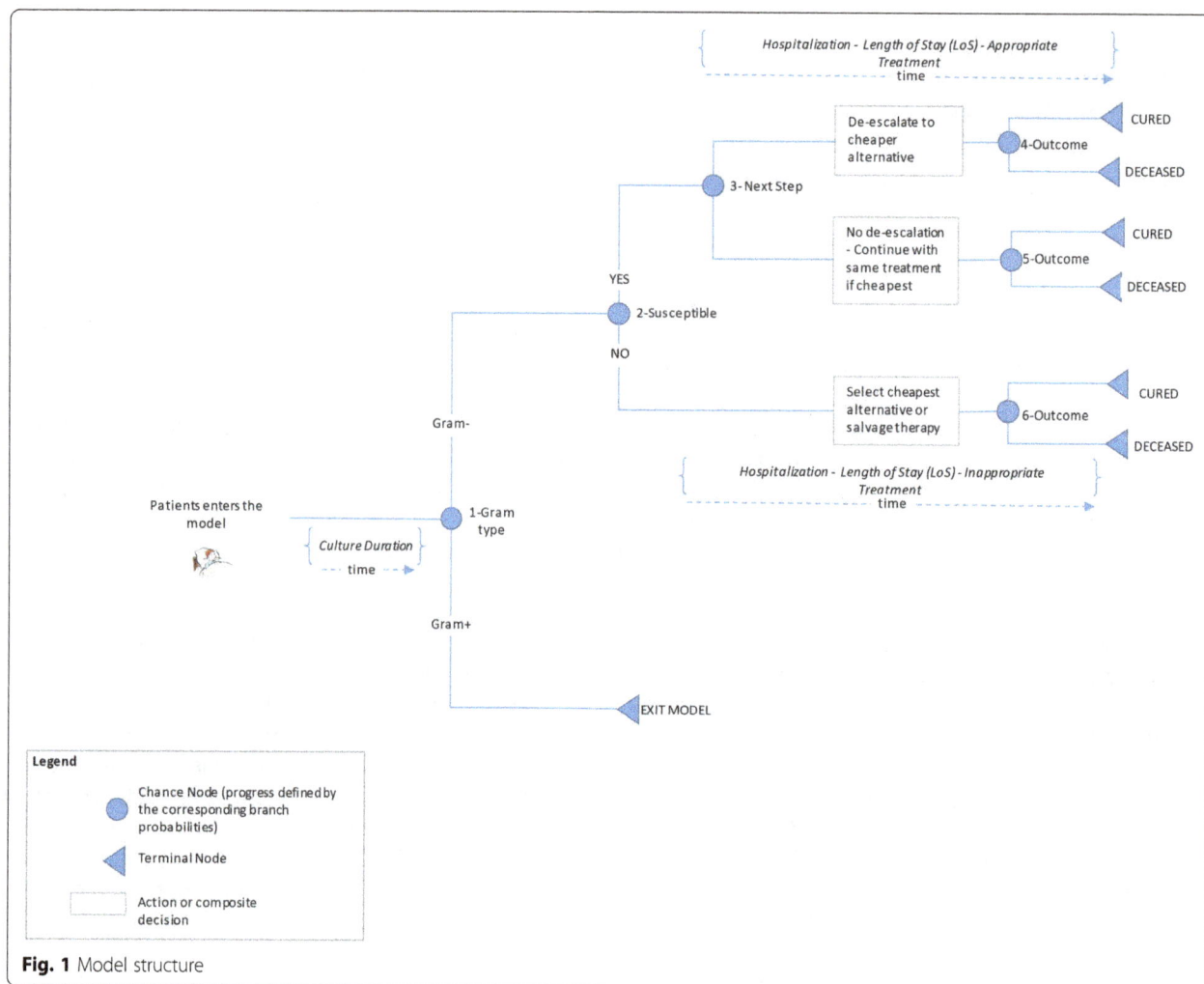

Fig. 1 Model structure

antimicrobial surveillance database. Each intra-abdominal pathogen from the PACTS database represents a single patient in the micro-simulation. The types of pathogens can be chosen within the model to allow analyses to be tailored to the underlying pathogens for specific indications. Further details regarding PACTS are provided in Additional file 1.

Treatment pathway and disease progression are estimated using a decision-tree shown in Fig. 1, after the patient is selected. Patients continue empiric treatment until culture results are available. Once culture results are known, patients are switched to the least expensive therapy to which the causative pathogen is susceptible. If the pathogen is not susceptible to any of the modeled comparators, patients are switched to salvage therapy (combination of meropenem and colistin).

The appropriateness of initial antibiotic therapy influences each patient's length of hospital stay and treatment outcome. Mortality in the model is dependent upon whether the patient experiences IAAT or IIAT (higher mortality rate applied for patients experiencing IIAT).

For patients who survive, we assume that they live a normal length of life based on their life expectancy, and incur health care expenditure comparable to those of the average person their age [18].

Patients with gram-positive pathogens exit the model because they may not be treated by either comparator drugs. We assume that patients incur similar outcomes and costs on either arms if they are gram-positive and therefore economic incremental impact on ceftolozane/tazobactam arm is likely to be negligible.

The model allows us to compute undiscounted and discounted costs and QALYs for each arm, the incremental costs, incremental QALYs and the incremental cost-effectiveness ratio.

Inputs

Susceptibility: Customizing PACTS database to represent cIAI patients

The in-vitro surveillance data from the PACTS database represents the only source of patient-level, real-world data reflecting IAI patients at risk of resistant infection in the US, includes isolate susceptibility to ceftolozane/tazobactam. Isolates obtained from US sites from 2011 to 2013 were included in this analysis. The following organisms were included in line with the approved label for ceftolozane/tazobactam and encompass the major pathogens involved in cIAIs: [2] *Enterobacter cloacae*, *Escherichia coli*, *Klebsiella oxytoca*, *Klebsiella pneumoniae*, *Proteus mirabilis* and *Pseudomonas aeruginosa*.

One limitation of the PACTS database is that it does not differentiate between complicated and uncomplicated IAI. In order to overcome this limitation, isolates in the PACTS database were sampled in proportion to the pathogen distribution for cIAI in a real-world setting found in the Premier hospital discharge database, [19] a complete census of inpatients and hospital-based outpatients from geographically diverse hospitals in the US. More information regarding Premier database is provided in Additional file 1. An algorithm based on a set of ICD-9 diagnosis codes and current procedural terminology (CPT) procedure codes was used to identify cIAI patients from the Premier database between January 1, 2009 and March 31, 2013. The cIAI cohort consisted of 10,159 abdominal isolates, the mean age was 55 ± 22 years (median age: 59 years), and most patients with positive cultures were above 50 years. The resulting pathogen distribution used in the model was 26.6% for *Escherichia coli*, 16.0% for *Klebsiella pneumonia*, 13.5% for *Pseudomonas aeruginosa*, and 9.0% for *Enterobacter cloacae*. The gram-negative pathogens that occurred in less than 5% of patients were grouped together and made up the remaining 5.8%. The percentage of patients with gram-positive pathogens in the cohort was 29.1% [2].

Susceptibility breakpoints
The susceptibility is evaluated using Clinical and Laboratory Standards Institute (CLSI) breakpoints. A breakpoint of 2 mg/L was used for *Enterobacteriaceae* and a susceptibility breakpoint of 4 mg/L was used for *Pseudomonas spp.* [20].

Drugs used for the model
The empiric treatments used in the model are ceftolozane/tazobactam + metronidazole for one arm and piperacillin/tazobactam for another, which are consistent with the approved therapies and international cIAI treatment guidelines [14, 15]. The following additional drugs were considered for switching upon pathogen confirmation: aztreonam, cefepime, ceftazidime, ceftriaxone, ciprofloxacin, doripenem, imipenem, levofloxacin, meropenem and tigecycline.

Clinical inputs
The key clinical inputs are summarized in Table 1. Mortality rates and length of stay were based on Edelsberg et al., where patients who received IIAT spent 4.6 more days in the hospital (11.6 vs. 6.9 total days) [13]. Duration of empiric therapy was assumed to be 3 days. US life-tables were used for the prediction of life expectancy [21]. The percentage of cIAI patients requiring re-intervention has been reported at approximately 8–9% [22, 23]. While most published studies examining the impact of IIAT on treatment outcomes in cIAI did not report re-intervention rates, there is evidence from at least one study that IIAT may increase the risk of re-intervention (relative risk ratio, 5.1; 95% CI, 1.7–15.4) [24]. As the Krobot et al. study [24] was relatively small and conducted over a decade ago, the analysis conservatively assumed that there was no differential impact of IIAT on re-intervention. Similarly, any costs associated with re-intervention, such as imaging, were excluded from the model since those costs did not vary by empiric treatment option.

An assumed utility value of 0.85 was applied to cured patients for the remainder of their lives (Table 1). This was a conservative estimate based on a utility value of 0.9 proposed by Jansen et al. [25]. QALYs were discounted at a rate of 3% per annum [26].

Economic inputs
Hospitalization costs per day (Table 1) were derived from the 2013 Healthcare Cost and Utilization Project (HCUP) [27] and inflated to 2015 values using the Gross Domestic Product (GDP) price index [28]. Hospitalization costs were based on primary diagnoses for cIAI (ICD-9 code 540.0, 540.1, 567.0, 567.21, 567.22, 567.23, 567.29, 567.31, 567.89, 567.9, and 569.5) [27]. The average cost per hospital day for cIAI patients, inflated to 2015 values, was $2558.55.

Daily drug costs (Table 1) were calculated for the duration of hospitalization based on wholesale acquisition cost at labeled doses [29].

For healthy survivors, lifetime health care expenditure was calculated using average annual age-adjusted values [18] inflated to 2015 values using the Gross Domestic Product (GDP) price index (Table 1) [28].

Hospitalization and daily drug costs were not discounted as all costs were incurred within the first year, given the acute nature of cIAI. A discount rate of 3% per annum was applied to lifetime health care expenditure for health survivors.

Analysis
A lifetime time horizon was applied to capture the costs and utility of healthy survivors over their lifetime. The model compared ceftolozane/tazobactam + metronidazole with piperacillin/tazobactam from the healthcare perspective.

To compare the two treatment strategies the following outcomes were estimated from the model: proportion of patients appropriately and inappropriately treated (sensitive/resistant to empiric therapy, cost per QALY saved, drug costs, hospitalization costs, proportion of cases by pathogen, total costs, total QALYs). Differences in these

Table 1 Clinical and economic inputs

Input Parameters	Mean	Lower bound	Upper bound	Source
Mortality rate with appropriate empiric treatment	0.013	0.012	0.014	Edelsberg et al. [13]
Mortality rate with inappropriate empiric antibiotic	0.095	0.086	0.105	Edelsberg et al. [13]
Duration of empiric therapy	3 days	3 days	3 days	Assumption
Total LOS for IAAT (inc. empiric therapy)	6.9 days	6.8 days	7 days	Edelsberg et al. [13]
Total LOS for IIAT (inc. empiric therapy)	11.5 days	11.3 days	11.9 days	Edelsberg et al. [13]
Health utility for survivors	0.85	0.70	1.00	Assumption based on Jansen et al. [25]
Discount rate	3.0%	3.0%	3.0%	AMCP [26]
Hospital cost per day (average)	$2558.55	$2046.84	$3070.26	HCUP [27]
Drug acquisition costs per day				
Ceftolozane/tazobactam plus metronidazole	$253.20			Analy$ource [29]
Aztreonam	$84.24			Analy$ource [29]
Cefepime	$23.04			Analy$ource [29]
Ceftazidime	$36.66			Analy$ource [29]
Ceftriaxone	$6.40			Analy$ource [29]
Ciprofloxacin	$5.26			Analy$ource [29]
Doripenem	$125.22			Analy$ource [29]
Imipenem	$73.12			Analy$ource [29]
Levofloxacin	$6.24			Analy$ource [29]
Meropenem	$81.51			Analy$ource [29]
Piperacillin/tazobactam	$43.08			Analy$ource [29]
Tigecycline	$238.34			Analy$ource [29]
Salvage[a]	$164.31			Analy$ource [29]
Health care expenditure incurred per year				
<25 years	$477			Basu [18]
25 to 34 years	$790			Basu [18]
35 to 44 years	$947			Basu [18]
45 to 54 years	$1422			Basu [18]
55 to 64 years	$2106			Basu [18]
65 to 74 years	$2758			Basu [18]
75 years and above	$3100			Basu [18]

[a]Salvage therapy consists of meropenem + colistin for cost purposes

LOS Length of stay, IAAT Initial appropriate antibiotic therapy, IIAT Initial inappropriate antibiotic therapy

outcomes of interest were estimated, along with the incremental cost-effectiveness ratio (ICER) based on total cost per QALY gained.

One-way sensitivity analyses (OWSA) and probabilistic sensitivity analysis (PSA) were performed to quantify the uncertainty in the model outcomes based on the uncertainty of the input parameters. The model assessed the sensitivity of the model results to all the input data for which uncertainty has been defined one parameter at a time by means of OWSA. The parameters with the greatest impact were summarized with tornado diagrams.

Ten thousand samples were taken to estimate ranges for the PSA. Input parameter values were sampled from the defined distributions for efficacy, safety, and costs. Lognormal distributions were used for odds ratios, beta distributions for utilities, and for gamma distributions for resource use and costs.

For each treatment strategy, the probability of cost-effectiveness was expressed with cost-effectiveness acceptability curves, calculated as the number of iterations out of the total number of iterations for which the net monetary benefit (NMB) was greatest for a given treatment strategy out of all strategies.

The NMB was calculated as the QALYs multiplied by a willingness to pay (WTP) ratio minus the costs, where the WTP is the amount decision makers were willing to pay per additional QALY gained. An amount of US $100,000 was used as a WTP threshold [30].

Risk factors associated with infection due to resistant pathogens (vs. susceptible pathogens) have been identified in the literature [31, 32]. Information regarding a portion of these risk factors for cIAI was available for patients in the PACTS dataset, including (a) nosocomial infection, (b) age ≥ 65 years, and (c) ICU stay.

Scenario analyses were performed firstly using all available isolates for high risk patients aged ≥65 years and requiring an ICU stay, and secondly using only nosocomial isolates for high risk patients aged ≥65 years and requiring an ICU stay.

An additional scenario was also performed excluding lifetime health care expenditure for healthy survivors.

Results

Base case results

In the cohort of 1000 patients, the average age was 67.1 years ranging from 21 to 100 years.

The key results from the model are summarized in Table 2. Under the base case scenario, ceftolozane/tazobactam + metronidazole arm resulted in lower total costs than the piperacillin/tazobactam arm ($44,226 per patient vs. $44,811). The ceftolozane/tazobactam + metronidazole arm also experienced a greater number of QALYs than the piperacillin/tazobactam arm (12.85 per patient vs. 12.70 per patient). This resulted in ceftolozane/tazobactam + metronidazole dominating piperacillin/tazobactam with 0.63 hospitalization days saved per patient.

In patients with a gram-negative infection receiving ceftolozane/tazobactam + metronidazole as empiric therapy, 6.1% were resistant compared with 19.7% in patients receiving piperacillin/tazobactam. Since 29.1% of pathogens were gram-positive, overall, 35.2% were not susceptible to ceftolozane/tazobactam + metronidazole compared with 48.8% for piperacillin/tazobactam. There were 41.8 deaths (4.2%) in the ceftolozane/tazobactam + metronidazole arm compared with 53.0 (5.3%) in the piperacillin/tazobactam arm. Amongst those who died, a larger proportion was resistant to initial therapy in the piperacillin/tazobactam arm than the ceftolozane/tazobactam + metronidazole arm. Ceftolozane/tazobactam + metronidazole reduced overall mortality by 1.1% versus piperacillin/tazobactam.

When examining the QALY results in more detail, the ceftolozane/tazobactam + metronidazole arm generated 0.15 more QALYs (discounted) per patient. The average number of QALYs (discounted) experienced by patients in the ceftolozane/tazobactam + metronidazole arm were 12.85 and 12.70 for ceftolozane/tazobactam + metronidazole and piperacillin/tazobactam, respectively.

Lifetime health care expenditure was the largest contributor to total costs in both treatment arms followed by hospital costs. The average lifetime health care expenditure per patient in the ceftolozane/tazobactam + metronidazole arm was higher than in the piperacillin/tazobactam arm ($27,940 vs. $27,546). The average hospital cost per patient in the ceftolozane/tazobactam + metronidazole arm was lower than in the piperacillin/tazobactam arm ($15,468 vs. $17,069, respectively).

Table 2 Results

Summary of results	Ceftolozane/ tazobactam + metronidazole	Piperacillin/tazobactam	Incremental Ceftolozane/tazobactam + metronidazole - Piperacillin/tazobactam
Total costs per patient	$44,226	$44,811	-$585
Total life years per patient (undiscounted)	21.75	21.50	0.25
Total QALYs per patient (undiscounted)	18.49	18.27	0.22
Total QALYs per patient (discounted)	12.85	12.70	0.15
Incremental Cost Effectiveness Ratio (Cost per discounted QALY saved)	–	–	Dominant
Hospitalization days saved per-patient	–	–	0.63
Distribution of patients based on empiric treatment			
Resistant to initial therapy (%)	35.2	48.8	–
Susceptible to initial therapy (%)	64.8	51.2	–
Costs			
Hospital costs per patient	$15,468	$17,069	-$1601
Drug costs per patient	$818	$196	$622
Lifetime health care expenditure per patient	$27,940	$27,546	$394

QALY Quality Adjusted Life Year, *IAAT* Initial appropriate antibiotic therapy, *IIAT* Initial inappropriate antibiotic therapy

Per-patient drug costs in the ceftolozane/tazobactam + metronidazole arm were slightly higher than in the piperacillin/tazobactam arm ($818 vs. $196, respectively).

All of the patients in the ceftolozane/tazobactam + metronidazole arm who received IAAT were able to switch to a less expensive therapy after 3 days (following culture results). For 1.0% of patients in the piperacillin/tazobactam arm who received IAAT, empiric therapy with piperacillin/tazobactam was the least expensive treatment option. In patients who received IIAT, an equal number of patients in each arm (n = 19, 1.9%) required salvage therapy with meropenem + colistin.

One-way sensitivity analysis

The results of the one-way sensitivity analysis are presented in a tornado graph (Fig. 2). Varying the average cost per hospital day resulted in the largest impact on the resultant ICER. The other input parameters which impacted the model results when varied were: resistance to piperacillin/tazobactam, resistance to ceftolozane/tazobactam, mortality rate with IIAT, the utility value applied to survivors, and the mortality rate with IAAT. Varying the additional length of stay associated with IIAT had very little impact on the ICER. In all instances, ceftolozane/tazobactam + metronidazole remained the dominant option versus piperacillin/tazobactam.

Probabilistic sensitivity analysis

The distribution of ICER estimates from the PSA show that in all instances, ceftolozane/tazobactam + metronidazole is more effective and less costly than piperacillin/tazobactam.

Subsequently, ceftolozane/tazobactam has a 100% probability of being cost-effective compared with piperacillin/tazobactam at a willingness-to-pay threshold of $100,000/QALY gained.

Scenario analyses

Seventy-four percent of patients from the US PACTS dataset were aged ≥65 years and 4% of patients required an ICU stay. Thirty-eight percent of patients had isolates from nosocomial sources. Amongst these patients, 37% were aged ≥65 years and 5% of patients required an ICU stay. Patients could be associated with more than one risk factor.

Results of the scenario analyses are presented in Table 3. Overall, the cost-effectiveness of ceftolozane/tazobactam + metronidazole improves versus piperacillin/tazobactam in high risk patients (≥65 years and requiring an ICU stay) and high risk patients with nosocomial infections. Differences in costs and the number of hospitalization days are larger in both of the subgroups explored, with a larger difference in total QALYs (discounted) seen in the high risk patients with nosocomial infections.

In the scenario where lifetime health care expenditure was excluded, the total costs per patient were considerably lower and the incremental cost between ceftolozane/tazobactam + metronidazole and piperacillin/tazobactam was larger. Ceftolozane/tazobactam + metronidazole remained the dominant choice.

Discussion

The objective of this analysis was to evaluate the use of ceftolozane/tazobactam + metronidazole compared with piperacillin/tazobactam in the empiric treatment of US patients with cIAI at risk of infection due to a resistant gram-negative pathogen. The ability of either ceftolozane/tazobactam + metronidazole or piperacillin/tazobactam to provide appropriate empiric coverage is an important concept in the model and the source of economic differentiation between the two therapies. Ceftolozane/tazobactam + metronidazole provides a greater

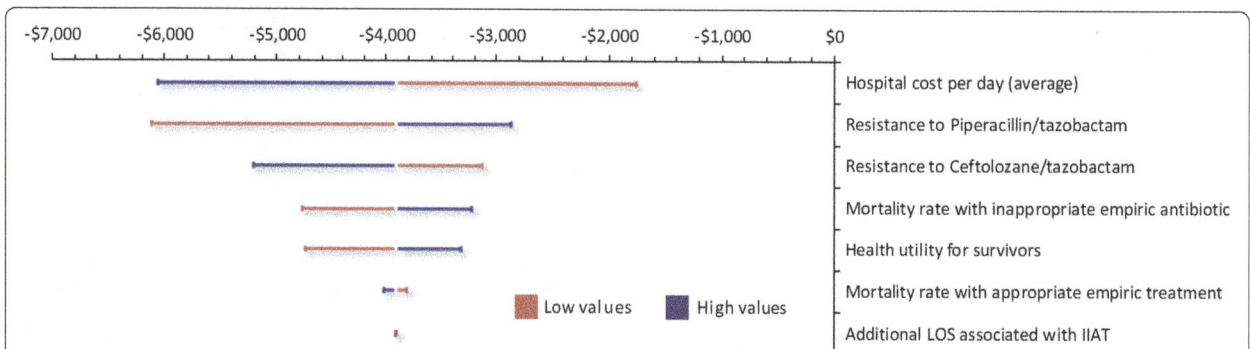

Fig. 2 Ceftolozane/tazobactam vs. piperacillin/tazobactam: influence of variables on ICER (cost per discounted QALY). ICER = Incremental cost-effectiveness ratio; QALY = Quality Adjusted Life Year

Table 3 Scenario analyses results

Results for high risk patients (aged 65 years and requiring an ICU stay) using all available isolates	Ceftolozane/tazobactam + metronidazole	Piperacillin/ tazobactam	Incremental Ceftolozane/tazobactam + metronidazole - Piperacillin/tazobactam
Total costs per patient	$41,838	$42,501	-$662
Total QALYs (discounted) per patient	11.38	11.24	0.14
Incremental Cost Effectiveness Ratio (Cost per discounted QALY saved)	–	–	Dominant
Results for high risk patients (aged 65 years and requiring an ICU stay) using nosocomial isolates	Ceftolozane/ tazobactam + metronidazole	Piperacillin/ tazobactam	Incremental Ceftolozane/tazobactam + metronidazole - Piperacillin/tazobactam
Total costs per patient	$42,979	$44,403	-$1424
Total QALYs (discounted) per patient	11.75	11.53	0.22
Incremental Cost Effectiveness Ratio (Cost per discounted QALY saved)	–	–	Dominant
Results when lifetime health care expenditure for health survivors is excluded	Ceftolozane/ tazobactam + metronidazole	Piperacillin/ tazobactam	Incremental Ceftolozane/tazobactam + metronidazole - Piperacillin/tazobactam
Total costs per patient	$16,286	$17,265	-$978
Total QALYs (discounted) per patient	12.85	12.70	0.15
Incremental Cost Effectiveness Ratio (Cost per discounted QALY saved)			Dominant

QALY Quality Adjusted Life Year

degree of appropriate empiric coverage than piperacillin/tazobactam, as demonstrated by the PACTS data.

We have presented a novel approach utilizing surveillance data to evaluate the cost-effectiveness of two empiric therapy options. A similar approach to ours was used in the study by Sader et al., where they used the SENTRY Antimicrobial Surveillance Program, a large multinational data source on pathogen prevalence and antimicrobial susceptibility, to estimate the effectiveness of tigecycline in complicated skin and skin structure infections [33]. Although this study only considered effectiveness and not costs.

The findings of our analysis suggest that the use of ceftolozane/tazobactam + metronidazole as initial (empiric) treatment may result in substantial cost-savings compared to piperacillin/tazobactam. Additionally, use of ceftolozane/tazobactam + metronidazole may save an average of 0.63 hospital days per patient.

IIAT is a key driver to the model and contributes to the differentiation between ceftolozane/tazobactam + metronidazole and piperacillin/tazobactam. The impact of IIAT is further emphasized in our two high risk scenarios. In both scenarios, susceptibility rates to ceftolozane/tazobactam + metronidazole remain largely unchanged, however, susceptibility rates to piperacillin/tazobactam are lower compared to the base case.

Cost savings are a function of several model parameters including duration of empiric therapy, susceptibility among comparators, and the increase in length of stay due to IIAT. Furthermore, differences in costs derive solely from

differences in antimicrobial activity between ceftolozane/tazobactam + metronidazole and piperacillin/tazobactam.

The inclusion of lifetime health care expenditures in our base case analysis reduced the incremental costs by approximately 50%. For our analysis, ceftolozane/tazobactam + metronidazole remained the dominant option, however, inclusion of lifetime healthcare expenditure may have a potential impact on comparisons which are borderline cost-effective or cost-saving.

We have shown how data from national surveillance data set can be used to guide the choice of cost-effective empirical therapy. Clinical trials are often conducted in a variety of different geographic locations/settings and the patients enrolled may not necessarily reflect the specific populations who will receive these treatments in real life. In practice, patient outcomes can be improved through improvements in the collection of local surveillance data and the use of local antibiograms in decision making and guideline development.

Limitations

An important limitation is that the model does not account for further treatment changes after any initial de-escalation/escalation, with patients assumed to be fully cured or dead at the end of hospitalization.

Additionally, recurrence and/or re-admission were not incorporated in this model. For readmission rates, we assumed that these were the same for patients with IAAT and IIAT, and subsequently did not have any economic impact. If patients with IIAT have a higher rate of readmission, the subsequent analysis would further improve results favoring the ceftolozane/tazobactam arm.

The model assumes that the duration of therapy, whilst shorter for IAAT compared with IIAT, is not directly impacted by the different drugs used following culture results. In practice, some treatments may shorten/prolong hospital length of stay.

The PACTS dataset was not designed to focus on resistant or complicated IAI. Therefore it did not contain enough information to specifically target complicated IAI (vs. uncomplicated IAI) patients and may under-represent pathogen resistance in the target population of cIAI. We attempted to overcome this limitation by sampling isolates in the PACTS database in proportion to the pathogen distribution for cIAI in a real-world setting found in the Premier hospital discharge database. PACTS is the only source of patient level, real-world data reflecting IAI patients at risk of resistant infection in the US that includes isolate susceptibility to ceftolozane/tazobactam. Our sample had 294 isolates from patients with IAIs. To conduct an analysis representative of local settings, more data at a local level may be needed. Also, within the PACTS database, only one isolate per patient infection was included in the surveillance whereas in clinical practice you are likely to encounter more than one isolate per patient.

Additional limitations are the exclusion from the model of bacterial resistance over time and costs of antibiotic preparation and administration, monitoring, and adverse events. These costs were assumed to be similar across treatments and/or minor. Similarly, dose adjustments were not considered.

The model only considers gram-negative aerobes, when in practice, gram-positive aerobes and anaerobes (both gram-positive and gram-negative) are frequently implicated. The proportion of patients with gram-positive infections in our cohort was based on the distribution of gram-positive bacteria identified from intraoperative samples reported by Sartelli et al. [2]. This figure may not be entirely accurate due to the fact that patients can harbor more than one type of bacteria, affecting that actual distribution of gram-positive bacteria amongst patients.

Conclusion

Economic models utilizing surveillance data can help to identify the appropriate choice of empiric therapy for the treatment of cIAI. The results of this cost-effectiveness model indicate that cost-savings and improvements in QALYs may be achieved by the empiric use of ceftolozane/tazobactam + metronidazole instead of piperacillin/tazobactam in US cIAI patients at risk of resistant infection.

Abbreviations

cIAI: complicated intra-abdominal infection; CLSI: Clinical and Laboratory Standards Institute; CPT: Current procedural terminology; GDP: Gross Domestic Product; HCUP: Healthcare Cost and Utilization Project; IAAT: Initial appropriate antibiotic therapy; ICD-9: International Classification of Diseases, Ninth Edition; ICER: Incremental cost-effectivness ratio; ICU: Intensive care unit; IDSA: Infectious Diseases Society of America; IIAT: Initial inappropriate antibiotic therapy; LOS: Length of stay; NMB: Net monetary benefit; PACTS: Program to Assess Ceftolozane/Tazobactam Susceptibility; QALYs: Quality-adjusted life years; US: United States; WTP: Willingness to pay

Acknowledgements
Dimitris Kabranis was involved in the development of the original model.

Authors' contributions
VP, JS, GM, RB, TK, BM, SS and AB were involved in the conception and design. VP, GM, JF, RB, TK, BM and SS were involved in data collection. VP, JS, GM, JF, TK, BM, SS and AB were involved in data interpretation. VP, JF and TK were involved in writing the manuscript. All authors read and approved the final manuscript.

Funding
Financial support for this study was provided by Merck & Co., Inc. The funding agreement ensured the authors' independence in designing the study, interpreting the data, writing, and publishing the report.

Consent for publication
Not applicable.

Competing interests
VP and SS report other conflicts of interest from Merck & Co., Inc., during the conduct of the study. JS reports personal fees from Merck & Co., Inc., outside the submitted work. GM has nothing to disclose. JF reports personal fees from Merck & Co., Inc., during the conduct of the study. RB reports that she is an employee of Merck & Co., Inc., and holds stocks in Merck & Co. Inc., outside the submitted work. TK and BM were full-time employees of Merck at the time of the study. AB reports personal fees from Merck & Co. Inc., outside the submitted work.

Author details
[1]Merck & Co., Inc., Kenilworth, NJ, USA. [2]University of Cincinnati College of Medicine, Cincinnati, OH, USA. [3]Mapi Group, Houten, The Netherlands. [4]Baxalta US Inc., Boston, MA, USA. [5]Shire, Lexington, MA, USA. [6]Pharmaceutical Outcomes Research and Policy Program, University of Washington, Seattle, WA, USA. [7]Center for Observational and Real World Evidence (CORE), Merck & Co., Inc., 2000 Galloping Hill Road, Kenilworth, NJ 07033, USA.

References
1. Menichetti F, Sganga G. Definition and classification of intra-abdominal infections. J Chemother (Florence, Italy). 2009;21(Suppl 1):3–4.
2. Sartelli M, Catena F, Ansaloni L, Coccolini F, Corbella D, Moore EE, Malangoni M, Velmahos G, Coimbra R, Koike K, et al. Complicated intra-abdominal infections worldwide: the definitive data of the CIAOW study. World J Emerg Surg : WJES. 2014;9:37.
3. Solomkin JS, Mazuski JE, Bradley JS, Rodvold KA, Goldstein EJ, Baron EJ, O'Neill PJ, Chow AW, Dellinger EP, Eachempati SR, et al. Diagnosis and management of complicated intra-abdominal infection in adults and children: guidelines by the surgical infection society and the Infectious Diseases Society of America. Clin Infect Dis. 2010;50(2):133–64.
4. Turner RM, Wu B, Lawrence K, Hackett J, Karve S, Tunceli O. Assessment of outpatient and inpatient antibiotic treatment patterns and health care costs of patients with complicated urinary tract infections. Clin Ther. 2015;37(9):2037–47.
5. Yang CC, Shao PL, CY L, Tsau YK, Tsai IJ, Lee PI, Chang LY, Huang LM. Comparison of acute lobar nephronia and uncomplicated urinary tract

infection in children. J Microbiol Immunol Infect. 2010;43(3):207–14.

6. MacVane SH, Tuttle LO, Nicolau DP. Impact of extended-spectrum beta-lactamase-producing organisms on clinical and economic outcomes in patients with urinary tract infection. J Hosp Med. 2014;9(4):232–8.

7. Osthoff M, McGuinness SL, Wagen AZ, Eisen DP. Urinary tract infections due to extended-spectrum beta-lactamase-producing gram-negative bacteria: identification of risk factors and outcome predictors in an Australian tertiary referral hospital. Int J Infect Dis. 2015;34:79–83.

8. Mauldin PD, Salgado CD, Hansen IS, Durup DT, Bosso JA. Attributable hospital cost and length of stay associated with health care-associated infections caused by antibiotic-resistant gram-negative bacteria. Antimicrob Agents Chemother. 2010;54(1):109–15.

9. Farrell DJ. Surveillance of ceftolozane/tazobactam antimicrobial activity tested against gram-negative organisms and streptococci (selected) isolated in the United States (13-CUB-02-USA/CXA.087.MC). In.: cubist. Pharmaceuticals. 2013;

10. Sader HS, Farrell DJ, Flamm RK, Jones RN. Ceftolozane/tazobactam activity tested against aerobic gram-negative organisms isolated from intra-abdominal and urinary tract infections in European and United States hospitals (2012). J Infect. 2014;69(3):266–77.

11. Sader HS, Farrell DJ, Castanheira M, Flamm RK, Jones RN. Antimicrobial activity of ceftolozane/tazobactam tested against Pseudomonas Aeruginosa and Enterobacteriaceae with various resistance patterns isolated in European hospitals (2011-12). J Antimicrob Chemother. 2014;69(10):2713–22.

12. Walkty A, Adam H, Baxter M, Denisuik A, Lagace-Wiens P, Karlowsky JA, Hoban DJ, Zhanel GG. Vitro activity of plazomicin against 5,015 gram-negative and gram-positive clinical isolates obtained from patients in canadian hospitals as part of the CANWARD study, 2011-2012. Antimicrob Agents Chemother. 2014;58(5):2554–63.

13. Edelsberg J, Berger A, Schell S, Mallick R, Kuznik A, Oster G. Economic consequences of failure of initial antibiotic therapy in hospitalized adults with complicated intra-abdominal infections. Surg Infect. 2008;9(3):335–47.

14. Solomkin JS, Mazuski JE, Bradley JS, Rodvold KA, Goldstein EJ, Baron EJ, O'Neill PJ, Chow AW, Dellinger EP, Eachempati SR, et al. Diagnosis and management of complicated intra-abdominal infection in adults and children: guidelines by the surgical infection society and the Infectious Diseases Society of America. Surg Infect. 2010;11(1):79–109.

15. Eckmann C, Dryden M, Montravers P, Kozlov R, Sganga G. Antimicrobial treatment of "complicated" intra-abdominal infections and the new IDSA guidelines ? A commentary and an alternative European approach according to clinical definitions. Eur J Med Res. 2011;16(3):115–26.

16. Zhanel GG, Chung P, Adam H, Zelenitsky S, Denisuik A, Schweizer F, Lagace-Wiens PR, Rubinstein E, Gin AS, Walkty A, et al. Ceftolozane/tazobactam: a novel cephalosporin/beta-lactamase inhibitor combination with activity against multidrug-resistant gram-negative bacilli. Drugs. 2014;74(1):31–51.

17. Kauf TL, Prabhu VS, Medic G, Borse RH, Miller B, Gaultney J, Sen SS, Basu A. Cost-effectiveness of ceftolozane/tazobactam compared with piperacillin/tazobactam as empiric therapy based on the in-vitro surveillance of bacterial isolates in the United States for the treatment of complicated urinary tract infections. BMC Infect Dis. 2017;17(1):314.

18. Basu A. Estimating Costs and Valuations of Non-Health Benefits in Cost-Effectiveness in Health and Medicine. Second edition (Neumann PJ, Sanders GD, Russell LB, Siegel JE, Ganiats TG, eds.) New York, NY: Oxford University Press; 2016.

19. Cubist Pharmaceuticals. Premier - study on prevalence and susceptibility of gram-negative infections version 1.0. Cubist Pharmaceuticals: Data on file; 2014.

20. Natale RBT, Greco S, Thomas FA, Tsai M, Sunpaweravong CM, Ferry P, Mulatero D, Whorf C, Thompson R, Barlesi J, Langmuir F, Gogov P, Rowbottom S, Goss JA, G. D. Phase III trial of vandetanib compared with erlotinib in patients with previously treated advanced non - small-cell lung cancer. J Clin Oncol. 2011;29(8):1059–66.

21. United States Life Tables, 2011 [http://www.cdc.gov/nchs/products/life_tables.htm].

22. Sartelli M, Catena F, Ansaloni L, Leppaniemi A, Taviloglu K, van Goor H, Viale P, Lazzareschi DV, Coccolini F, Corbella D, et al. Complicated intra-abdominal infections in Europe: a comprehensive review of the CIAO study. World J Emerg Surg: WJES. 2012;7(1):36.

23. Sturkenboom MC, Goettsch WG, Picelli G, in 't Veld B, Yin DD, de Jong RB, Go PM, Herings RM: Inappropriate initial treatment of secondary intra-abdominal infections leads to increased risk of clinical failure and costs. Br J Clin Pharmacol 2005, 60(4):438–443.

24. Krobot K, Yin D, Zhang Q, Sen S, Altendorf-Hofmann A, Scheele J, Sendt W. Effect of inappropriate initial empiric antibiotic therapy on outcome of patients with community-acquired intra-abdominal infections requiring surgery. Eur J Clin Microbiol Infect Dis. 2004;23(9):682–7.

25. Jansen JP, Kumar R, Carmeli Y. Cost-effectiveness evaluation of ertapenem versus piperacillin/tazobactam in the treatment of complicated intraabdominal infections accounting for antibiotic resistance. Value Health. 2009;12(2):234–44.

26. Academy of Managed Care Pharmacy: The AMCP Format for Formulary Submissions Version 3.1. In.; December 2012.

27. 2013 Healthcare Cost and Utilization Project (HCUP). [http://hcupnet.ahrq.gov/].

28. Using appropriate price indices for analyses of health care expenditures or income across multiple years. [http://meps.ahrq.gov/about_meps/Price_Index.shtml].

29. Liu JBC, Yuan CX, Liu LF, Gao W, Shi CH, Tang SP, Shao HJ, Z. J. Gemcitabine combined with ifosfamide as second-line chemotherapy in advanced non-small cell lung cancer. [Chinese]. Chinese J Cancer Prev Treat. 2011;18(8):624–5.

30. Framework Summary [http://icer-review.org/wp-content/uploads/2016/02/Value-Assessment-Framework-One-Pager.pdf].

31. Marchaim D, Gottesman T, Schwartz O, Korem M, Maor Y, Rahav G, Karplus R, Lazarovitch T, Braun E, Sprecher H, et al. National multicenter study of predictors and outcomes of bacteremia upon hospital admission caused by Enterobacteriaceae producing extended-spectrum beta-lactamases. Antimicrob Agents Chemother. 2010;54(12):5099–104.

32. Aloush V, Navon-Venezia S, Seigman-Igra Y, Cabili S, Carmeli Y. Multidrug-resistant Pseudomonas Aeruginosa: risk factors and clinical impact. Antimicrob Agents Chemother. 2006;50(1):43–8.

33. Sader HS, Mallick R, Kuznik A, Fritsche TR, Jones RN. Use of in vitro susceptibility and pathogen prevalence data to model the expected clinical success rates of tigecycline and other commonly used antimicrobials for empirical treatment of complicated skin and skin-structure infections. Int J Antimicrob Agents. 2007;30(6):514–20.

9

The social biography of antibiotic use in smallholder dairy farms in India

Abhimanyu Singh Chauhan[1,2], Mathew Sunil George[3,4], Pranab Chatterjee[1,5], Johanna Lindahl[6,7,8], Delia Grace[6] and Manish Kakkar[1*]

Abstract

Background: Antimicrobial resistance (AMR) has been identified as one of the major threats to global health, food security and development today. While there has been considerable attention about the use and misuse of antibiotics amongst human populations in both research and policy environments, there is no definitive estimate of the extent of misuse of antibiotics in the veterinary sector and its contribution to AMR in humans. In this study, we explored the drivers ofirrational usage of verterinary antibiotics in the dairy farming sector in peri-urban India.

Methods and materials: The study was conducted in the peri-urban belts of Ludhiana, Guwahati and Bangalore. A total of 54 interviews (formal and non-formal) were carried out across these three sites. Theme guides were developed to explore different drivers of veterinary antimicrobial use. Data was audio recorded and transcribed. Analysis of the coded data set was carried out using AtlasTi. Version 7. Themes emerged inductively from the set of codes.

Results: Findings were presented based on concept of 'levels of analyses'. Emergent themes were categorised as individual, health systems, and policy level drivers. Low level of knowledge related to antibiotics among farmers, active informal service providers, direct marketing of drugs to the farmers and easily available antibiotics, dispensed without appropriate prescriptions contributed to easy access to antibiotics, and were identified to be the possible drivers contributing to the non-prescribed and self-administered use of antibiotics in the dairy farms.

Conclusions: Smallholding dairy farmers operated within very small margins of profits. The paucity of formal veterinary services at the community level, coupled with easy availability of antibiotics and the need to ensure profits and minimise losses, promoted non-prescribed antibiotic consumption. It is essential that these local drivers of irrational antibiotic use are understood in order to develop interventions and policies that seek to reduce antibiotic misuse.

Keywords: Antimicrobial use, Antimicrobial resistance, Dairy farm, Dairy farmer, Veterinary, Qualitative, India

Background

India is the global leader in the production of milk and dairy products, accounting for 18.5% of the global output, with an annual output of 146 million tons [1]. The tremendous growth in the demand for milk and other animal-source foods has been accompanied by a corresponding increase in small-scale ventures, characterised by farms that typically occupy less than one hectare, employ within-family labour, and function with minimal input costs by adopting intensive, industry style rearing of livestock [2]. Over 80% of all cattle holdings in India are in smallholder farms, which cover over 45% of agricultural land and account for over half of total production [2, 3].

India has witnessed unprecedented growth in the urban population over the past decade [4]. Peri-urban fringes, developing in the shadows of India's growing cities, play an increasingly important role in ensuring food security including dairy farms [5]. To maintain production levels, these farms, which often function in jurisdictional grey zones, with minimal quality control, infrastructure, support and oversight, practise which may result in adverse public health impacts [6, 7]. One such practice, which may have long-term adverse effects, is the non-therapeutic, irrational use of antibiotics in farm animals [8, 9].

Antibiotics are arguably the single most important and widely used medical intervention of our times. They

* Correspondence: manish.kakkar@phfi.org
[1]Public Health Foundation of India, Plot 47, Sector 44, Gurgaon, Haryana 122002, India
Full list of author information is available at the end of the article

have been rampantly used not only in human medicine but also in agricultural system(s), specifically in livestock production. Antibiotics are used therapeutically to treat sick animals, as well as prophylactically and metaphylactically to prevent infection and as growth promoters [10]. Emergence of infectious agents which are resistant to commonly used antimicrobial agents threatens the advances made by modern medicine, and AMR organisms have rapidly become one of the primary public health challenges the world over, but especially in developing and low- and middle-income countries like India [11].

Multiple studies in India, beginning with exploratory studies in the 1980s, have consistently shown that a large proportion of the tested milk samples contain antibiotic residues [12–15]. A recent study undertaken in the organised as well as organised dairy farms has reported tetracycline, oxytetracycline, sulfadimidine and sulfamethoxazole above MRL in milk samples [16]. Similarly, antimicrobial residues was reported in 23.3% dairy farm in the settings similar to the current study [17]. However, there remains a dearth of evidence about the drivers and determinants of antibiotic use in dairy farms in India, especially with respect to vulnerable areas like peri-urban areas [18]. This study was conducted to understand the practices and drivers related to the veterinary use of antibiotics in peri-urban smallholder dairy farms in selected sites of India.

Methods
Study setting
The study was conducted among smallholding dairy farmers in peri-urban areas of Guwahati,east of India, (26.1445° N, 91.7362° E); Ludhiana, north of India (30. 9010° N, 75.8573° E); and Bangalore, south of India (12. 9716° N, 77.5946° E). Like any developing country, peri-urban areas of a typical city encompass a wide range of economic activities, including farming (dairy, poultry etc.), husbandry and, small and medium scale industries, land speculation, residential suburbanization and waste disposal [19]. Definition of Peri-urban is still context specific and varies from city to city, it's difficult to estimate the exact population. However, large proportion of people from rural to urban migration settles in peri-urban fringes of the cities [19]. The background review of literature, the formative phase, and a formal consultation with experts enabled us to identify relevant stakeholders in each of the sites, whilst allowing us to refine the topic guides that we used for data collection. The main phase of data collection was preceded by a formative phase that included scoping interviews with key informants at each site, as well as a pilot testing of instruments. Fieldwork was carried out between1st February 2015 to 30th September 2015 across all three study sites.

Sampling and data collection
Data collection at each of the field sites was carried out in successive phases.. The dual strategies of purposive sampling and snowballing were employed to identify potential respondents with the help of the local partners in each of the field sites. This enabled us to not only identify those stakeholders whom knew to be relevant to this study, but also identify specific stakeholders at each site, who were involved, in some capacity, with smallholder dairy farmers (eg: traders and veterinary field assistants in Guwahati, informal treatment providers in Ludhiana, and the Karnataka Milk Federation officials in Bangalore). At each of the sites, we identified areas where most dairy farms were clustered and fitted the project definition of a smallholding dairy farm (A farm with up-to 10 cattle, at-least one milking and contributing to a minimum of 25% of the total family income). From this list we then selected farms that were spread across various locations, thus ensuring representation of farms from across the various clusters (i.e., north, south, east and west). Using a phasic, cyclical strategy for the fieldwork, data collection was stopped on reaching saturation point across the various key themes of inquiry.

The health related interviews were conducted by ASC (male) and MSG (male). Both the interviewers were practicing public health researchers with over five years experience in qualitative data collection and held graduation in public health (MPH) at the time of field work. Face to face interviews with farmers were conducted at their homes, whereas those with other stakeholders were typically conducted at their places of employment (like, veterinary hospital, pharmacy etc.). Local NGO facilitated the scheduling of interviews as per the time convenient to farmers. An appointment was sought with the government functionaries in advance and almost all interviews were conducted in the office premises. Most interviews with farmers and traders were conducted in the local language (Hindi, Punjabi and Kannada at Guwahati, Ludhiana and Bangalore site, respectively). However, government officials were comfortable in interacting in English. In order to ensure that the mediator did not introduce bias and followed the topic guide faithfully, mock interviews and training were carried out prior to the actual field visit. A typical interview lasted between 45 min to 1 h. All interviews were audio-recorded, transcribed, translated into English, and crosschecked against the original recordings.

Data management and analysis
Data analyses was done using inductive approach and content analyses. The translated transcripts were then coded using the software package AtlasTi 7.2°, utilizing a reflexive and inductive approach to allow codes and categories to emerge from within the data. The initial list of codes was compared with newer codes, enabling refinement of the

coding framework, which was utilised to guide the coding process. Coding was done by two coders and coding disagreements was sorted in consultation with senior researchers of the study (MK and DG).

In addition to the interview recordings, each researcher maintained detailed field notes in field diaries. This enabled capturing of details related to the key issues that emerged in each location, concerns regarding the fieldwork, as well as any potential trends that emerged from the participant responses. The field diary provided us with adequate details to discuss during the daily review carried out at the end of the day's work and plan for subsequent data collection. The field diaries also helped in identifying early patterns as well as assessing attainment of saturation of responses.

At the end of each phase, data management and analysis of the previous site was completed, and summary results prepared. This enabled further probing of specific areas. This iterative process ensured that the data collected was grounded, rich in details, and saturation obtained prior to termination of data collection.

Quality assurance

Interviews were conducted by trained investigators. They were monitored for completeness, correctness, and comprehensive transcription and translation of responses with appropriate labelling of recordings. Thirty per cent of the interviews from every site were randomly rechecked for transcription and translation. Due to inherent limitations of interpretation of qualitative data from different parts of the country, we undertook regular consultations with the steering group (comprising of seven experts across the fields of medical, veterinary and social sciences) about the data and its interpretations.

It was ensured that interviews were conducted in place where only interviewee and interviewer was present. The study followed the COnsolidated criteria for REporting Qualitative research (COREQ) for reporting the findings of this qualitative research study [20].

Results

A total of 54 interviews (formal and non-formal) were conducted across the three sites (Table 1). These included dairy farmers, veterinary officers, veterinary field assistants, pharmacists, drug distributors and civic officials. Site-specific stakeholders were also identified through the snowballing process. Traders, who procured milk from

farmers and sold to sweet shops and households, were interviewed in Guwahati. Officials of Karnataka Milk Federation (KMF), a cooperative with a membership base of around 90% of the smallholder dairy farmers in periurban Bengaluru, were also interviewed. Those who were approached, none of them refused to participate in the study.

The results are presented as three core themes that emerged from insights of the different stakeholders: 1. Self-treatment and peer learning; 2. Limited systems support, outreach and oversight; 3. Limited regulatory framework to regulate use, market pressures and distribution of veterinary antibiotics. Details of sub-themes and domains are listed in Table 2.

Themes could be further grouped into drivers operating at three levels of the system: individual, health systems, and market or policy levels. The system, in this case, was defined as the smallholder dairy farm in periurban settings and its associated veterinary antibiotic use practices. The concept of a "system" allowed us to study the linkages and interactions between the sub-themes and core themes that operate at different levels. For the purpose of this study, individual/community level drivers were defined as practices at the level of farm owners, labourers, family members, community, traders and others players who can influence antimicrobial usage. Health systems drivers were defined as those associated with systems stakeholders like veterinary doctors, veterinary field assistants, laboratory staff and others who could possibly contribute to the dynamics of antimicrobial usage in small holding dairy farms. Policy level drivers included the drivers that were associated with the government, national as well as local, and policies affecting the use of antimicrobials in smallholding dairy farms.

CORE THEME I - Self-treatment and peer learning: Individual and community level drivers for irrational usage of veterinary antibiotics

Self-treatment of animals by farmers and peer learning were significant determinants of antibiotic usage, which emerged as the core theme at the community/individual level. These core themes further comprised of limited knowledge, self-treatment, and peer-learning as sub themes.

Sub-theme I – Knowledge about veterinary antibiotics

Majority of the farmers across three sites were unaware of the word 'antibiotic'. No local name existed specifically for

Table 1 Details of the stakeholders interviewed

Study sites	Dairy farmer	Veterinary/ Ext. officer	Veterinary field assistant	Trader	Pharmacist/Drug Distr.	Civic official Or Union
Guwahati	7	5	3	3	3	3
Bangalore	4	6	2	N/A	2	3
Ludhiana	4	2	2	N/A	2	3

Table 2 Core themes and sub-themes emerged from the inductive data analyses

Sl. No.	Domain	Core themes	Sub-themes
1	Community and Individual	Self-treatment and peer learning	Limited knowledge about antibiotics and their use
			Self-treatment using veterinary antibiotics
			Peer learning and self-treatment
2	Veterinary health system support	Limited system support, outreach and oversight.	Shortage of veterinary doctors
			Laboratory support to diagnose diseases and make informed prescription
			Support from extension services
			Shortage of pharmacists
3	Policy and market scenario	Limited regulatory framework on usage, market pressures and distribution of veterinary antibiotics	Absence of regulation for veterinary antibiotics
			Direct marketing of veterinary antibiotics to consumer
			Compulsion of milking - Market demand and competition.

the term either. Most of the farmers could not differentiate between antibiotics and non-antibiotic, allopathic medicines. However, the interviewed veterinarians reported that many farmers administer antibiotics to the farm cattle irrespective of the disease being infectious or not. Veterinarians also mentioned that choice of drug is based mostly on the ease of availability and the experience of the farmers with the drug while treating similar symptoms on previous occasions, some of which could be undertaken at the advise of a veterinarian. Fin.

Sub-theme II - Self-treatment using veterinary antibiotics

Most information on how farmers prefer medicines that give them 'quick results' came from pharmacists. Sick animals are treated with broad-spectrum antibiotics on the basis of prior experience. This experience could be that of the concerned farmer or be obtained through by social peer learning networks (like elders or influential farmers who had previously treated their cattle successfully; more details in the next subsection). Intergenerational transfer of this information also played a significant role. Additionally, nearly all the veterinarians reported that by the time a farmer brings his animal to a licensed veterinarian, the farmer would have already tried out several treatment strategies, none of which were successful in curing the affected animal.

"We are trying this medicine for last three days but not seeing much improvement; we will wait a bit and see, and if we do not see any improvements, we will try to call a doctor." (Dairy farmer, Ludhiana).

"If I know what the problem is then I try to manage it. Sometimes it will be the same problem that another cow had, so I will buy and give the same

medicines that the doctor prescribed last time." (Dairy farmer, Guwahati).

One of the reasons stated for self-treatment was the cost of getting a veterinarian to come to the farm, especially in Guwahati. While this was not an issue among well-established farms, smallholding farmers found this to be barrier.

"My biggest problem is if my animals fall sick. Getting a veterinarian to come to my farm is costly and I can't afford it. I give the animal what I can". (Dairy farmer, Guwahati).

Sub- theme III - Peer learning and self-treatment

Many field veterinarians, as well as a few dairy farmers, reported that they follow the advice of the local elders, influential persons, or village heads ('*Gaon budha*' (Guwahati) and '*sarpanch*' (Ludhiana)) for advice related to medication. Most of these opinion leaders are commercial dairy farmers with farms having more than 50 heads of cattle. They usually enjoy a good relationship with pharmaceutical representatives and drug distributors.

CORE THEME II - limited system support, outreach and oversight

Limited systems support, outreach and oversight were significant reasons of antibiotic usage and emerged as the core theme at the veterinary health systems level. These core themes further could be split into the following factors: a shortage of licensed veterinarians and a profusion of informal prescribers; laboratory support to diagnose diseases and plan appropriate therapeutic strategies; inadequate IEC (Information, Education and Communication) support through extension services; and a shortage of veterinary pharmacists with a profusion of informal drug distributors.

Sub-theme I: Shortage of veterinary doctors and active informal prescribers

All three levels of stakeholders in the three sitesreported that there was an acute shortage of trained veterinarians. Stakeholders, including veterinary doctors and state officials, also reported that veterinary field assistants and informal prescribers attempt to fill the gap. This results in a cadre of untrained caregivers with a propensity to overprescribe, leading to irrational prescription and usage of antibiotics. These informal prescribers are also known as 'private doctors' among the dairy farmers.

"How it is possible for a doctor to visit 30,000 cows? So definitely, if you call me and someone else calls me at the same time and there is a distance of 10 KM between the two houses, it is not possible for me to attend to both the cases simultaneously. I will definitely have to send somebody to attend the other patient. So what I do is that I send the VFA and tell him to go and check on the patient, and consult me over the phone. Mobiles are extensively used now, so it is possible. I do not go for visits nowadays, yet I have the information that I need to know. I think non-availability [of enough trained and licensed veterinarians] is one of the reasons, and because of that, slowly they (the VFAs) are emerging as the first point of care consultant; the other reason is that if they call the VFA then the fees will be much lower than that of a veterinarian, I think that might also be one of the reasons" (Veterinary doctor, Guwahati).

"The private doctors, they keep visiting farms and are very busy. In fact, they are occupied from early in the morning to late evenings everyday. They are not really doctors but that's what they are known as. They treat a lot of animals in these farms" (Pharmacist, Ludhiana).

Sub theme II: Laboratory support to diagnose diseases and make informed prescription

Senior government officials' perspective Across the three sites, senior officials in the animal husbandry department pointed out that labs and diagnostic support services were functional and provided value addition to the work of field veterinarians. However, when asked specifically about testing and screening facility for various infections in cattle, very few veterinarians mentioned regular testing done at the smallholder or commercial dairy farms. None of the state level officials reported any

disease screening programs specifically directed at cattle in smallholder dairy farms.

Field veterinarians' perspective Veterinarians reported that they do not depend on lab reports to treat any sick animals. Most treatment plans were based on case history and symptomatic assessments. Lab support was only sought when the treatment administered to the animal did not give the desired results. Two reasons were stated by veterinarians for not seeking lab support: First, by the time a farmer reaches the veterinarian the farmer has already spent time and money in trying out other alternatives and the veterinarian has to begin some treatment almost immediately to save the cattle. Secondly, even if labs do exist, most of them are not adequately equipped; if they are equipped, it would be expensive and unaffordable to access their services, and hence it was not considered to be practical to utilize them.

"If the lab is in working condition we don't have a microbiologist, if the microbiologist is there then there is no proper equipment. So how do I make use of it? On paper it is all there but practically it is not possible. If I need a lab report, then I ask them to go to the university or to some private labs to get a report." (Veterinarian, Ludhiana).

"Look, we treat primarily from the case history of the sick animal and after some years of experience you know that an animal which is in this condition, is suffering from this problem, and needs this treatment. Other than that not much to do for us." (Veterinarian, Guwahati).

Sub theme III: Support from extension services in context to veterinary use of antibiotics

Dairy farmers' perspective It was striking that none of the farmers across the three sites referred to benefitting from any extension services. They perceived services to be of poor quality. Also, according to them, these services were conducted more out of the need to demonstrate activities to students, and were not particularly concerned with the welfare of a farmer or their animals.

"What services are you talking about? There is such a big college here and they can't even provide us with proper semen." (Dairy farmer, Guwahati).

"No we do not get anything from the department or college." (Dairy farmer, Ludhiana).

Many of those who attended demonstration sessions and meetings happened to be owners of commercial dairy farms. These were individuals who had no prior experience of dairying and had entered the sector recently.

"The department does organise activities from time to time when they want to train their students. Other than that such activities are not focused on the small farmers and their farms."(Dairy farmer, Guwahati).

Extension department officials' opinion Extension departments are functional and claimed to offer relevant services to local dairy farmers on a regular basis. These services include sessions on the updated management practices in dairy farming, inputs on fodder management, disease management, breeding techniques, shed design, to name a few. Most services were offered completely free of charge so that local dairy farmers belonging to the lower socioeconomic strata could reap the benefits. However, when asked about the specific activities related to the use of antibiotics and their role in maintaining the health of animals, the interviewed stakeholders (state-level officials and veterinarians) failed to mention any particular programs.

"Regular meetings are organized by the department and we have sessions taken by experts to give them [dairy farmers] *the latest know-how on various issues on how to manage a dairy farm."* (Senior extension department official, Ludhiana).

Many veterinarians reported that farmers often chose to not attend these sessions. According to them, this is due to the farmers' belief and reliance on traditional knowledge, which is often handed down generations. In contrast, relatively new commercial dairy farmers, were more open to learning and behaviour modification in relation to dairy farming practices.

Sub-theme IV: Shortage of pharmacists and presence of informal drug distributors

Some veterinary officers and state level officials reported the scarcity of trained pharmacists in the peri-urban areas; this was especially notable in Guwahati. According to them, most of the drugs were distributed by drug distributors. Even if a pharmacist is present, prescription-based purchase is minimal in all the studied settings. They forwarded this as one of the reasons for the irrational use of veterinary antibiotics.

CORE THEME III: Limited regulatory framework on usage and distribution of veterinary antibiotics, and market pressure: Policy and market level drivers

Limited legislative frameworks to regulate the use and distribution of veterinary antibiotics, and mitigate market pressures are significant determinants of antibiotic over usage. These emerged as the core theme at the policy level. These core themes could further be split into: absence of regulation for the prudent use of veterinary antibiotics, Direct-to-Consumer Marketing of Veterinary Antibiotics (DTCMVA) and compulsion to maintain productivity to meet market demands in the face of stiff economic competition.

Sub theme I: Absence of regulation for the prudent use of veterinary antibiotics

Nearly all veterinary doctors and senior state level officials expressed the need to deploy potent regulations to deal with the situation of antibiotic growth promoters and non-therapeutic use of antibiotics. Many of the senior officials also reported the absence of evidence-based guidelines related to the prudent use of veterinary antibiotics; even when they were present, they were constrained by the complete absence of a strategy to operationalize the recommendations and monitor their implementation.

Sub theme II: Direct to consumer Marketing of Veterinary Antibiotics (DTCMVA)

"While visiting a village in Guwahati to capture the insights from small holder dairy farmers related to veterinary use of antibiotics, we observed a Medical Representative (MR) from a renowned pharmaceutical company visiting the most learned and influential (village leader) dairy farmer in the village. He was carrying boxes with a range of medicines - concentrates, calcium supplements as well as veterinary antibiotics. When asked about the content and why he has been keeping these items at the leader's house, we were informed by the dairy farmers that this was the 'drug depot' of the village. All farmers could access and purchase these medicines as and when required. Pharmacies are too far away and a significant cost is incurred when visiting them. Older members of the village informed that the depot holder received financial incentives from the MR as well as a supply of medicines at a discounted rate. As the depot holder is comparatively more qualified and influential, dairy farmers often consult him for the medicines and treatment. We discussed and validated these responses with local veterinarian and state level officials."
[Excerpt from field diary, 13th March 2015, Guwahati, Description of DTCMVA phenomena].

During field observations in Guwahati, we observed that the antibiotics are directly marketed in the village. The most influential or community leader or commercial dairy farmer acts as mediator between MR and smallholder dairy farmers. The relationship is mutually beneficial as the farmer gets the drugs at a discounted rate and without having to travel to a distant pharmacy; in return, this helps the pharmaceutical representatives to meet their sales targets. For the village elders or opinion leaders, this offers a position of relative power, which further consolidates their status in the community. Some smallholder farmers also reported that the depot holder was often offered medicines at a discounted rate by the pharmaceutical representative.

Sub theme III: Compulsion of milking - market demand and economic compulsion

Nearly all the stakeholders reported that the business of smallholding dairy farms operates at razor thin profit margins and to keep their livelihood intact the farmers need to maintain productivity in their animals on a daily basis. A majority of the farmers were unaware about the concept of withdrawal period following antimicrobial chemotherapy. However, even those who were aware of the importance of the withholding period reported that it was impractical due to high economic implications to their business. Additionally, famers also reported that they faced competition from milk cooperatives and private companies. This resulted in dwindling demands for non-packaged milk in the urban areas. As a result withholding milking and not supplying milk even for a day or two could result in an irreversible loss of customers which would have a significant adverse impact on their business. In absence of a formal system of incentives or disincentives, it was virtually impossible to practise the withholding. Health system level stakeholders also reinforced these concerns. According to them, withholding should be incentivised to prevent milk tainted with antimicrobial residues from entering into the food chain.

"Who will pay for the milk I throw out?. Each cow gives an average of 10 litres of milk everyday. I have four milking cows, and if one is on treatment and milking is withheld, it translates into a loss of INR 300 minimum. We need to continuously feed the animal, irrespective of whether we are selling the milk or not. From where will I get money for this?" (Dairy farmer, Guwahati)

"We need to take appropriate measures. How can we expect a poor farmer to discard the milk? The Government should identify certain incentives so that these farmers comply with the policy." (Senior official, Guwahati)

"Monetary loss for a day is just one way of looking at it. What about the customers we lose? Who is going to explain to them the reason behind why we are not providing the milk to them?" (Dairy farmer, Bangalore)

Behavioural model of drivers and determinants of non-prescribed use of antibiotics in smallholder periurban dairy farms

We developed a conceptual framework explaining the interplay of factors leading to non-prescribed usage of veterinary antibiotics using The theory of planned behaviour (Fig. 1) [21]. We mapped these factors to address the reasoned action for non-prescribed or self-administered use of veterinary antibiotics in the peri-urban smallholder dairy farms. This was determined by: [1] attitude towards irrational use of antibiotics, [2] subjective belief about the irrational use of antibiotics at the community level, and [3] the perceived control exerted over the act of irrational antibiotic use in livestock. Subjective belief is the perceived social pressure to perform or not to perform the behaviour and perceived control is an individual's beliefs about the presence of factors that may facilitate or hinder performance of the behaviour. We classified the drivers operational at the community, the system, and the market and policy levels. These drivers, in combination, resulted in the practice of self-administered use of antibiotics in livestock. The conceptual model, shown in Fig. 1, indicates a closely knit, inter-related, web of factors with recursive and reversible relationships. It is essential to disrupt this chain at the critical linkages to make a meaningful reduction in the irrational and non-prescribed consumption of veterinary antibiotics in the peri-urban smallholder dairy farms of India.

Discussion

This qualitative study adds to the growing body of evidence related to the issue of antimicrobial consumption. The study explicitly dealt with the non-prescribed and self-administered veterinary antibiotic usage in the smallholder dairy farms in peri-urban areas. Through in-depth-interviews across various stakeholders, this paper attempts to elucidate the complexities of antimicrobial usage in the smallholder dairy farming sector in peri-urban India. Each core theme was further explained under sub themes.

Antibiotic use practices in small holder dairy farms

In dairy farming, practices, knowledge and beliefs handed down from one generation to the next [22, 23]. Experienced dairy farmers have traditionally managed animal health issues using ethnoveterinary practices rooted in the use of indigenous medicinal herbs, utilising the Indian Systems of Medicine [24, 25]. The current generation has retained the self-reliance to manage livestock diseases on their own, and supplemented the traditional knowledge with their understanding of modern medicine. This self-reliance, in combination with market pressures and economic compulsions, has resulted in the widespread practice of self-administration of antibiotics in livestock for therapeutic, prophylactic and metaphylactic purposes,

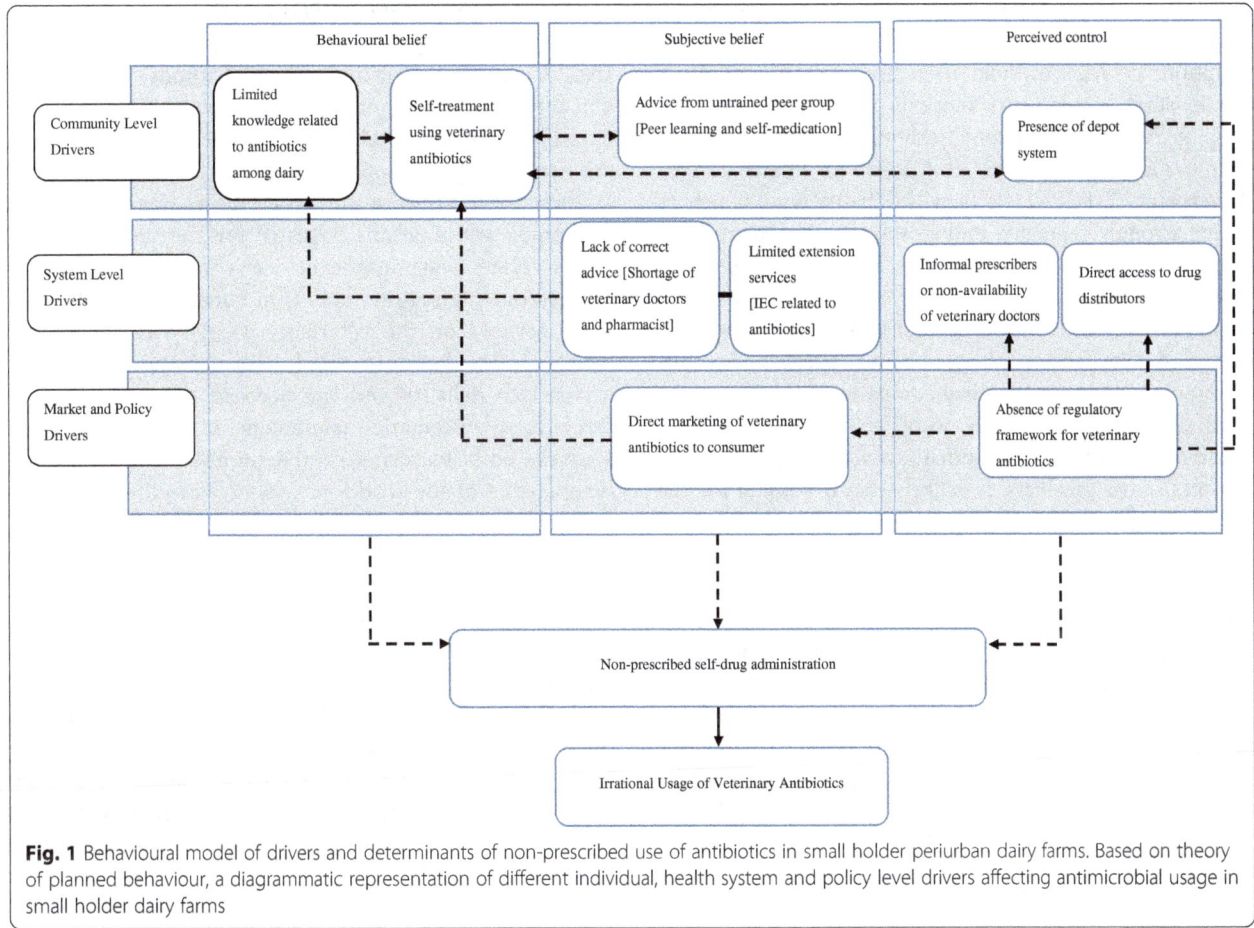

Fig. 1 Behavioural model of drivers and determinants of non-prescribed use of antibiotics in small holder periurban dairy farms. Based on theory of planned behaviour, a diagrammatic representation of different individual, health system and policy level drivers affecting antimicrobial usage in small holder dairy farms

thus augmenting the risk of emergence of AMR (Fig. 2). Along with easy over-the-counter access to antibiotics, often without any prescriptions, or with invalid prescriptions, or with prescriptions from unlicensed practitioners, there is a fertile socioeconomic backdrop encouraging irrational use of antibiotics in livestock held by peri-urban smallholder farmers. Irrational use of antibiotics is further fuelled by veterinarians who are more influenced by social expectations than by scientific reasoning, as has been the case with human antibiotics prescribing practices [26].

Drivers of antibiotic usage in Peri-urban smallholder dairy farms

The following key drivers directly influence the irrational usage of veterinary antibiotics: (a) direct marketing of veterinary antibiotics to consumer; (b) enabling of informal prescribers and caregivers to fill the gap created by inadequate coverage of veterinary services; (c) failure to regulate informal antibiotic supply chains in the community through drug depots and unfettered access to drug distributors; and (d) low literacy levels and poor awareness of antibiotics and the role they play in animal and human health.

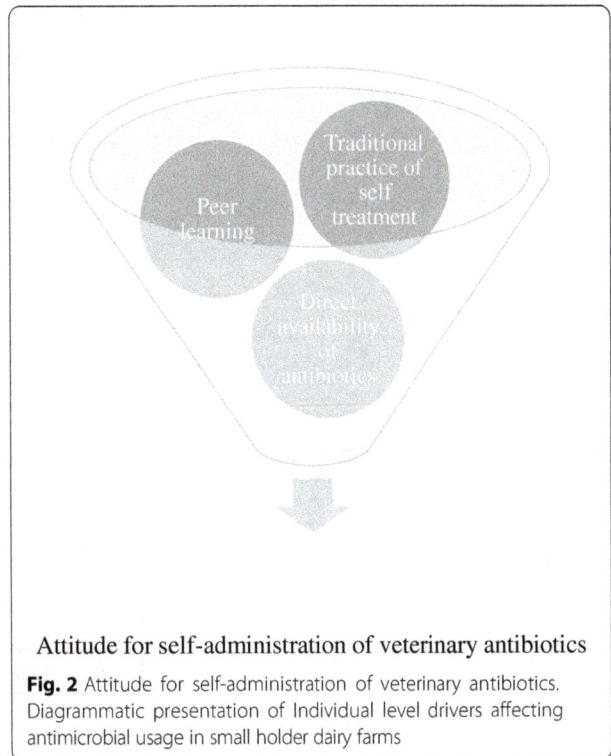

Attitude for self-administration of veterinary antibiotics

Fig. 2 Attitude for self-administration of veterinary antibiotics. Diagrammatic presentation of Individual level drivers affecting antimicrobial usage in small holder dairy farms

a. Direct Marketing of Veterinary Antibiotics to consumer

Although direct marketing and selling drugs without prescriptions is illegal in India, there are several loopholes in the existing regulatory provisions which have failed to keep up with the changing technological and socioeconomic milieu [27]. Direct-to-Consumer Pharmaceutical Advertising (DTCPA) is a heavily debated issue which remains strongly regulated and closely monitored in developed countries [28]. In the present study, some interesting facets with elements of DTCPA emerged as drivers of antibiotic use in livestock. Several veterinarians, pharmacists, and dairy farmers reported being approached by representatives of pharmaceutical companies advertising their products, some of which were veterinary antibiotics. Additionally, several respondents reported receiving free samples of the products. It is likely that bypassing the formal drug value chain (Fig. 3) by using informal channels of drug distribution, geared towards building a user base, further resulted in an irrational drug distribution (Fig. 4), increased the profit margins for the individual representatives who are usually required to meet time-bound sales targets [29, 30]. A previous study reported that the pharmaceutical companies do not impose the same influence in veterinary practice as in human [31]. However, the evidences from the current study strongly suggests pharmaceutical companies as potential influencer behind non-prescribed use.

b. Lack of qualified veterinarians and the role of informal caregivers

Use of veterinary antimicrobials without veterinarian consultation was reported in past with 87% and 38% among urban and rural farmers, respectively [32]. However, study did not report the drivers responsible for this. In the current study, a universal finding was the scarcity of trained veterinarians to cater for the animal health needs. There was significant convergence of all stakeholders on this matter. This is in concurrence with previous reviews on the veterinary capacity in the nation, which clearly demonstrated India's constrained veterinary service delivery and the need to meet the scarcity through a systematic assessment of the human resources, both in terms of the number as well as the competence of the workforce, followed by the establishment of new veterinary colleges and other institutions to bridge the human resources gap [33–35].

In addition to the perceived shortage of veterinarians, in the present study, informal interactions also revealed that the veterinarians are more interested in private veterinary practice, which is oriented towards treating pet animals (Mostly, dogs, cats, rabbits and birds.), in contrast to the government sector facilities which had a stronger focus on livestock. This is likely to be a factor promoting the informal or unauthorized (para-vet/veterinary field assistants etc.) prescriber network, which endeavours to

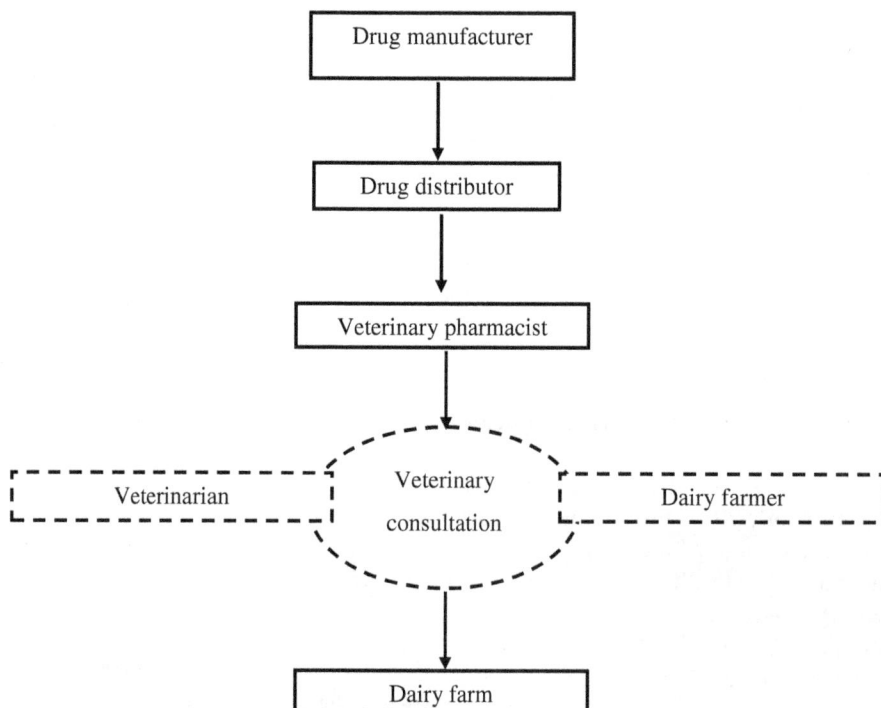

Fig. 3 A typical formal drug distribution channel. Flow chart represents a formal and rational drug delivery system

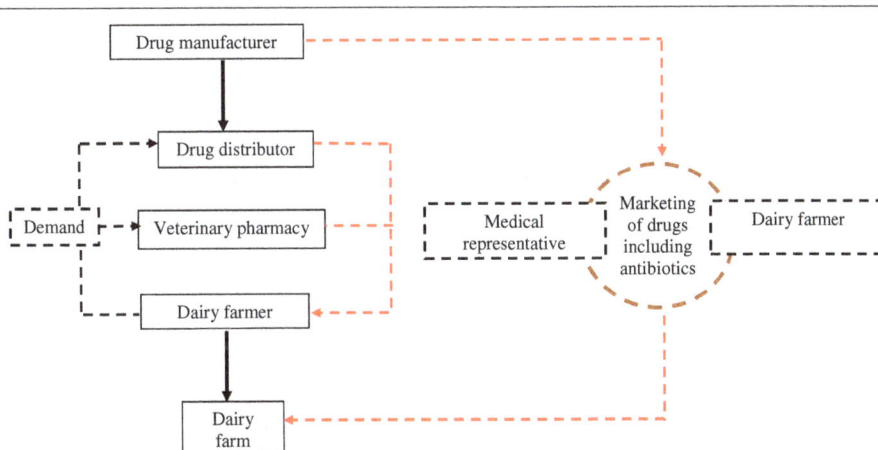

Fig. 4 Informal channels of introduction of veterinary antibiotic in dairy farms

reach the underserved population. Similar finding was reported in an earlier study conducted among veterinary doctors in south eastern part of India [31]. Study reported that veterinary doctors perceives that prior prescription by unqualified prescribers was influencing antimicrobial prescriptions for animals. Recent study in northern India reported low level of knowledge among para-vet about antibiotic resistance and its public health impact [36]. The use of antibiotics not prescribed by a veterinarian, or the use of antibiotics from non-accredited sources was frequently reported in different parts of the world [37]. However, no single study has explained the interplay of different drivers at different levels potentially responsible for the non-prescribed usage of veterinary antimicrobials.

The shortage of trained and licensed pharmacists was also identified to be an issue by some state-level stakeholders. The pharmacist has a vital role to play in limiting access to antibiotics and providing proper guidance to care-seeking farmers. It is essential to incorporate them within the ambit of community-based antibiotic stewardship efforts to reduce the unintended consequences of overuse and abuse of veterinary antibiotics [38–40]. The absence of adequately trained pharmacists could contribute to the nexus between non-licensed distributors and representatives of pharmaceutical companies. According to a report based on a survey conducted in the WHO European Member States, adequately trained pharmacists can act as gatekeepers to rational drug usage interventions and are uniquely positioned to influence prudent antibiotic consumption [41]. The shortage of such a vital component of the healthcare delivery system is, therefore, of special concern.

c. Easy access through informal antibiotic supply chains
The depot system, direct accessibility of community opinion leaders to pharmaceutical representatives, and easy access to over-the-counter antibiotics represents an informal supply chain through which the dairy farmers may access antibiotics and other veterinary drugs. The dairy farmers preferred this informal supply chain as well, since it provides direct access to medications perceived to be effective, without the accompanying costs, both in terms of money and time, of consulting a veterinarian. Similar findings were reported in a study from Peru where farmers preferred prescription as well as purchase of drug from other channels such as direct purchase from pharmacies and feed-store vendors [42]. Consequently, the farmers often contacted the pharmaceutical representatives directly when they needed to explore options for treating their animals.

Another phenomenon which raised concerns is the depot system. An elderly or experienced farmer, who often happened to be the opinion leader in the community, was approached by the pharmaceutical representatives, and provided sample medications to distribute to neighbouring farmers. The possibility remained that such informal routes, in addition to encouraging irrational use, could also promote multi-drug use or use of supra-therapeutic doses, as the elderly farmers would want to ensure clinical success and consolidate their position in the social hierarchy. A further consequence of the unregulated access to the supply chain of veterinary antibiotics is the repeated use of the same drug for different clinical conditions even if the underlying pathophysiology is different and warrants a different therapeutic approach.

d. Poor literacy, low level of education and low level of awareness
Access to information has been cited to be an important factor in promoting equity in healthcare [43, 44]. Building awareness about antibiotics has been identified as one of the key strategic objectives espoused by the World Health Organization (WHO) in its global action plan to contain AMR [45]. In the present study, an additional layer of

complexity was added to irrational antibiotic use by peri-urban smallholder dairy farmers because of the relatively low levels of literacy and awareness, which has been previously reported by studies conducted in similar settings [46, 47]. This implies that the farmers might be unable to interpret complex medical information even if they have access to it. This assertion receives endorsement from the veterinarian input that farmers are often unable to comprehend why a drug is inappropriate for a given clinical scenario, even when symptoms mimic a previous episode where the same drug was prescribed.

The veterinarians also admitted that there is a definite "pull" from farmers who insist on antibiotics for illnesses where they may not be recommended; they preferred a shorter course of more expensive or newer antibiotics over a recommended, longer regimen. Similar findings were reported in a previous study from New Zealand, where 22% of the veterinary doctors admitted that their prescribing decision was influenced by non-clinical reasons such as farmers' preferences [48]. Similarly, veterinarians reported 'external pressures', such as pressure from clients, legislation and public perception, strongly influence their antimicrobial prescribing behaviour [49]. Limited or no evidence is available to compare the findings in this context from India. Farmers interacted more often with pharmaceutical representatives or informal practitioners, who are likely to be more amenable to giving in to such demands. This could potentially lead to a vicarious pressure on veterinarians to prescribe per the farmers' wishes to retain their patients. Longer duration of therapy could result in adverse economic implications for the farmers, hence, when such a course is recommended at government hospitals or licensed veterinarians, they risk losing their credibility with the farmers unless the farmers are adequately informed and counselled. These perverse financial forces could distort prescription practices even in the formal clinical systems, resulting in inappropriate use or overuse of antibiotics.

Though there is limited evidence related to the market pressures on smallholder dairy farmers contributing to compulsion to milking and overlooking the issue of withholding, the current study indicates that in the absence of quality-based incentives, farmers have no motivation to withhold milking cattle undergoing antimicrobial chemotherapy. Nearly all farmers reported a very small profit margin and the compulsion of milking to ensure solvency. There is a small, but growing body of published evidence, advocating for incentives to ensure milk quality. These incentives should be deployed in addition to IEC activities focussing on the improvement of mammary health, milk hygiene and safety was envisaged [50].

The lack of outreach activities, targeting the information needs of the community further deepened the crisis of misinformation in the farmers. This pattern of antibiotic misuse was further stimulated by the sense of control that most traditional dairy farmers felt they had on the farming process (unpublished findings, "Stakeholder mapping and analysis in peri-urban dairy farms of India", Manish Kakkar). A typical finding was the creation of a depot system. This was seen to be a recursive issue, since the presence of a depot system encouraged farmers to self-administer antibiotics, and the depots were sustained by the continued interest of farmers in having quick access to medications, by-passing the somewhat onerous conventional animal healthcare system. This also created a perverse peer-support group, which functioned to propagate the misinformation about antibiotics and their utility, further ensuring their entrenchment in the community [51]. National Livestock Mission (NLM) could be a platform to engage the dairy farm owners to raise awareness related to prudent use of veterinary antimicrobials [52]. The mission has national presence and is supported by the central government. The current objective of the sub-mission in context to IEC involves increased awareness among all stakeholders involved in the animal husbandry sector regarding scientific methods of rearing, susceptibility to disease, vaccination, breed improvement, animal nutrition, schemes implemented by various agencies and support for Livestock Extension at various levels. An evidence-based intervention package related to knowledge on antibiotics, need for using prescribed antibiotics, adherence to prescribed therapy and observing withholding period can be incorporated in the revised NLM IEC strategies [52].

In addition to the centrally run schemes and missions, there are schemes under the state governments which aim to attract smallholders into the supply cycle to provide increased returns for their produce, thus stimulating production and encouraging the uptake of improved technologies. Inclusion of rational use of veterinary antibiotics as an objective under the awareness programme might result in changing the risk practices of dairy farmers with respect to veterinary antimicrobial consumption [53]. Similarly, other programmes like the National Programme for Bovine Breeding and Dairy Development (NPBBD), which was initiated in February 2014, could be used as a platform to raise awareness related to veterinary antimicrobial use among smallholder dairy farmers, as well as strengthening the laboratory screening facility of residues in [54].

Limitations of the study

A very small number of state-level civic officials were involved in this study. Notwithstanding this, the limited number provided rich and meaningful data as the respondents who participated had decades of experience in animal husbandry and veterinary medicine. IDI with dairy farmers were performed in the local languages and then translated into English. Despite the rigorous verification process, some subtle nuances might have been missed during the verbatim transcribing.

Conclusion

The current study identifies several factors which come together to determine the use of antibiotics in the small-holding dairy farms located in peri-urban fringes of Indian cities. The qualitative nature of the enquiry provides us with unique insights which are difficult to identify using the traditional quantitative surveillance approaches. In this study we explore the social biography of antibiotics, as they find their way through formal and informal routes, into the peri-urban smallholder dairy farms, often in the form of irrational, non-therapeutic, sub- or supra-therapeutic usage.

The study concludes that in the presence of weak veterinary care infrastructures with limited outreach activities, severe human resource limitations, poor legislative and regulatory oversight, and limited knowledge and awareness of the role of antibiotics in consumers, it would be difficult to combat the issue of emergent antibiotic resistance. Interventions such as community awareness programmes related to veterinary antibiotics, establishing an effective drug distribution policy, imposing penalties on defaulters, and strengthening of veterinary human resources both in terms of quantity as well as competence is required to address the issue adequately.

Abbreviations
AMR: Antimicrobial Resistance; DTCMVA: Direct to Consumer Marketing of Veterinary Antibiotics; DTCPA : Direct to consumer pharmaceutical advertising; IEC : Information Education Communication; MR : Medical Representative; VFA : Veterinary Field Assistants; WHO : World Health Organization

Acknowledgements
We thank site partners (Assam Agriculture University, Karnataka Veterinary Animal and Fisheries Sciences University and Guru Angad Dev Veterinary and Animal Sciences University) for facilitating the field interviews. We would also like to thank team members of Centre for Rural Development (CRD) and BHOOMI sustainable development society, non-governmental organizations for coordination and facilitating the field interviews.

Funding
This study was part of a larger project supported by International Development Research Centre, Canada grant (No.107344–001).

Authors' contributions
MK, DG, MSG and ASC conceived the study design. ASC and MSG contributed in acquisition of data. ASC, MSG, PC and JL contributed in analysis and interpretation of data. ASC, MSG, MK, PC contributed in drafting the manuscript. All authors read, reviewed and approved the final manuscript.

Competing interests
The authors declare that they have no competing interests.

Author details
[1]Public Health Foundation of India, Plot 47, Sector 44, Gurgaon, Haryana 122002, India. [2]Department of Public Health Sciences, Faculty of Medicine, University of Liège - Hospital District, Hippocrates Avenue 13 - Building 234000, Liège, Belgium. [3]Indian Institute of Public Health, Gurgaon, Haryana 122002, India. [4]Centre for Research and Action in Public Health (CeRAPH), University of Canberra, Building 22, Floor B, University Drive, Bruce ACT 2617, Australia. [5]Indian Council of Medical Research, Division of Epidemiology, National Institute of Cholera and Enteric Diseases, Kolkata 700010, India. [6]International Livestock Research Institute, Nairobi 30709-00100, Kenya. [7]Zoonosis Science Laboratory, Uppsala University, Po Box 582, Uppsala SE-751 23, Sweden. [8]Department of Clinical Sciences, Swedish University of Agricultural Sciences, PO Box 7054, Uppsala SE-750 07, Sweden.

References
1. Ministry of Finance. Prices, agriculture and food management. Economic survey volume II. 1st ed. New Delhi: Government of India; 2015. p. 89–123.
2. Singh R, Kumar P, Woodhead T. Smallholder contributions to agriculture: Smallholder farmers in India: Food security and agricultural policy. Thailand: RAP publications; 2002. p. 5.
3. Agricultural Census Division. Agriculture Census 2010–2011: All India report on number and area of operational holdings. New Delhi: Agricultural Census 2010–11; 2014.
4. Census of India. Government of India. India: Office of the Registrar General & Census Commissioner. Available from: http://www.censusindia.gov.in/2011census/PCA/A2_Data_Table.html.
5. Chatterjee P, Kakkar M, Biswas T. Cities: new fringes to act as safety nets. Nature. 2016;540(7631):39–9.
6. Wolfenson KDM. Coping with the food and agriculture challenge: smallholders' agenda preparations and outcomes of the 2012 United Nations conference on sustainable development (Rio+20). Rome: Food and Agriculture Organization; 2013.
7. Arias P, Hallam D, Krivonos E, Morrison J. Smallholder integration in changing food markets. Rome: Food and Agriculture Organization; 2013.
8. WHO. Antimicrobial Resistance: Global Report on surveillance [Internet]. World Health Organization. Geneva; 2014. Available from: http://apps.who.int/iris/bitstream/handle/10665/112642/9789241564748_eng.pdf?sequence=1
9. Marshall BM, Levy SB. Food animals and antimicrobials: impacts on human health. Clin Microbiol Rev. 2011;24(4):718–33.
10. Center for Disease Dynamics Economics and Policy, Global Antibiotic Resistance Partnership. Antibiotic Use and Resistance in Food Animals: Current policy and recommendations. Washington DC; 2016.
11. Kakkar M, Walia K, Vong S, Chatterjee P, Sharma A. Antibiotic resistance and its containment in India. Br Med J. 2017;358:j2687.
12. Ramakrishna Y, Singh R. Residual streptomycin in milk. A survey. Indian J Dairy Sci. 1985;38:148–9.
13. Unnikrishnan V, Bhavadassan MK, Nath BS, Ram C. Chemical residues and contaminants in milk: a review. Indian J Anim Sci. 2005;75(5):592-8.
14. Chand R, Bhavadasan M, Vijya G. Antimicrobial drugs in milk from southern India. Indian Dairym. 2003;55(3):154.
15. Grover CR, Bhavadesan M. Antibiotic residues in milk: a public health concern. In: National Conference on Food Safety and Environmental TOxins New Delhi: Centre for Science and Environment; 2013. p. 47.
16. Nirala RK, Anjana K, Mandal KG, Jayachandran C. Persistence of Antibiotic Residue in Milk under Region of Bihar, India. Int J Curr Microbiol Appl Sci. 2017;6(3):2296-9.
17. Dinki N, Balcha E. Detection of antibiotic residues and determination of microbial quality of raw milk from milk collection centres. Adv Anim Vet Sci. 2013;1(3):80–3.
18. Venkatasubramanian P, Islam MA, Van 't Hooft KE, Groot MJ. The hidden effects of dairy farming on public and environmental health in the Netherlands, India, Ethiopia, and Uganda, considering the use of antibiotics and other agro-chemicals. Front Public Heal. 2016;4(4):123389–12.
19. Narain V, Anand P, Banerjee P. Periurbanization in India: a review of the literature and evidence [internet]. Rural to Urban Transitions and the Peri-urban Interface, SaciWATERs. 2013. Available from: http://www.saciwaters.org/east-west-center/pdf/status-paper.pdf.
20. Tong A, Sainsbury P, Craig J. Consolidated criteria for reporting qualitative research (COREQ): a 32-item checklist for interviews and focus groups. Int J Qual Heal Care. 2007;19:349–57.

21. Ajzen I. From intentions to actions: a theory of planned behavior. In: Kuhl J, Beckmann J, editors. Action control: from cognition to behavior. 1st ed. berlin, Heidelberg. New York: Springer-Verlag; 1985. p. 11–39.

22. Brandth B, Overrein G. Resourcing children in a changing rural context: fathering and farm succession in two generations of farmers. Sociol Ruralis. 2013;53(1):95–111.

23. Bowen S, De Master K. New rural livelihoods or museums of production? Quality food initiatives in practice. J Rural Stud. 2011;27(1):73-82.

24. Balaji S, Chakravarthi V, Manager 1 Product, Product A. Ethnoveterinary practices in India – a review. Vet World 2010;3(12):549–551.

25. Phondani PC, Maikhuri RK, Kala CP. Ethnoveterinary uses of medicinal plants among traditional herbal healers in Alaknanda catchment of Uttarakhand, India. African J Tradit Complement Altern Med. 2010;7(3):195–206.

26. Paredes P, et al. Factors influencing physicians' prescribing behavior in the treatment of childhood diarrhoea: knowledge may not be the clue. Soc Sci Med. 1996;42(42):1141–53.

27. Lal A. Pharmaceutical drug promotion: how it is being practiced in India? J Assoc Physicians India. 2001;49:266–73.

28. Humphreys G. Direct-to-consumer advertising under fire. Bull World Health Organ. 2009;87(8):576–7.

29. Fugh-Berman A, Melnick D. Off-label promotion, on-target sales. PLoS Med. 2008;5(10):e210.

30. Fischer MA, Keough ME, Baril JL, Saccoccio L, Mazor KM, Ladd E, et al. Prescribers and pharmaceutical representatives: why are we still meeting? J Gen Intern Med. 2009;24(7):795–801.

31. Sahoo KC, Tamhankar AJ, Johansson E, Lundborg CS. Antibiotic use, resistance development and environmental factors: A qualitative study among healthcare professionals in Orissa, India. BMC Public Health [Internet]. 2010; 10(1):629. Available from: http://www.biomedcentral.com/1471-2458/10/629.

32. Sudershan RV, Bhat RV. A survey on veterinary drug use and residues in milk in Hyderabad. Food Addit Contam. 1995;12(5):645–50.

33. Rao SV e. Improving the delivery of veterinary services in India. Rev Sci Tech. 2015;34(3):767–77.

34. Chatterjee P, Kakkar M, Chaturvedi S. Integrating one health in national health policies of developing countries: India's lost opportunities. Infect Dis Poverty. 2016;5(1):87.

35. Kakkar M, Abbas SS, Kumar A, Hussain MA, Sharma K, Bhatt PM, et al. Veterinary public health capacity- building in India: a grim reflection of the developing world's underpreparedness to address zoonotic risks. WHO South-East Asia J Public Heal. 2013;2(3–4):187–91.

36. Kumar V, Gupta J. An analytical study to assess the awareness level of Para-veterinarians about antibiotic resistance in eastern Haryana. India Int J Curr Microbiol Appl Sci. 2017;6(10):1819–26.

37. Manishimwe R, Nishimwe K, Ojok L. Assessment of antibiotic use in farm animals in Rwanda. Trop Anim Health Prod. 2017;49(6):1101–6.

38. Drew RH. Antimicrobial stewardship programs: how to start and steer a successful program. J Manag Care Pharm. 2009;15(2 Supp A):18–23.

39. Septimus EJ, Owens RC. Need and potential of antimicrobial stewardship in community hospitals. Clin Infect Dis. 2011 Aug;53(Suppl 1(suppl 1)):S8–14.

40. MacDougall C, Polk RE. Antimicrobial stewardship programs in health care systems. Clin Microbiol Rev. 2005;18(4):638–56.

41. World Health Organization Regional Office for Europe. The role of pharmacist in encouraging prudent use of antibiotics and averting antimicrobial resistance: a review of policy and experience. Copenhagen: WHO; 2014.

42. Redding LE, et al. The role of veterinarians and feed-store vendors in the prescription and use of antibiotics on small dairy farms in rural Peru. J Dairy Sci. 2013;96(11):7349–54.

43. Bhaumik S, Pakenham-Walsh N, Chatterjee P, Biswas T. Governments are legally obliged to ensure adequate access to health information. Lancet Glob Heal. 2013;1(3):e129-30.

44. Chatterjee P, Datta TBA, Sriganesh V. Healthcare information and the rural primary care doctor. SAMJ South African Med J. 2012;102(3):138–9.

45. World Health Organization. Global action plan on antimicrobial resistance. Geneva: WHO; 2015.

46. Katakweba A, Mtambo M, Olse J, Muhairwa A. Awareness of human health risks associated with the use of antibiotics among livestock keepers and factors that contribute to selection of antibiotic resistance bacteria within livestock in Tanzania. Livest Res Rural Dev. 2012;24(10):1–9.

47. Robinson TP, Bu DP, Carrique-mas J, Fèvre EM, Gilbert M, Grace D, et al. Antibiotic resistance is the quintessential one health issue. Trans R Soc Trop Med Hyg. 2016;110(7):377–80.

48. Mcdougall S, Compton C, Botha N. Factors influencing antimicrobial prescribing by veterinarians and usage by dairy farmers in New Zealand. N Z Vet J [Internet]. 2017;65(2):84–92. Available from: https://doi.org/10.1080/00480169.2016.1246214

49. Coyne LA, et al. Understanding antimicrobial use and prescribing behaviours by pig veterinary surgeons and farmers: a qualitative study. Vet Rec [Internet]. 2014;175(23):593. Available from: http://www.ncbi.nlm.nih.gov/pubmed/25200432.

50. Cristina L, Picinin A, Toaldo IM, Hoff RB, Souza FN, Leite MO, et al. Milk quality parameters associated with the occurrence of veterinary drug residues in bulk tank milk. Sci Agric. 2017;74(3):195–202.

51. Bose SP. The diffusion of a farm practice in Indian villages. Rural Sociol. 1964;29(1):53.

52. Government of India. Ministry of Agriculture and Farmers Welfare. National Livestock Mission [Internet]. 2016. Available from: http://dahd.nic.in/sites/default/filess/REVISED%20GUIDELINES%20OF%20NLM%2027.04.16.pdf.

53. Government of Assam. Directorate of dairy development. Schemes and Projects State Owned Priority Development (SOPD) : Under State Government [Internet]. 2017 [cited 2017 Nov 13]. p. 11–4. Available from: http://diarydev.webcomindia.org/sites/default/files/G2G%20B%20Operational%20Guidelines%20for%20formation%20of%20DCS%2001-06-17.docx.

54. Government of India. Ministry of Agriculture. National Programme for Dairy Development (NPDD). [Internet]. 2014 [cited 2017 Nov 12]. Available from: http://dahd.nic.in/sites/default/filess/NPBB%20Details%20and%20Scheme.pdf.

10

An electronic trigger tool to optimise intravenous to oral antibiotic switch: a controlled, interrupted time series study

Marvin A. H. Berrevoets[1*], Johannes (Hans) L. W. Pot[2], Anne E. Houterman[2], Anton (Ton) S. M. Dofferhoff[3], Marrigje H. Nabuurs-Franssen[4], Hanneke W. H. A. Fleuren[2], Bart-Jan Kullberg[1], Jeroen A. Schouten[5] and Tom Sprong[3]

Abstract

Background: Timely switch from intravenous (iv) antibiotics to oral therapy is a key component of antimicrobial stewardship programs in order to improve patient safety, promote early discharge and reduce costs. We have introduced a time-efficient and easily implementable intervention that relies on a computerized trigger tool, which identifies patients who are candidates for an iv to oral antibiotic switch.

Methods: The intervention was introduced on all internal medicine wards in a teaching hospital. Patients were automatically identified by an electronic trigger tool when parenteral antibiotics were used for >48 h and clinical or pharmacological data did not preclude switch therapy. A weekly educational session was introduced to alert the physicians on the intervention wards. The intervention wards were compared with control wards, which included all other hospital wards. An interrupted time-series analysis was performed to compare the pre-intervention period with the post-intervention period using '% of i.v. prescriptions >72 h' and 'median duration of iv therapy per prescription' as outcomes. We performed a detailed prospective evaluation on a subset of 244 prescriptions to evaluate the efficacy and appropriateness of the intervention.

Results: The number of intravenous prescriptions longer than 72 h was reduced by 19% in the intervention group ($n = 1519$) ($p < 0.01$) and the median duration of iv antibiotics was reduced with 0.8 days ($p = <0.05$). Compared to the control group ($n = 4366$) the intervention was responsible for an additional decrease of 13% ($p < 0.05$) in prolonged prescriptions.
The detailed prospective evaluation of a subgroup of patients showed that adherence to the electronic reminder was 72%.

Conclusions: An electronic trigger tool combined with a weekly educational session was effective in reducing the duration of intravenous antimicrobial therapy.

Keywords: Decision support system, Antimicrobial stewardship, Iv-oral switch, Quality of care

* Correspondence: Marvin.Berrevoets@radboudumc.nl
[1]Department of Internal Medicine and Infectious Diseases, Radboudumc, Nijmegen, the Netherlands
Full list of author information is available at the end of the article

Background

Most patients with an infection that requires inpatient treatment initially receive empirical intravenous (iv) antimicrobial therapy. When the patient clinically improves within 48 h and results from microbiology cultures and other tests become available these iv antibiotics may be switched to oral therapy, with the exception of certain clinical conditions that necessitate prolonged iv treatment (e.g. *Staphylococcus aureus* bacteremia, endocarditis, meningitis). Previous studies have shown that a timely switch from intravenous to oral therapy is safe and reduces risk of complications related to intravenous treatment, healthcare costs and duration of hospitalization [1–6].

A Dutch study found that for patients with community-acquired pneumonia, a switch to oral antibiotics was possible in 46% of the patients on day 3 of treatment, but was not performed in 40% of eligible switch opportunities [7]. Barriers that preclude switching include misconceptions, practical considerations and organizational factors [7, 8]. Different approaches have been deployed to incorporate switch therapy into daily practice. However, the major conversion programmes evaluated in the literature were labour intensive interventions [3, 4] and not aimed at solving the barriers to timely switching therapy from iv to oral [5]. Previous research showed that introducing switch therapy into daily practice by a computerized trigger tool was effective in promoting iv to oral switch therapy [9, 10]. However, these reminders were produced with low specificity, were only performed for a limited number of antibiotics or had a low adherence rate.

The goal of this study was to evaluate the effect of a combined intervention targeting different barriers that preclude switching. The first intervention, a computerized reminder, was chosen to target both practical and organisational factors, while continuous education and feedback on iv-oral switch practice and promoting the use of a so called 'switch card' aimed to improve misconceptions about switching. The computerized reminder relies on an electronic trigger tool, which identifies patients who are candidates for antibiotic switch therapy.

With this combined intervention we aimed to improve the rate of safe iv to oral antibiotic switch on internal medicine wards.

Methods

This controlled intervention study was performed at the Canisius-Wilhemina Hospital, Nijmegen, the Netherlands, a 455-bed non-academic teaching hospital. The study was performed during a 26-month period. The pre-intervention period was defined as the first 13 months of the study period and the post-intervention period was defined as the last 13 months of the study period. The intervention was carried out at the internal medicine wards. The control wards included all other hospital wards.

Intervention
Computerised reminders

The multidisciplinary Antimicrobial Stewardship team (AST) (comprised of an infectious disease specialist, microbiologist and clinical pharmacist) created an automatic warning system that identifies candidates who are eligible for iv-oral switch therapy. The tool was based on the Dutch National Antibiotic Switch guidelines [3] and was developed in Crystal Reports® using data from the hospital pharmacy database and the clinical chemistry department.

Patients were identified as eligible for iv-oral switch therapy when antibiotic treatment had been prescribed 48 to 72 h previously. To alert the physician of the possibility of iv-oral switch an automated reminder was sent on day 3 of the treatment. This trigger tool automatically checked whether the following clinical or pharmacological conditions precluded switch therapy: (i) increase in CRP during iv treatment; (ii) neutrophils $<0,5*10^9$/ml; (iii) leukocytes $<1*10^9$/ml; (iv) usage of parenteral medication only or total parenteral nutrition, as an inability for oral intake predictor; (v) specific or high dose antibiotic suggesting severe infection (e.g. endocarditis, meningitis) (Additional file 1: Appendix 1). Patients meeting one or more of these criteria were not selected for switch therapy. If a single patient received more than one antibiotic, each single prescription (given for more than 48 h) was checked by the trigger tool to determine eligibility for iv-oral switch. Every morning, for each eligible patient, a written notice was automatically generated and sent out to the department secretary. This form contained identifying data of the patient, the antibiotic(s) that were eligible to be switched, and possible oral options or alternatives for these antibiotics. The form was presented to the attending physician during ward rounds by the department secretary. The decision whether to switch or not was made by the physician, based on the clinical situation of the patient. For each patient the physician was asked to fill in a form on which considerations concerning the switch were listed (ability to switch, impeding reasons). Reasons precluding iv-oral switch were categorized as 'clinical instability', no oral intake possible, severe infection (e.g. *Staphylococcus aureus* bacteremia, meningitis, endocarditis) or resistant micro-organisms for which no oral therapy is available.

A second reminder was sent when the iv medication order was started 96 to 120 h before and no oral switch had yet been performed, based on the same algorithm as mentioned earlier. To prevent alert fatigue a maximum of two reminders per medication order per patient was chosen.

Due to organizational factors no switch forms were distributed during the weekend.

Educational program

The start of the intervention was preceded by an educational program. Pocket cards with the switch protocol were presented to each physician. The hospital protocol (Additional file 2: Appendix 2) recommends to choose an oral antibiotic based on culture results. When no oral formulation of the iv antibiotic eligible for switch is available and culture results are negative, an oral antibiotic covering a similar spectrum as the empirically started iv antibiotic is recommended (e.g. ceftriaxon should be switched to oral amoxicillin/clavulanic acid).

To optimize adherence, direct feedback and education was given to the physicians working on the intervention wards regarding the returned switch forms in a weekly short meeting.

During this 15-min meeting (called "Switch of the week") one or more of the completed switch forms were selected by an infectious disease specialist (T.S.) and the content was presented to the physicians. Both appropriate and inappropriate decisions of the physicians were discussed and feedback was given on the decisions made.

Prospective observational study to assess the effectiveness of the intervention

To determine the effectiveness of the intervention in promoting iv-oral switch therapy, data of all iv antibiotic prescriptions was collected from the hospital pharmacy database for the whole study period. The intervention group was represented by patients from the internal medicine wards, while the control group was represented by patients in the same hospital during the same period from all other wards. The intervention was carried out at the internal medicine wards during the last 13 months of the study period. The percentage of intravenous prescriptions that exceed 72 h (% > 72 h) and median treatment duration in days of intravenous therapy on the intervention wards were calculated and compared to the control period and the control wards.

Detailed prospective evaluation of a subset of prescriptions to assess appropriateness

During the first 4 months of the intervention period, antibiotic prescriptions selected by the trigger tool were included in a detailed analysis to evaluate the efficacy and appropriateness of the intervention. The following patient data were collected to categorize the switch: patient's age and gender, source of infection, time of hospitalization, antimicrobial treatment, starting date, dose, body temperature, blood leukocyte count, blood neutrophil count, culture results and reasons which impeded the switch, based on the returned switch-forms. The appropriateness of the iv to oral switch was evaluated by an infectious disease specialist (TS). Options to categorize the conversion were: 'appropriate switch', 'inappropriate switch', 'appropriate continuation of iv therapy' and 'inappropriate continuation of iv therapy.

Categorization was based on the following switch criteria: no indication for prolonged iv antibiotic treatment (e.g. *Staphylococcus aureus* bacteremia, endocarditis, meningitis), improving vital signs, susceptible micro-organism (if cultured) for oral antibiotics, and the presence of a functional tractus digestivus. A patient who fulfilled these 4 switch criteria and who was switched to oral antibiotic therapy was categorized as an appropriate switch (Additional file 2: Appendix 2 – Table S3).

Endpoints
The primary endpoints were the change in percentage of iv treatment exceeding >72 h for all patients in both the intervention group and control group between the pre- and post-intervention period and the percentage of patients appropriately switched to oral therapy on day 3 of treatment. Secondary outcome was the change in median treatment duration.

Statistics
All data was analyzed using the IBM SPSS20 software package. We performed an interrupted time series analysis (ITSA), for which we used segmented linear regression to assess the significance of changes in level and slope of the regression lines before and after the introduction of the intervention for both the intervention and control groups [11, 12]. This methodology evaluates data collected at multiple time points before and after an intervention to detect whether the intervention had a greater effect than the expected secular trend. An abrupt intervention effect constitutes a change in the level of the outcome directly after the intervention is implemented. The slope represents a gradual change in the outcome parameter during the segment [12]. We divided the dataset into monthly periods (of which there were 26; 13 periods before the intervention started and 13 periods after the intervention started). The analysis was performed for the outcomes percentage of iv treatment >72 h, and median treatment duration in both the intervention and control group. We used a p-value of <0.05 as a threshold for all statistical tests.

Adherence to the intervention was determined by dividing the prescriptions that were appropriately switched (numerator) by the total amount of prescriptions eligible for switch (denominator).

Ethics statement
As iv to oral antibiotic switch therapy is proven to be safe and effective and is an essential element of many antimicrobial stewardship programs we considered timely switch as a standard of care, and our study is an evaluation of a new method to promote this standard of care. Patient data were collected anonymously. This study does not fall within the remit of the Medical Research involving

Human Subjects Act (WMO). Therefore the study can be carried out in the Netherlands without an approval by an accredited research ethics committee and without explicit informed consent of the participants.

Results
Baseline characteristics
During the whole study period, 1519 patients on the intervention wards and 4366 patients on the control wards received intravenous antibiotics (Table 1). At baseline, on the intervention wards 50.5% of prescriptions were given for >72 h versus 49.8% on the control wards.

Prospective observational study to assess the effectiveness of the intervention
Using interrupted time-series analysis, we compared the percentage of iv antibiotic prescriptions >72 h in the pre-intervention and post-intervention periods. There was a significant decrease (reduction 19.3%, $p < 0.001$; Table 2, Fig. 1) in the intervention group. We observed a significant but smaller decrease in the control group as well (reduction 6.1%, $p < 0.05$; Table 2, Fig. 1). The difference between the intervention and control group showed a significant additional reduction of intravenous antibiotic usage of 13.2% ($p = 0.014$) in favour of the intervention group.

During the post-intervention period, a non-significant increase in % of prescriptions >72 h was observed in the intervention-group (solid line in the white area, slope of +0.48% / month, $p = 0.43$; Fig. 1) and a non-significant decrease in the control group (dashed line in the white area, slope of –0.26% /month, $p = 0.46$; Fig. 1), with no significant difference between these groups.

Median duration of antibiotic usage on the intervention wards was decreased by 0.8 day (4.0 to 3.2, $p = 0.015$) (Table 2) after the intervention was introduced. There was no significant decrease observed on the control wards or between the intervention and control wards.

Detailed prospective evaluation of a subset of prescriptions to assess appropriateness
During a 4-month period there were 244 unique antibiotic medication orders for which the intervention was activated, 21 prescriptions were excluded, since these patients left the hospital on the day of the possible iv-oral switch. This resulted in 223 medication orders for a detailed analysis (Fig. 2).

Of all medication orders, 116 were eligible for switch. Of these, 84 were switched correctly (72%) and 32 (28%) were incorrectly not switched. A total of 78 orders were not eligible for switch. For 29 orders there was no evaluation possible, either because the switch order was generated in the weekend or there was no form filled in. Most of the patients with medication orders that were candidates for conversion had pneumonia (24.7%). The mean age was 71 years and most patients were female (53%). Table 3 shows data about the infections treated, and antibiotics prescribed during this phase of the study. The antibiotic agent that was most often eligible for switch was cefotaxime (27.5%).

During the detailed prospective evaluation, the digital switch forms were generated at two points in time. In case the first form did not result in a switch, a second form was generated from 96 to 120 h after therapy initiation. This resulted in 56 switch forms generated of which 20 lead to a correct switch and no incorrect switches, 31 were not eligible for iv-oral switch and 5 were indicated as incorrectly not switched (Fig. 2).

This detailed analysis showed that no patients were inappropriately switched.

Discussion
A computerized intervention in combination with an educational and feedback program, safely reduces the percentage of prolonged intravenous antibiotic use in hospital wards with 19%.

Many studies have demonstrated that iv-oral switch therapy is associated with a reduced length of iv therapy and low clinical failure rate [6]. In most studies an investigator identified cases eligible for switch by manual data extraction. This is time consuming and has limited feasibility in daily practice.

In this study, a simple automated trigger tool in our clinical pharmacy database, selected patients eligible for switch. An automated reminder was printed and sent to the ward prompting the physician to perform an iv-oral switch.

Table 1 Baseline characteristics of patients on the intervention wards and controls wards during the pre-intervention and post-intervention periods

Characteristic	Intervention wards		Control wards	
	Pre-intervention period	Post-intervention period	Pre-intervention period	Post-intervention period
Patients	771	748	2154	2212
Hospital admissions	880	835	2458	2478
Medication orders (iv antibiotics)	1781	1534	4769	4294
Mean age [range]	68.3 [16–101]	68.4 [17–101]	54.8 [1–100]	54.1 [0–98]
Female (%)	405 (53%)	371 (50%)	1029 (48%)	1073 (49%)

Table 2 Change in percentage of iv antibiotic prescriptions >72 h and median antibiotic duration (days) during the pre-intervention and post-intervention period and comparison between the intervention and control group using interrupted time series analysis

	Slope during the pre-intervention period (SE)	P	Change in level after intervention[a] (SE)	P	Slope during the post-intervention period[b] (SE)	P
Percentage of iv antibiotic prescriptions >72 h (%)						
Intervention group	−0.03 (0.42)	0.94	−19.30 (4.41)	<0.01	0.48 (0.59)	0.43
Control group	−0.36 (0.25)	0.16	−6.12 (2.61)	<0.05	−0.26 (0.35)	0.46
Difference between intervention and control group	0.33 (0.48)	0.50	−13.17 (5.13)	<0.05	0.74 (0.68)	0.29
Median duration of iv antibiotics (days)						
Intervention group	−0.02 (0.03)	0.49	−0.77 (0.29)	0.015	0.02 (0.04)	0.63
Control group	−0.38 (0.03)	0.16	−0.15 (0.28)	0.59	0.04 (0.04)	0.32
Difference between intervention and control group	0.02 (0.04)	0.62	0.62 (0.41)	0.14	−0.02 (0.05)	0.72

[a]Measures the immediate impact of the intervention
[b]Measures the long-term impact over time of the intervention

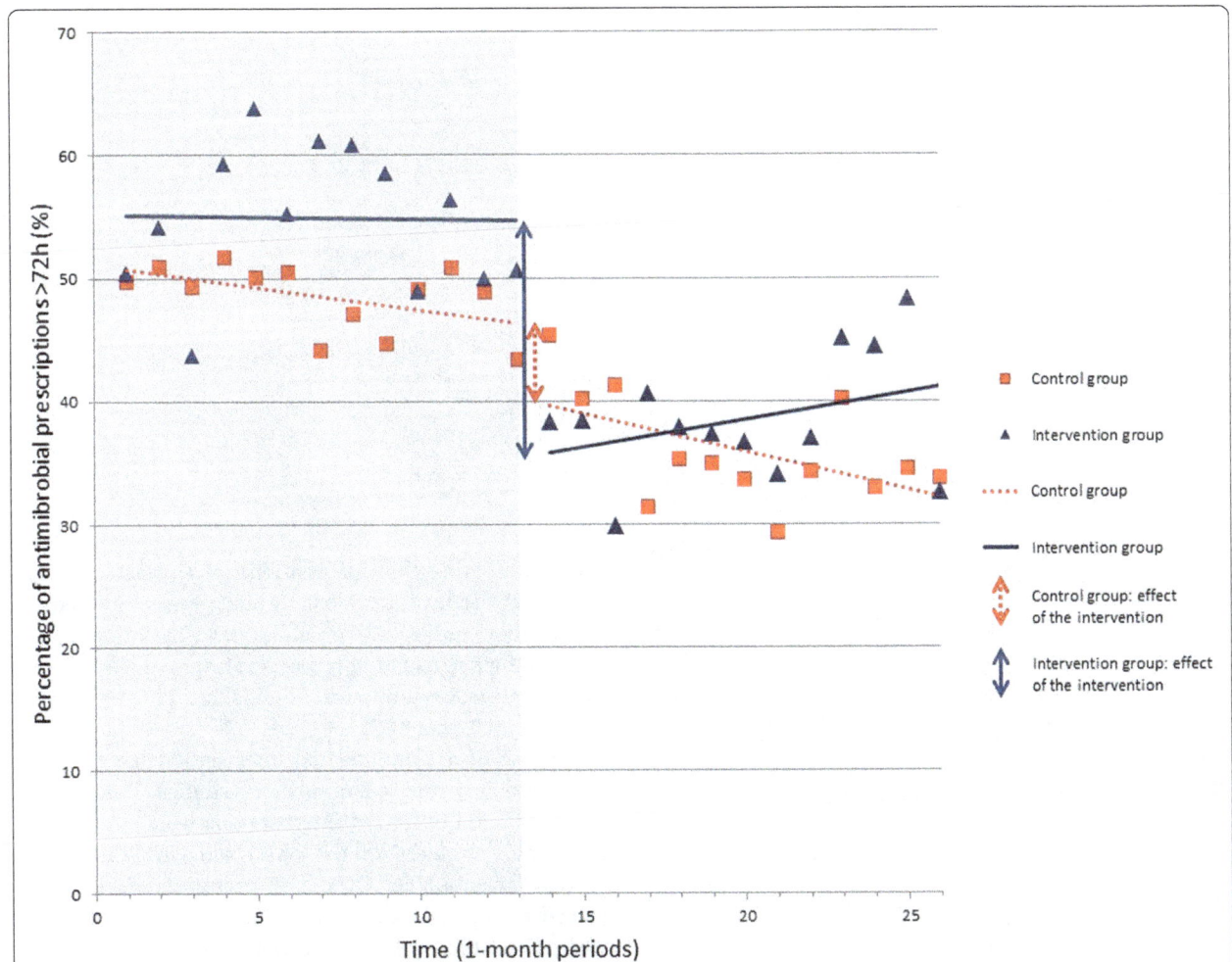

Fig. 1 Interrupted time series analysis of percentage of iv antimicrobial prescriptions >72 h. The grey area in the chart represents the pre-intervention period, the white area the post-intervention period. The squares represent the control group, where the triangles represent the intervention group. A trend line has been drawn through the data points for each group during the pre- and post-intervention period. The time series analysis demonstrated a significant decrease in the percentage of antimicrobial prescriptions in the intervention group (solid lines and solid double arrow, reduction 19.3%; $p < 0.01$) and in the control group (dashed lines and dashed double arrow, reduction 6.1%; $p < 0.05$), with an additional reduction of 13.2% ($p < 0.05$) in favour of the intervention group

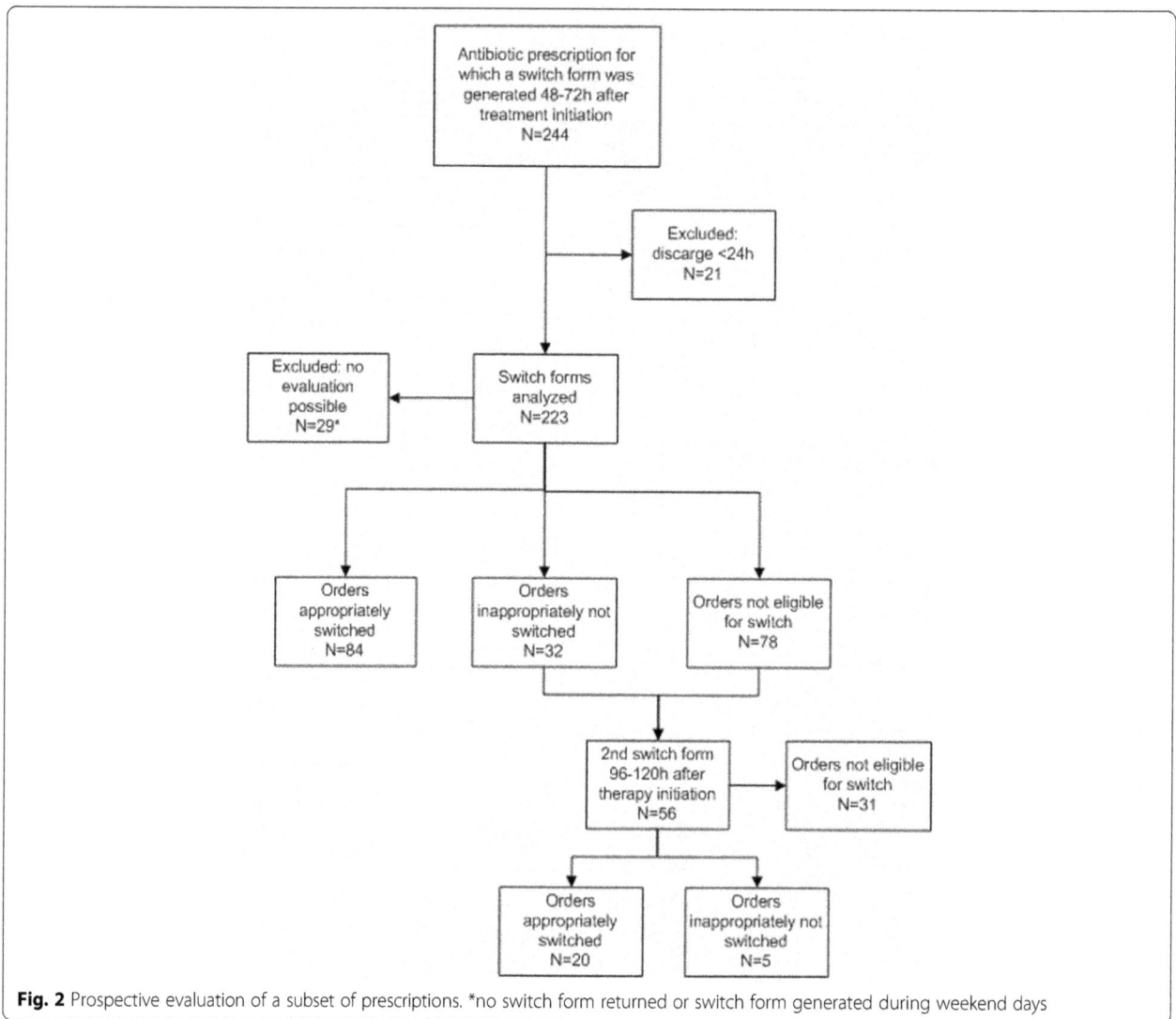

Fig. 2 Prospective evaluation of a subset of prescriptions. *no switch form returned or switch form generated during weekend days

Table 3 Detailed prospective analysis; indications and antibiotics prescribed for 244 analysed switch forms

Indication		Antibiotic	
Pneumonia	24.7%	cefotaxim	27.5%
Sepsis	20.4%	ciprofloxacin	19.0%
Pyelonephritis/urosepsis	18.6%	amoxicillin	16.2%
Abdominal infection	17.6%	metronidazole	15.0%
Skin and soft tissue infection	11.5%	cefazolin	12.1%
Unknown indication	2.5%	penicillin	4.5%
Gastro-enteritis	2.5%	clindamycin	4.0%
Bone and joint infection	1.1%	fluconazole	0.8%
Other	1.1%	ceftriaxone	0.4%
		flucloxacillin	0.4%

By automating the intervention, we were able to systematically reduce workload, which was a problem in many other studies [13]. In addition, we gave direct feedback to the participating physicians improving adherence to the national iv-oral switch guideline. This resulted in a high switch-rate of 72%.

The use of a computerized intervention has been investigated in a limited number of studies. Fisher et al. developed computerized interventions which automatically sent reminders to the physician, when an iv-oral switch was possible. Of the iv orders 21.6% were replaced by an oral agent, and 14% of the selected orders were discontinued [10]. However, this intervention was initiated on only 5 different categorized target drugs and adherence was low. Another study showed a decrease of iv use of levofloxacin and ciprofloxacin when displaying electronic alerts [9].

Beeler et al. [14] performed a prospective, controlled trial using an electronic reminder to stimulate iv-oral switch. Their study resulted in a decrease of total iv duration of 17.5% in the intervention group, and a switch-rate of 26.6%. Unfortunately, they did not report on the amount of patients who were not eligible for switch, which could explain the difference with the adherence rate in our own study.

Our study has several strengths. First, we used a large patient population and physician response to the switch reminder was high (72%). The advantage of our switch intervention lies in the possibilities of automatically identifying patients eligible for switch and alerting the physician. Besides the distribution of the switch-forms by the department secretary, no man-power is required for the continuous operation of the trigger tool, furthermore the educational program only takes 15-min a week. This enables antimicrobial stewardship teams to focus on other stewardship activities. The implementation of more sophisticated electronic health record systems (EHRS), which provide electronic alerts, could contribute to an additional reduction of workload [14, 15].

A recent survey conducted in France showed that human resources needed to implement AST activities were estimated at 3.6 full-time equivalent (FTE) positions/1000 acute care beds for antibiotic/infectious disease lead supervisors, at 2.5 FTE/1000 beds for pharmacists, and at 0.6 FTE/1000 beds for microbiologists [16]. Most hospitals in the Netherlands have restricted manpower for AST and can only focus on a limited number of stewardship activities. Our intervention is free and effective and can contribute to a simple and successful implementation of an iv-oral switch program.

Second, our controlled, interrupted time series analysis design is more robust than (un)controlled before and after analyses or uncontrolled interrupted time series designs used in most stewardship studies [17]. We were able to identify a significant difference in intravenous usage of antibiotics >72 h on the intervention wards (reduction 19%). However, in the control wards a significant effect (reduction 6%) was also found. This effect could possibly be contributed to the nationwide and local hospital attention for antimicrobial stewardship during the time of the study. Nevertheless, our iv-oral switch intervention was responsible for an additional effect of 13% reduction in iv antibiotic usage >72 h in favor of the intervention wards.

Our study has some limitations. First, baseline characteristics of the intervention and control groups were not comparable. The intervention was implemented at internal medicine wards and the control wards represented all other hospital wards; the baseline percentage of intravenous antibiotic use for >72 h was higher (+0.7%) in the intervention group. Therefore, the effect of our intervention may not be transferable to all hospital wards. Second, our intervention was not fully effective, from all antibiotics

eligible for switch, 28% were incorrectly not switched and due to organizational factors we were not able to implement the intervention during the weekend. This indicates that there is still ample room for improvement. Since physicians were asked to fill in reasons for not switching, these will be used to improve the educational program. Third, patients who received solely iv antibiotics could have been incorrectly excluded, while they may have been candidates for iv-oral switch therapy. Nowadays, with modern EHRS, more sophisticated algorithms that are based on general accepted switch criteria, and that incorporate both clinical, pharmaceutical and laboratory details could be developed.

Finally, this was a single center study, therefore, results may not be widely generalizable. However, the iv-oral switch algorithm was designed based upon commonly used clinical and laboratory criteria. With the help of an information technician the implementation in other hospitals with an electronic prescribing system should be possible.

Conclusion

This study showed the efficacy of an electronic trigger tool combined with targeted education on iv-oral switch. The intervention significantly decreased the amount of intravenously administered antibiotics used for >72 h by 19%.

This trigger tool enables hospital ASTs to implement a feasible and effective stand-alone iv-oral switch strategy, winning them valuable time to address more complicated issues of antimicrobial prescribing in daily practice.

Abbreviations
AST: Antimicrobial stewardship teams; EHRS: Electronic health record systems; FTE: Full-time equivalent; ITSA: Interrupted time series analysis; IV: Intravenous

Acknowledgements
Not applicable.

Funding
Not applicable.

Authors' contributions
MB and JP analyzed and interpreted the patient data and wrote the manuscript. AH, AD, MN and HF were involved in developing the electronic trigger tool, implementing the intervention in the hospital, and data collection. TS and JS coordinated the study team. TS, JS and BJK were a major contributor in writing the manuscript. All authors edited, read and approved the manuscript.

Consent for publication
Not applicable.

Competing interests
The authors declare that they have no competing interests.

Author details
[1]Department of Internal Medicine and Infectious Diseases, Radboudumc, Nijmegen, the Netherlands. [2]Department of Clinical Pharmacy, Canisius-Wilhelmina Hospital, Nijmegen, the Netherlands. [3]Department of Internal Medicine, Canisius-Wilhelmina Hospital, Nijmegen, the Netherlands. [4]Department of Medical Microbiology and Infectious Diseases, Canisius-Wilhelmina Hospital, Nijmegen, the Netherlands. [5]Department of Intensive Care, Canisius-Wilhelmina Hospital, Nijmegen, the Netherlands.

References
1.   Ahkee S, Smith S, Newman D, Ritter W, Burke J, Ramirez JA. Early switch from intravenous to oral antibiotics in hospitalized patients with infections: a 6-month prospective study. Pharmacotherapy. 1997;17:569–75.
2.   Athanassa Z, Makris G, Dimopoulos G, Falagas ME. Early switch to oral treatment in patients with moderate to severe community-acquired pneumonia: a meta-analysis. Drugs. 2008;68:2469–81.
3.   Sevinc F, Prins JM, Koopmans RP, Langendijk PN, Bossuyt PM, Dankert J, et al. Early switch from intravenous to oral antibiotics: guidelines and implementation in a large teaching hospital. J Antimicrob Chemother. 1999;43:601–6.
4.   Handoko KB, van Asselt GJ, Overdiek JW. Preventing prolonged antibiotic therapy by active implementation of switch guidelines. Ned Tijdschr Geneeskd. 2004;148:222–6.
5.   Oosterheert JJ, Bonten MJ, Schneider MM, Buskens E, Lammers JW, Hustinx WM, et al. Effectiveness of early switch from intravenous to oral antibiotics in severe community acquired pneumonia: multicentre randomised trial. BMJ. 2006;333:1193.
6.   Schuts EC, Hulscher ME, Mouton JW, Verduin CM, Stuart JW, Overdiek HW, et al. Current evidence on hospital antimicrobial stewardship objectives: a systematic review and meta-analysis. Lancet Infect Dis. 2016;16(7):847–56.
7.   Engel MF, Postma DF, Hulscher ME, Teding van Berkhout F, Emmelot-Vonk MH, Sankatsing S, et al. Barriers to an early switch from intravenous to oral antibiotic therapy in hospitalised patients with CAP. Eur Respir J. 2013;41:123–30.
8.   Schouten JA, Hulscher ME, Natsch S, Kullberg BJ, van der Meer JW, Grol RP. Barriers to optimal antibiotic use for community-acquired pneumonia at hospitals: a qualitative study. Qual Saf Health Care. 2007;16:143–9.
9.   Hulgan T, Rosenbloom ST, Hargrove F, Talbert DA, Arbogast PG, Bansal P, et al. Oral quinolones in hospitalized patients: an evaluation of a computerized decision support intervention. J Intern Med. 2004;256:349–57.
10.   Fischer MA, Solomon DH, Teich JM, Avorn J. Conversion from intravenous to oral medications: assessment of a computerized intervention for hospitalized patients. Arch Intern Med. 2003;163:2585–9.
11.   Wagner AK, Soumerai SB, Zhang F, Ross-Degnan D. Segmented regression analysis of interrupted time series studies in medication use research. J Clin Pharm Ther. 2002;27:299–309.
12.   Kontopantelis E, Doran T, Springate DA, Buchan I, Reeves D. Regression based quasi-experimental approach when randomisation is not an option: interrupted time series analysis. BMJ. 2015;350:h2750.
13.   Buyle FM, Metz-Gercek S, Mechtler R, Kern WV, Robays H, Vogelaers D, et al. Prospective multicentre feasibility study of a quality of care indicator for intravenous to oral switch therapy with highly bioavailable antibiotics. J Antimicrob Chemother. 2012;67:2043–6.
14.   Beeler PE, Kuster SP, Eschmann E, Weber R, Blaser J. Earlier switching from intravenous to oral antibiotics owing to electronic reminders. Int J Antimicrob Agents. 2015;46:428–33.
15.   Kim M, Song KH, Kim CJ, Song M, Choe PG, Park WB, et al. Electronic alerts with automated consultations promote appropriate antimicrobial prescriptions. Plos One. 2016;11:e0160551.
16.   Le Coz P, Carlet J, Roblot F, Pulcini C. Human resources needed to perform antimicrobial stewardship teams' activities in French hospitals. Med Mal Infect. 2016;46:200–6.
17.   McGregor JC, Furuno JP. Optimizing research methods used for the evaluation of antimicrobial stewardship programs. Clin Infect Dis. 2014; 59(Suppl 3):S185–92.

11

Anti-bacterial efficacy of alcoholic hand rubs in the Kenyan market, 2015

Missiani Ochwoto[1*], Lucy Muita[1], Keith Talaam[1], Cecilia Wanjala[1], Frank Ogeto[1], Faith Wachira[1], Saida Osman[1], James Kimotho[1] and Linus Ndegwa[2]

Abstract

Background: Hand hygiene is known to be effective in preventing hospital and community-acquired infections. The increasing number of hand sanitizer brands in Kenyan hospitals and consumer outlets is of concern. Thus the main aim of this study was to evaluate the anti-bacterial efficacy and organoleptic properties of these hand sanitizers in Kenya.

Methods: This was an experimental, laboratory-based study of 14 different brands of hand sanitizers (coded HS1-14) available in various retail outlets and hospitals in Kenya. Efficacy was evaluated using standard non-pathogenic *Escherichia coli* (ATCC 25922), *Staphylococcus aureus* (ATCC 25923) and *Pseudomonas aeruginosa* (ATCC 27853) as per the European Standard (EN). The logarithmic reduction factors (RF) were assessed at baseline and after treatment, and log reduction then calculated. Ten and 25 healthy volunteers participated in the efficacy and organoleptic studies respectively.

Results: Four (28.6%) hand sanitizers (HS12, HS9, HS13 and HS14) showed a 5.9 reduction factor on all the three bacteria strains. Seven (50%) hand sanitizers had efficacies of <3 against all the three bacteria strains used. Efficacy on E. Coli was higher compared to the other pathogens. Three hand sanitizers were efficacious on one of the pathogens and not the other. In terms of organoleptic properties, gel-based formulations were rated far higher than the liquid based formulations brands.

Conclusion: Fifty percent (50%) of the selected hand sanitizers in the Kenyan market have efficacy that falls below the World Health Organization (WHO) and DIN EN 1500:2013. Of the 14 hand sanitizers found in the Kenyan market, only four showed efficacies that were comparable to the WHO-formulation. There is a need to evaluate how many of these products with <3 efficacy that have been incorporated into the health system for hand hygiene and the country's policy on regulations on their usage.

Keywords: Hand rubs, Hand sanitizer, Efficacy, Organoleptic, Reduction factor

Background

Globally, the prevalence of hospital associated infections (HAIs) ranges from 4 to 10% in developed countries, and has been reported as being more than 20% in developing countries [17]. Studies by Ndegwa et al. [12] established an overall incidence of respiratory HAIs in three major hospitals in Kenya to be 9.2 per 10,000 patient days, with the highest incidence being in the Intensive Care Units (ICUs).

Hand hygiene is known to be effective in preventing hospital and community-associated infections, and a number

of studies have demonstrated the benefits of hand sanitizers in both community and hospital settings [5, 10, 15, 16].

Alcohol-Based Hand Rubs (ABHRs) are the most widely used hand sanitizers [16]. They may contain additional active ingredients such as quaternary ammonium compounds (QAC), povidone-iodine, triclosan or chlorhexidine that mainly serve to contribute to the efficacy of formulations [1, 8, 14]. Alcohols act by denaturing proteins, and are most effective at concentrations of 60–80%. Concentrations higher than 80% alcohol are less potent because proteins are not easily denatured in the absence of water [9]. Alcohols manifest a good in vitro germicidal activity against Gram-positive and Gram-negative vegetative bacteria as well as various strains of fungi. However, they have minimal

* Correspondence: omissiani@kemri.org
[1]Production Department, Kenya Medical Research Institute, P. O. Box 54840-00200, Nairobi, Kenya
Full list of author information is available at the end of the article

activity against bacterial spores, protozoan oocytes and some non-enveloped (non-lipophilic) viruses [9]. The reference standard against which ABHRs are compared is 60% isopropanol [4]. In most cases, the efficacy of ethanol and isopropanol are comparable, though ethanol has been found to have better efficacy profile against viruses [6]. Some studies have demonstrated that ethanol gel formulations, unless they have been specially formulated and tested, are less efficacious than ethanol solution formulations [2, 7]. There are a number of hand sanitizers sold to the Kenyan market with labels on their package that claim that the handrub can kill 99.9% of germs. The objective of this study was to evaluate the anti-bacterial efficacy and organoleptic properties of the hand sanitizers available in the Kenyan market, to help set the standards required for hand sanitizers in the country.

Methods
Study design
This study was an experimental, laboratory-based study that was carried out at the technology development and production facility of the Kenya Medical Research Institute (KEMRI) in Nairobi, Kenya.

Sample size
Fourteen (14) available brands of hand sanitizers (Fig. 1) were picked from various retail outlets and hospitals in Kenya. The total number of hand sanitizers, in the market was not available at the time of the study, therefore, the investigators regularly picked up to four different batches of the each hand sanitizer that was in the market from September 2014 to July 2015. Thirty-five healthy volunteers participated in the study: 10 for efficacy and 25 for organoleptic studies.

Efficacy testing
The number of viable bacterial microbes present after application of the hand rub was used to calculate the efficacy of the hand rub. A hand rub with the ability to reduce the microbes by 50% (equivalent to Log reduction below 3) was considered efficacious. Efficacy testing was carried out step by step as described in the European Standard (EN) 1500:2013; briefly, the standard non-pathogenic *Escherichia coli* (ATCC 25922), *Staphylococcus aureus* (ATCC 25923), and *Pseudomonas aeruginosa* (ATCC 27853) were incubated overnight in a sterile broth suspension.

Ten staff members of KEMRI volunteered to participate in the study and verbal informed consent was sought. The hand rub/sanitizer (HS) samples were fully concealed to the participants; the containers of HS were wrapped with identical opaque papers leaving only the cap of the HS open with codes labelled HS1-14.

All the participants were expected to test all the different batches of HS for all the three pathogens. The initial procedure required the participants to thoroughly wash their hands with soap and water and drying them with paper towels. This was followed by contaminating of 4 fingers in a 10 ml 0.5 Mac Farland suspensions of bacteria (A) prepared as per the method described by the National Committee for Clinical Laboratory Standards [11]. A second set of sterile broth (B) was used to determine the post-value Colony Forming Units (CFU) after sanitizing with respective hand sanitizer. All the hand washing and sanitation were done as described in WHO Hand Hygiene: Why, How & When - brochure of 2009 [18]. Ten microliter (10 μl) of each of suspension was inoculated on Tryptic Soy Agar (TSA) and incubated at 37 °C overnight for pre-value and post-value colony-forming unit (CFU) count respectively. Logarithmic reduction factors (RF) were assessed based on the baseline and after treatment with the HS and the results of each HS were compared with the reference standard (60% IPA). The logarithmic reduction factor was then expressed as a percent reduction. Log reduction was calculated as $\log_{10}(A) - \log_{10}(B)$ and the percent reduction was calculated as (A-B)/A% where; where A = number of

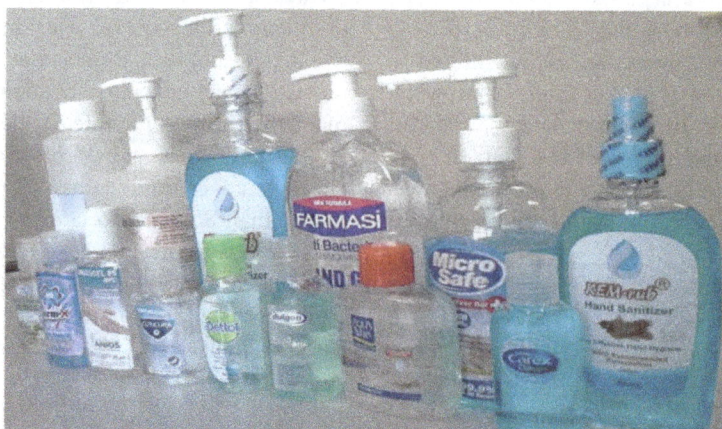

Fig. 1 A photograph of hand sanitizers in the Kenyan market that were used in the study

viable microorganism at baseline and B = number of viable microorganism after treatment [4, 18].

Organoleptic test

A questionnaire was designed to test organoleptic properties of the hand sanitizers in the Kenyan market. The organoleptic properties tested using the questionnaires were: general appearance and feeling of the hand after use and ease-of-use. The 25 selected participants were requested to score the hand sanitizers: 5 as "excellent", 4 as "good", 3 as "fair", 2 as "poor" and 1 as "very poor" and a mean product rating was calculated. During the testing process, the identity of the hand sanitizers was concealed to the participants, by wrapping the containers with opaque papers, leaving only the cap of HS open. This made it difficult for the participants to recognize or speculate the product.

Results

All hand sanitizer products sampled listed ethanol or isopropyl alcohol as its active ingredient either in single form or in combination with other compounds. We did not do any chemical analysis of the hand sanitizers. Those hand sanitizers that were in single form had different ethanol concentration (70–75%) and they include HS2, HS3, HS4, HS5, HS6, HS7, and HS13 (Table 1). Among ethanol-based hand sanitizers that were in combination with other compounds, there were four different compounds used triclosan (HS1), aloe barbadensis (HS8), chlorhexidine (HS9) and hydrogen peroxide (HS12). Only one hand sanitizer with

isopropyl as the active ingredient was in single form (HS14) and the rest were in combination form with triclosan (HS10) and hydrogen peroxide (HS11) (Table 1).

Active ingredients and effectiveness of the hand sanitizers

Each of the two main active ingredients (ethanol and isopropyl alcohol) had at least one product which demonstrated 99.9% bacterial reduction. Among the ethanol group, only one product with 70% ethanol (HS13) demonstrated a reduction factor of 5.9. The remaining alcohol products (HS2, HS3, HS4, HS5, HS6 and HS7) did not mention the alcohol concentration in the product ingredient list and these products were poorly effective with an overall bacterial reduction factor of less than 3 (Table 1). HS7 was more effective against *Pseudomonas aeruginosa* than the other poorly effective sanitizers whereas HS4 was more effective against *Escherichia coli* than the rest (5.1 and 4.8 bacterial reduction factors respectively) (Table 1).

Among the combined alcohol formulation, two products demonstrated 5.9 overall reduction factor, one combined with chlorhexidine (HS9) and the other combined with hydrogen peroxide (H_2O_2) (HS12) (Table 1). On the other hand, one product with alcohol and tricosan (HS1) was effective against *Escherichia coli* (5.9 reduction factor), but was not effective against the other two micro-organisms *Staphylococcus aureus* and *Pseudomonas aeruginosa*; 3.1 and 3.8 respectively. One product with a combination of ethyl alcohol and aloe (HS8) was the least effective among all the products sampled with an overall reduction factor of

Table 1 Log reduction values of various hand Sanitizers in the Kenyan market

Serial No.	Active ingredient	Form	*Escherichia coli* Reduction Factor	*Staphylococcus aureus* Reduction Factor	*Pseudomonas aeruginosa* Reduction Factor
HS 1	Alcohol [a]and Triclosan	Gel	6.0	3.1	3.8
HS 2	Alcohol[a]	Gel	2.1	1.9	3.0
HS 3	Alcohol[a]	Gel	2.9	1.9	3.0
HS 4	Ethyl Alcohol	Gel	4.8	1.9	3.1
HS 5	Ethyl Alcohol	Gel	3.2	2.1	2.3
HS 6	Alcohol[a]	Gel	3.1	2.3	2.2
HS 7	Alcohol[a]	Gel	3.5	2.9	5.1
HS 8	Ethyl Alcohol and aloe barbadensis	Gel	1.0	0.9	1.5
HS 9	Alcohol and Chlorhexidine	Solution	6.0	5.9	6.1
HS 10	Isopropyl alcohol and Triclosan	Gel	2.3	2.0	2.8
HS 11[b]	Isopropyl alcohol and Hydrogen Peroxide	Gel	1.0	2.1	2.6
HS 12[b]	Ethyl Alcohol and Hydrogen Peroxide	Gel	6.0	5.9	6.1
HS 13	70% Denatured alcohol	Gel	6.0	5.9	6.1
HS 14[b]	75% Isopropyl alcohol	Solution	6.0	5.9	6.1
	70% ethanol	Solution	6.0	5.9	6.1
60% Ref	60% IPA	Solution	3.0	3.0	3.0

[a]Type of alcohol not specified
[b]Locally produced HS

less than 3. One product (HS14) out of three that contained isopropyl as the only active ingredient had 5.9 reduction factor as compared to those with isopropyl and tricosan (HS10) and isopropyl and hydrogen peroxide (HS11) (Table 1).

Only those hand sanitizers that showed high reduction factor when using the three bacteria strains were considered to be the best and most effective. Based on WHO Requirements for ABHRs (WHO Guidelines on Hand Hygiene in Health Care [17] and (EN) 1500:[4]), seven out of 14 hand sanitizers (50%) had very low efficacy of less than 3 reduction factor, against all the three bacteria strains; *Escherichia coli*, and *Pseudomonas aeruginosa* as compared to *Staphylococcus aureus*.

Four hand sanitizers (HS12, HS9, HS13 and HS14) showed 5.8 reduction factor on all three micro-organisms. These results were comparable to those of the World Health Organization (WHO) standard formula. Of these, two were solution formulations and the two were gel formulations, having active ingredients of either alcohol with chlorhexidine or hydrogen peroxide (Fig. 2). A quarter of the hand sanitizers were effective against only one bacteria strain, for example, HS1 and HS4 were so effective on *E. coli*; 5.8 and 4.8 respectively. Whereas HS7 was effective on *P. aeruginosa* (4.8) (Fig. 2). Other sanitizers were not effective in any bacteria, and HS8 was the least effective with *E. coli*; 1.0, *S. aureus*; 0.9 and *P. aeruginosa* 1.5 (Fig. 2). Ethanol-based gel formulations demonstrated higher efficacy profiles than isopropyl alcohol based-gel formulation.

Organoleptic properties of the hand sanitizers

There were three organoleptic parameters tested in this study; ease-of-use, general appearance and feeling on the hand after use.

HS11 and HS12 were rated "very good" with a mean of value of 4.1 ± 0.2 and 4.2 ± 0.2 respectively. Most hand sanitizers (9/15) were rated as "good" with a mean range

of 3.0–3.9; these were hand sanitizers HS1, HS2, HS4, HS5, HS7, HS9, HS10 and HS13, in the descending order (Fig. 3). Four products were rated as "poor", with a mean range of 2.0–3.0 and they were hand sanitizer HS3, HS8, HS6 and HS14 (Fig. 3).

Generally, in easy to use, hand sanitizer HS12 and HS11 was rated the highest whereas hand sanitizer HS6 and HS14 was rated the least (Fig. 3).

None of the hand sanitizer had a mean of greater than 4. Almost all hand sanitizers (13/15) were rated between 3.0 and 3.9. HS12 had the highest mean of 3.9 ± 0.2 followed by hand sanitizer HS2 with a mean of 3.8 ± 0.2. In the lower bracket, HS14 and HS9 had the least average rates of 2.19 ± 0.1 and 2.92 ± 0.2 respectively (Fig. 3). There was only one hand sanitizer (HS12) that scored "very good" (4.04 ± 0.2) based on how it felt on the hand after using it.

Comparing all the hand sanitizers and the parameters, it was observed that HS1, HS2, HS10, HS11 and HS12 had average rates that were more than 3.5 of all the three parameters (Fig. 3). Some hand sanitizers had contrasting mean of parameter, with one being poor and the other good. For instance, HS6 in easy to use scored poorly whereas in general appearance it was good. Similarly, HS14 scored very poorly on easy to use, poor on general appearance and good on feeling on the hand after use (Fig. 3).

In general, when the three parameters were averaged and compared, HS12 was rated very good with a score of 4.1 and it was followed by HS11 with a score value of 3.9. The lowest were HS 14, 3, 6 and 8 (Fig. 3).

Discussions

Use of hand sanitizers has gained popularity in Kenya in the recent past. This has led to the development, production and importation of several hand sanitizers by various companies with the aim of commercialization as well as supporting the health care system in preventing transmission of pathogens.

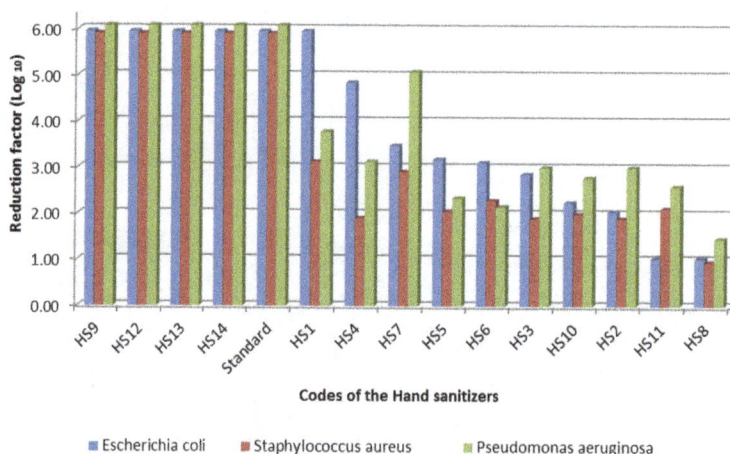

Fig. 2 Log reduction of all hand sanitizers against the three bacteria strains

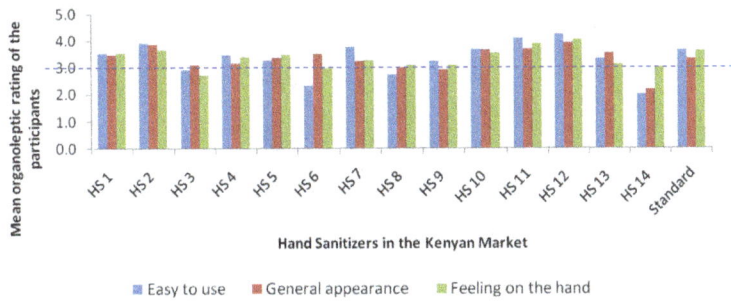

Fig. 3 Mean organoleptic comparison of different hand sanitizers in the market

Four out of 14 (28%) hand sanitizers (HS12, HS9, HS13 and HS14) that were subject of this study showed efficacy profiles that were above the 60% IPA Reference Standard. The four achieve the required high log reduction rate. Seven out of 14 hand sanitizers (50%) had very low efficacy of less than 3.0 against all the three bacteria and hence failing to meet the Health Canadian Requirements for ABHRs of log reduction of ≥3 using EN or ASTM methods [3]. All the poor performing were gel formulations. This finding is in concordance with those of the studies by Kramer et al. [7] and Dharan et al. [2] who established that ethanol gel formulations, unless they have been specially formulated and tested, are less efficacious than ethanol solution formulations. Edmond and Macinga [3] reported a study in Canada that demonstrated that formulation of ABHRs had far greater influence on efficacy than alcohol concentration alone. They established that products having concentration of 70% performed equally well and sometimes better than those with higher concentration. It is this concern that led to the development of solution-based alcohol formulations by WHO for local production in the willing health institutions [17]. However, as demonstrated in this study the solution-based alcohol formulations scored very poorly in terms organoleptic properties in comparison with gel-based alcohol formulations where the gel based brands HS11 and HS12 were rated as 'very good' while the WHO-formulation (HS14) was rated as being 'very poor'. It is notable that the gel-based brands HS12 achieved both high efficacy and desirable organoleptic properties.

The findings in this study that ethanol-based gel formulation (HS12) have higher efficacy than isopropyl alcohol based-gel formulations (HS11), this is contrary to what, has been observed by other studies that isopropyl alcohol solution has higher efficacy than ethanol solution [13].

The main limitation of this study is that we did not pick all known hand sanitizers in Kenya, may be because they were out of stock at the time of the study and the number of hand sanitizers in the market was unknown. To the best of our knowledge we tried as much as possible to sample all hand sanitizers available. Secondly, the EN1500

protocol required that Fingertips of each hand kneaded separately in 10 ml of broth with added neutralizers. We did not add the neutralizers because some HS already contained them. Not knowing the concentration of the active ingredients for many of the products limited our conclusion on the hand sanitizers that poorly performed.

Conclusion

In conclusion, this study established that 50% of the selected ABHRs in the Kenyan market have the efficacy values below that of International Reference Standard (60% Isopropyl alcohol) and that some of those ABHRs with the desired efficacy value have poor organoleptic characteristics. There is a need to evaluate how many of these products with <50% efficacy that have been incorporated into the health system for hand hygiene and the country's policy on regulations on their usage.

We recommend that similar experiments to be conducted to involve the other micro-organisms such as viruses and fungi. Additionally, the efficacy studies in relationship to the antimicrobial residual effect may be necessary too.

Abbreviations
µl: Microliter; ABHRs: Alcohol-based hand rubs; CDC: Centers for Disease Control and Prevention; CFU: Colony forming units; EN: European standard; HAIs: Hospital associated infections; HS: Hand sanitizer; HS1- HS14: Codes of hand sanitizers; ICUs: Intensive care units; IPA: Isopropyl alcohol; KEMRI: Kenya Medical Research Institute; RF: Bacterial logarithmic reduction factors; SSC: Scientific Steering Committee; TSA: Tryptic soy agar; WHO: World Health Organization

Acknowledgements
We would like to thank all the staff at KEMRI Production Department especially S. Muchiri, A. Mwangi, E. Kerubo, Doris Night and P. Kaiguri (retired), for the support they accorded us in carrying out this study. We would also like to thank Director KEMRI for providing the necessary moral and financial support to execute this study as well as the permission to publish this work. Finally, we acknowledge support from staff of the CDC Atlanta and Kenya for their great support.

Funding
This study was jointly funded by KEMRI and by the United States Government through the CDC- iFund project, which was awarded to Linus Ndegwa.

Authors' contributions

LM, KT, CJ, JH, MO (KEMRI) were all involved in conceptualization and project design, MO, LM, JH (KEMRI), LN (CDC), were project leaders, SO, FW, SM, KT, LM and MO performed the experiments. LM and KT prepared the samples, MO, JH, LM entered the data and analyzed. MO, JH, LM, KT and LN prepared the manuscript. MO submitted the manuscript. All authors read and approved the final manuscript.

Competing interests

This study was conducted as part of the authors' usual employment. No author received outside support or funding to conduct this study.

Consent for publication

The consent for publication was obtained from KEMRI publication committee (Ref. No. KEMRI/CBRD/PUB/001/01), CDC – Atlanta (CGH tracking #2016-084) and the study participants.

Disclaimer

The findings and conclusions in this report are those of the authors and do not necessarily represent the official position of the Centers for Disease Control and Prevention (CDC).

Author details

[1]Production Department, Kenya Medical Research Institute, P. O. Box 54840-00200, Nairobi, Kenya. [2]Centers for Disease Control and Prevention, Nairobi, Kenya.

References

1. Ayliffe GA, Babb JR, Davies JG, Lilly HA. Hand disinfection: a comparison of various agents in laboratory and ward studies. J Hosp Infect. 1988;11:226–43.
2. Dharan S, Hugonnet S, Sax H, Pittet D. Comparison of waterless hand antisepsis agents at short application times: raising the flag of concern. Infect Control Hosp Epidemiol. 2003;24:160–4.
3. Edmond S, Macinga DR. Meeting health Canada standard for alcohol based rub efficacy: formulation matters. 2011.
4. European standard DIN EN 1500. Chemical disinfectants and antiseptics. Hygienic handrub. Test method and requirements. Brussels: European Committee for Standardization; 2013.
5. Hammond B, Ali Y, Fendler E, Dolan M, Donovan S. Effect of hand sanitizer use on elementary school absenteeism. Am J Infect Control. 2000;28:340–6. doi:10.1067/mic.2000.107276.
6. Kampf G, Kramer A. Epidemiologic background of hand hygiene and evaluation of the most important agents for scrubs and rubs. Clinical Microbiology Review. 2004;17:863–93.
7. Kramer A, Rudolph P, Kampf G, Pittet D. Limited efficacy of alcohol-based hand gels. Lancet. 2002;359:1489–90.
8. Larson EL, Eke PI, Laughon BE. Efficacy of alcohol-based hand rinses under frequent-use conditions. Antimicrob Agents Chemother. 1986;30:542–4.
9. Larson EL, Morton HE. Alcohols. In: Block SS, editor. Disinfection, sterilization and preservation. 4th ed. Philadelphia: Lea & Febiger; 1991. p. 191–203.
10. Magill SS, Edwards JR, Bamberg W, et al. Multistate point-prevalence survey of health care-associated infections. N Engl J Med. 2014;370:1198–208.
11. National Committee for Clinical Laboratory Standards Performance standards for antimicrobial disk susceptibility testing. NCCLS document. 1999. M2-A6, M100-S9.
12. Ndegwa LK, Katz MA, McCormick K, Nganga Z, Mungai A, Emukule G, Kollmann MK, Mayieka L, Otieno J, Breiman RF, Mott JA, Ellingson K. Surveillance for respiratory health care-associated infections among inpatients in 3 Kenyan hospitals, 2010–2012. Am J Infect Control. 2014;42(9):985–90. doi:10.1016/j.ajic.2014.05.022.
13. Oke MA, Bello AB, Odebisi MB, Ahmed El-Imam AM, Kazeem MO. Evaluation of antibacterial efficacy of some alcohol-based hand sanitizers sold in Ilorin (North-Central Nigeria). IFE J Sci. 2013;15(1):111–7.
14. Rotter M. Hand washing and hand disinfection. In: Mayhall CG, editor. Hospital epidemiology and infection control. 2nd ed. Philadelphia: Lippincott Williams & Wilkins; 1999. p. 1339–55.
15. Sandora TJ, Taveras EM, Shih M-C, Resnick EA, Lee GM, Ross-Degnan D. Hand sanitizer reduces illness transmission in the home [abstract 106]. In: Abstracts of the 42nd annual meeting of the Infectious Disease Society of America; Boston, Massachusetts; 2004 Sept 30–Oct 3. Alexandria: Infectious Disease Society of America; 2004.
16. White C, Kolble R, Carlson R, Lipson N, Dolan M, Ali Y. The effect of hand hygiene on illness rate among students in university residence halls. Am J Infect Control. 2003;31:364–70. doi:10.1016/S0196-6553(03)00041.
17. WHO Guidelines for Hand hygiene in healthcare. First global patient safety challenge: clean care is a safer care. Geneva: WHO patient safety; 2009. http://apps.who.int/iris/bitstream/10665/44102/1/9789241597906_eng.pdf. Accessed 5 July 2013.
18. World Health Organization. Hand hygiene: Why, How & When? 2009. http://www.who.int/gpsc/5may/Hand_Hygiene_Why_How_and_When_Brochure.pdf. Accessed 5 July 2013.

12

Comparing appropriateness of antibiotics for nursing home residents by setting of prescription initiation

Michael Pulia[1]*, Michael Kern[2], Rebecca J. Schwei[1], Manish N. Shah[1,4], Emmanuel Sampene[3] and Christopher J. Crnich[4]

Abstract

Background: The pervasive, often inappropriate, use of antibiotics in healthcare settings has been identified as a major public health threat due to the resultant widespread emergence of antibiotic resistant bacteria. In nursing homes (NH), as many as two-thirds of residents receive antibiotics each year and up to 75% of these are estimated to be inappropriate. The objective of this study was to characterize antibiotic therapy for NH residents and compare appropriateness based on setting of prescription initiation.

Methods: This was a retrospective, cross-sectional multi-center study that occurred in five NHs in southern Wisconsin between January 2013 and September 2014. All NH residents with an antibiotic prescribing events for suspected lower respiratory tract infections (LRTI), skin and soft tissue infections (SSTI), and urinary tract infections (UTI), initiated in-facility, from an emergency department (ED), or an outpatient clinic were included in this sample. We assessed appropriateness of antibiotic prescribing using the Loeb criteria based on documentation available in the NH medical record or transfer documents. We compared appropriateness by setting and infection type using the Chi-square test and estimated associations of demographic and clinical variables with inappropriate antibiotic prescribing using logistic regression.

Results: Among 735 antibiotic starts, 640 (87.1%) were initiated in the NH as opposed to 61 (8.3%) in the outpatient clinic and 34 (4.6%) in the ED. Inappropriate antibiotic prescribing for urinary tract infections differed significantly by setting: NHs (55.9%), ED (73.3%), and outpatient clinic (80.8%), $P = .023$. Regardless of infection type, patients who had an antibiotic initiated in an outpatient clinic had 2.98 (95% CI: 1.64–5.44, $P < .001$) times increased odds of inappropriate use.

Conclusions: Antibiotics initiated out-of-facility for NH residents constitute a small but not trivial percent of all prescriptions and inappropriate use was high in these settings. Further research is needed to characterize antibiotic prescribing patterns for patients managed in these settings as this likely represents an important, yet under recognized, area of consideration in attempts to improve antibiotic stewardship in NHs.

Keywords: Antibiotic stewardship, Antimicrobial resistance, Emergency department, Long-term care, Nursing home, Outpatient clinic

* Correspondence: mspulia@medicine.wisc.edu
[1]BerbeeWalsh Department of Emergency Medicine, University of Wisconsin-Madison School of Medicine and Public Health, Madison, WI, USA
Full list of author information is available at the end of the article

Background

The pervasive, often inappropriate, use of antibiotics in healthcare settings has been identified as a major public health threat due to the resultant widespread emergence of antibiotic resistant bacteria [1]. In nursing homes (NH), as many as two-thirds of residents receive antibiotics each year and up to 75% of these are estimated to be inappropriate [2, 3]. This inappropriate use is in spite of existing guidelines released by the Infectious Disease Society of America that provide specific recommendations on how to evaluate and treat infection in NHs [4]. As a result, NHs can serve as reservoirs for resistant bacteria within a community [3, 5, 6].

Although commensurate attention has been given to improving antibiotic stewardship within NHs [7–10], little is known about the antibiotic prescribing for NH residents initiated in outpatient clinics or the emergency department (ED). For example, although at least 25% of NH residents visit the ED each year, the contribution and appropriateness of outpatient antibiotic therapy initiated in this setting is unknown [11]. Recent regulatory changes by the Centers for Medicare and Medicaid Services, a center within the United States Department of Health and Human Services that regulates NHs, now mandate antibiotic stewardship programs in NHs [12] and this raises an interesting dilemma for how to approach antibiotics initiated by outside providers. Understanding the burden of outside antibiotic prescribing and what documentation is required by the NH to justify ongoing treatment will be critical to guide future antibiotic stewardship efforts in this setting. As such, the aims of this study were to characterize the initiation of antibiotic therapy for NH residents by setting, infection type, and antibiotic class and then compare prescribing patterns and appropriateness between settings from the NH perspective.

Methods

Study design and setting

We conducted a detailed medical record extraction involving all NH residents at five southern Wisconsin facilities who had an antibiotic prescribing event from January 2013 through September 2014. Antibiotic events were identified from NH facility pharmacy records. Outpatient clinic and ED health records were reviewed when available. The location of the antibiotic start was determined by review of orders (which includes prescriptions sent from outpatient clinics or the ED), transfer documents, and documentation in the NH records. These NH facilities are required to document an assessment of any resident change-in-condition, regardless of whether they are transferred to another care setting. The change-in-condition documentation in ideal circumstances includes a detailed record of the signs and symptoms of the resident. The decision to seek care for a NH resident at an outpatient clinic or the ED could result from a wide variety of scenarios that range from patient or family member request to an acute change in condition that the NH cannot manage to routine follow up after a procedure. Most commonly this decision results from a shared decision making process that occurs between the NH staff, the resident, the resident's family and the resident's primary care provider.

All facilities were skilled nursing facilities located in Wisconsin, a state in the Midwest United States. Four of the facilities were located in Dane County which is the second largest County in Wisconsin with a total population of just over half a million residents and has 19 NHs [13]. One of the facilities was located in Rock County, the ninth largest County in Wisconsin with a population of 162,000 and 10 NHs [13]. The NHs in this sample had a mixture of long-term stay and post-acute care beds, and had an average of 106 beds ranging from 71 to 184. Four of the facilities had on-site nurse practitioners during regular hours and none of the facilities had a formal antibiotic stewardship program during the study period. While several of the facilities were part of a long-term care system that provided assisted living, we did not collect data in any assisted living facilities. At the time of data collection, none of these facilities used electronic prescribing and standard practice was to enact prescription orders from outpatient settings without requiring approval from a facility-associated provider. We selected facilities based on existing collaborations with the study investigators.

A trained research specialist entered health record abstraction data directly into an electronic, standardized report form in a REDCap™ database. In order to ensure consistency, the principle investigator abstracted the first 20 records and no discrepancies were observed. The local Health Sciences Minimal Risk Institutional Review Board approved all study activities.

Participants

Figure 1 is a flow chart describing how the final sample was determined. There were 1442 antibiotics initiated in the sample. As our focus was on comparing antibiotic starts in a NH facility with antibiotic starts in an outpatient clinic or the ED, we excluded prescriptions initiated at the time of discharge from an inpatient hospital unit as noted in the NH pharmacy order records. In order to focus on the most commonly encountered bacterial infections, we only included antibiotic starts associated with a diagnosis of LRTI, SSTI, or UTI. We also excluded prophylactic antibiotic prescriptions as they are not associated with change of condition documentation and the selected appropriateness criteria is specific for acute infections.

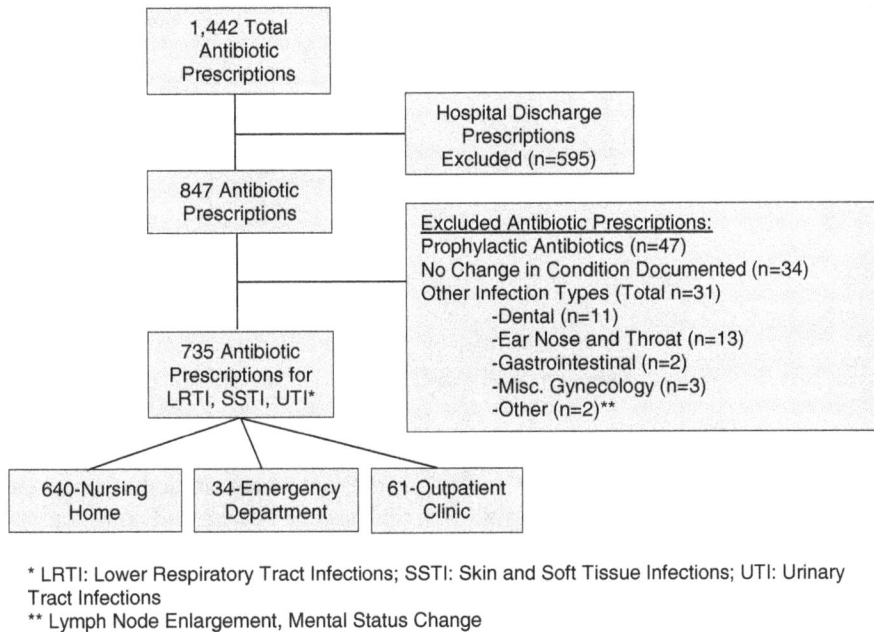

Fig. 1 Antibiotic prescribing event flow chart

Methods

Data extracted included setting of prescription initiation (NH, ED, outpatient clinic), indication for antibiotic (LRIT, SSTI, UTI), patient demographics (gender, age), vital signs on day of prescription, symptoms, and antibiotic prescribed. Antibiotic appropriateness (yes, no) was determined according the Loeb consensus criteria which proposes a minimum set of clinical criteria (symptoms and vital signs) that should be present before initiating empiric antibiotics for suspected, acute bacterial infections in NH residents [14].

For the purposes of this analysis, the 15% of patients who met 2 of 4 systemic inflammatory response syndrome (SIRS) [15] criteria or 2 of 3 quick Sepsis Related Organ Failure Assessment (qSOFA) [16] criteria were considered septic regardless of prescription setting. Although there is ongoing controversy about the optimal criteria for early sepsis determination, SIRS is currently utilized in the Centers for Medicare and Medicaid Services (CMS) quality reporting measure, SEP-1, which mandates antibiotic administration within 3 h of a patient meeting severe sepsis criteria in the ED [17]. Without access to additional clinical records to enable a more definitive determination about the presence of sepsis, all antibiotic starts that met these definitions of sepsis were characterized as appropriate. Failure to take this approach would inappropriately penalize antibiotic starts in settings with a higher relative percentage of systemically ill patients who meet federally defined sepsis criteria.

Data analysis

Differences in the frequency distributions of baseline covariates by setting were compared via Chi-square test for categorical variables and a one-way analysis of variance (ANOVA) for continuous variables. Covariates considered for all statistical approaches included age, gender, setting of antibiotic initiation and infection type. Frequency of antibiotic use by class was calculated and then ranked from most prescribed to least prescribed by setting and within each of the three infection types. The frequency of inappropriate antibiotic use by infection type and setting was also calculated.

A multivariable logistic regression was then performed to determine if any of the covariates were associated with inappropriate antibiotic use. The analytic strategy for selecting the final model was to investigate each predictor to the outcome through a univariate analysis process. After gaining inferences from the univariate analysis, interactions among the predictors were checked before proceeding to fit a full model. As the presence of sepsis criteria automatically resulted in antibiotic prescribing being characterized as appropriate, it was removed from the model due to collinearity. Since the interaction terms were not significant, our main effect model was used as our final model. All analyses are interpreted as odds ratios. Data analysis was preformed using *Stata Statistical Software: Release 14* (College Station, TX: StataCorp LP).

Results

Table 1 describes the patient demographics and infection type distribution of our sample across the different

Table 1 Characteristics of nursing home antibiotic prescriptions by infection type and location

	Overall (n = 735)		NH (n = 640)		ED (n = 34)		Clinic (n = 61)		P-Value*
	n	%	n	%	n	%	n	%	
Mean Age, (SD)	84.8 ± 9.9		85.2 ± 9.9		83.5 ± 10.4		81.1 ± 9.8		0.006[†]
Female	523	71.2	459	71.7	25	73.5	39	63.9	0.491
Lower Respiratory Tract	195	26.5	181	28.3	7	20.6	7	11.5	0.013[†]
Skin and Soft Tissue	175	23.8	135	21.1	12	35.3	28	45.9	< 0.001[‡]
Urinary Tract	365	49.7	324	50.6	15	44.1	26	42.6	0.394
Sepsis Criteria Met	109	14.8	99	15.5	5	14.7	5	8.2	0.327

NH, Nursing Home; ED, Emergency Department
*p-value tests for independence between covariate and location of antibiotic initiation
[†]Significant at p < .05
[‡]Significant at p < .001

settings. The mean age ± SD was 84.8 ± 9.9 years and with a majority of females (71.2%). There was a significant difference in the age of patients treated by setting, with slightly younger patients managed in the ED and outpatient clinics (p = .006). The majority of antibiotic prescriptions were initiated within the NH (85.2%). Overall, urinary tract infection (UTI) was the most commonly treated type of infection (49.7%). Lower respiratory tract infections comprised a significantly higher proportion of cases managed in the NH (p = .013) while SSTI comprised a higher proportion of cases managed in the ED and outpatient clinic settings (p < .001). We could not calculate SIRS or qSOFA scores for 2.5% (n = 18) of all subjects due to missing vital sign documentation.

Inappropriate antibiotic use by infection type and setting is displayed in Table 2. Across all settings and infection types, 48.8% of antibiotic prescriptions were deemed inappropriate. This included 58.4% of UTIs, 50.7% of lower respiratory tract infections and 26.9% of skin and soft tissue infections. Overall, inappropriate antibiotic use varied significantly by setting: NH (47.5%), ED (47.1%), and outpatient clinics (63.9%), P = .048. Inappropriate antibiotic prescribing for UTIs varied significantly by setting: NH (55.9%), ED (73.3%), and outpatient clinics (80.8%), P = .023. Inappropriate antibiotic prescribing for skin and soft tissue infections also varied significantly by setting: NH (21.5%), ED (25.0%), and clinics (53.6%), P = .002.

A detailed representation of antibiotic class prescribing frequency by setting and infection type is available in Table 3. Fluoroquinolones were the most commonly prescribed class of antibiotic for UTIs (35.6%) and lower respiratory tract infections (34.9%). Cephalosporins were the most often prescribed class for skin/soft tissue infections (61.7%). The ED and outpatient clinics utilized a higher frequency of fluoroquinolones for lower respiratory tract infections and UTIs as compared to the NHs.

In our multivariate analysis (Table 4), odds of inappropriate antibiotic prescribing did not vary based on each increased year of patient age or by gender. Patients who had an antibiotic initiated in an outpatient clinic had 2.98 (95% CI: 1.64–5.44) times increased odds of inappropriate use compared to antibiotic initiation in a NH, when controlling for other variables. Overall, there was a significant difference in odds of inappropriate antibiotic use by infection type. Patients with lower respiratory tract infection had 3.41 times increased odds (95% CI: 2.15–5.40) and patients with UTI had 4.47 times increased odds (95% CI: 2.96–6.77) of an inappropriate prescription when compared to SSTIs, when controlling for other variables.

Discussion
Through this cross sectional study of antibiotic prescribing events for NH residents, we have identified important differences in prescribing patterns between those initiated in-facility and other outpatient settings (clinic,

Table 2 Inappropriate antibiotic use stratified by location of antibiotic initiation and infection type (n = 735)

	Overall		NH		ED		Clinic		P-Value*
	n	%	n	%	n	%	n	%	
Inappropriate use across all Infection Types	359	48.8	304	47.5	16	47.1	39	63.9	0.048
Inappropriate for Lower Respiratory Tract Infections	99	50.7	94	51.9	2	28.6	3	42.9	0.437
Inappropriate for Skin and Soft Tissue Infections	47	26.9	29	21.5	3	25.0	15	53.6	0.002
Inappropriate for Urinary Tract Infections	213	58.4	181	55.9	11	73.3	21	80.8	0.023

*p-value tests for independence between covariate and location of antibiotic initiation
NH Nursing Home, ED Emergency Department

Table 3 Frequency of antibiotic classes prescribed by setting and infection type (n = 735)

	Overall		NH		ED		Clinic	
	n	%	n	%	n	%	n	%
Lower Respiratory Tract Infection	n = 195		n = 181		n = 7		n = 7	
Fluoroquinolones	68	34.9	60	33.2	5	71.4	3	42.9
Macrolides and Lincosamides	66	33.9	65	35.9	1	14.3	0	0
Penicillins and Beta-Lactamase	27	13.9	25	13.8	0	0	2	28.6
Cephalosporins	24	12.3	22	12.2	1	14.3	1	14.3
Tetracyclines	8	4.1	8	4.4	0	0	0	0
Other[a]	2	1.0	1	0.6	0	0	1	14.3
Skin/Soft Tissue	n = 175		n = 135		n = 12		n = 28	
Cephalosporins	108	61.7	87	64.4	8	66.7	13	46.4
All Penicillins/Beta-Lactamase	26	14.9	19	14.1	3	25.0	4	14.3
Fluoroquinolones	16	9.1	12	8.9	0	0	4	14.3
Tetracyclines	11	6.3	8	5.9	0	0	3	10.7
Macrolides and Lincosamides	8	4.6	4	3.0	0	0	4	14.2
Other[b]	6	3.4	5	3.7	1	8.3	0	0
Urinary Tract Infection	n = 365		n = 324		n = 15		n = 26	
Fluoroquinolones	130	35.6	112	34.6	8	53.3	10	38.5
Sulfonamides	78	21.4	73	22.5	1	6.7	4	15.4
Nitrofurantoin	66	18.1	59	18.2	2	13.3	5	19.2
Cephalosporins	58	15.9	50	15.4	3	20.0	5	19.2
All Penicillins/Beta-Lactamase	27	7.4	24	7.4	1	6.7	2	7.7
Other[c]	6	1.6	6	1.9	0	0	0	0

[a]Sulfonamides
[b]Sulfonamides, Metronidazole, Carbapenems
[c]Tetracyclines, Metronidazole, Aminoglycosides, Fosfomycin

ED) for this vulnerable population. Consistent with previously published data, overall we observed nearly 50% inappropriate antibiotic initiation for NH residents using the Loeb consensus criteria [3, 14]. Although this study was limited to 5 facilities in the state of Wisconsin, it

Table 4 Odds of inappropriate antibiotic use in a logistic regression model

	Model n = 735 Odds Ratio (95% CI)
Age	1.00 (0.98–1.01)
Female	1.25 (0.90–1.75)
Location Antibiotic Initiated	
Nursing Home	Ref
Emergency Department	1.17 (0.56–2.44)
Outpatient Clinic	2.98 (1.64–5.44)*
Infection Type	
Skin/Soft Tissue	Ref
Lower Respiratory Tract	3.41 (2.15–5.40)*
Urinary Tract	4.47 (2.96–6.77)*

*Significant at p < .001

does indicate the persistent nature of the challenge to improve judicious antibiotic use in NHs, even in the setting of increased efforts by the Centers for Disease Control (CDC) to address this issue [18]. Although the vast majority of antibiotic courses were initiated within the NHs themselves, nearly 13% (1 of 8) were initiated in either outpatient clinics or the ED. This highlights the need to consider interventions to improve prescribing not only within NHs, but also when these residents receive care outside of the facility.

When examining inappropriate prescribing in our regression model, prescriptions in the outpatient clinic setting were observed to have nearly 3 times the odds of being inappropriate. There were no increased odds with prescriptions initiated in the ED setting, which is consistent with results from several recently published reports [19–21]. Although our data do not provide insight into why the outpatient clinics might be particularly high risk for inappropriate antibiotic initiation, we hypothesize it is related to the well-established challenges associated with diagnosing acute infections in elders [22]. Providers in outpatient clinics and the ED may be significantly disadvantaged as they are often not familiar with a patient's baseline (e.g. chronic venous stasis dermatitis mimicking cellulitis) and are not afforded time to observe the individual's clinical trajectory that might emerge from serial examinations. However, ED providers have universal access to rapid diagnostic testing which can provide objective data and reduce diagnostic uncertainty (e.g. chest radiographs and urinalysis with microscopy). This finding highlights the need for increased efforts to establish outpatient clinic antimicrobial stewardship programs based on the CDC's recently published guidelines for this setting [23].

Another potential factor in the observed setting variability is disagreement between medical specialties when it comes to diagnosing infections in older adults. Caterino et al. observed that nearly 20% of ED patients admitted with suspected infection were not diagnosed as such by the inpatient physicians [24]. Additionally, emergency physicians were found to over diagnose pulmonary infections and underdiagnose UTIs relative to the inpatient team's determination [24]. This important finding highlights the need for interdisciplinary collaboration to enhance consensus in terms of diagnostic criteria and appropriate initiation of empiric antibiotics.

In addition to setting, infection type was also significantly associated with increased odds of inappropriate prescribing. UTIs increased the odds of inappropriate prescribing by nearly 4.5 times, which is consistent with prior literature highlighting the clinical uncertainty which surrounds the diagnosis of UTI in elders [24–27]. The vast majority of UTI related antibiotics were initiated in-facility with lower rates of inappropriate prescribing as compared to the ED and outpatient clinics. This perhaps reflects uptake of published methods to improve antibiotic prescribing for suspected UTI among NH residents [28]. There is also emerging evidence to suggest UTIs are often misdiagnosed in the ED setting resulting in unnecessary empiric antibiotic administration [29, 30]. A recent cohort study of elders admitted through the ED to general medical services found that 62% underwent urinalysis at the time of admission while 84% of these patients did not have symptoms of UTI [31]. Overuse of diagnostic testing, such as urinalysis, in the ED has recently come to the forefront of national discussions and certainly may play a role in the observed overtreatment of UTIs in this setting [32]. However, any attempt to improve diagnostic testing in the ED must consider both provider and system level factors such as protocol driven ordering of urinalysis in triage by nurses prior to physician evaluation [33].

Similar to UTI, LRTIs increased the odds of inappropriate prescribing by nearly 3.5 times in our regression model. This again reflects the diagnostic challenges specific to LRTIs in the older adult population. Previous literature suggests that nearly 75% of elders with pneumonia will not have fever and less than half report cough, with increased risk of atypical presentations among NH residents specifically [34–40]. Although the Loeb criteria for suspected LRTI offers five distinct sets of signs and symptoms to meet the minimum criteria to initiate antibiotics, we observed high rates of prescribing outside of these parameters. This is likely to indicate ongoing clinical concerns for atypical presentations among this high-risk population. The vast majority of LRTIs were managed in the NHs which is potentially indicative of practice patterns informed by a published clinical pathway that demonstrated similar clinical outcomes for NH residents with LRTIs treated in-facility as compared to those who were hospitalized [41].

Relative to UTIs and LRTIs, SSTIs had the lowest overall rate of inappropriate antibiotic prescribing and were therefore selected as the reference condition in the regression model. This is likely because the Loeb criteria for initiating of antibiotics for SSTIs focus more on signs of infection which are readily identified by conducting a basic physical exam as opposed to patient reported symptoms [14]. Despite this finding, antibiotic stewardship in the management of SSTIs should remain an area of great concern. This is emphasized by a recent study reporting that nearly 50% of empiric antibiotic use among NH residents with suspected SSTI failed to meet the Loeb criteria [42]. SSTIs made up a higher relative percentage of infections managed in the ED and outpatient clinics. Although the reason for this is unclear, we hypothesize that NH residents may be sent to these settings for advanced imaging if clinical uncertainty exists around the presence of a purulent SSTI. In addition, purulent SSTIs often require surgical drainage for source control, which may necessitate transfer out of the NH.

In comparing the classes of antibiotics between settings (Table 3), we observed areas of consistency and variation in practice patterns. The most common class of antibiotic used for UTIs in each care setting was fluoroquinolones, with the ED having the highest prescribing rate (53.3%). However, the second most common class used for UTIs differed by setting with NHs favoring sulfonamides while the ED and outpatient clinics favoring cephalosporins. Interestingly, these results conflict with a prior report out of Canada indicating nitrofurantoin was the most commonly used agent for treatment of UTIs in the NH setting [2]. Fluoroquinolones were also the most common class of antibiotic used for LRTIs, with the ED having the highest prescribing rate. Cephalosporins and penicillins were the two most common classes of antibiotics used for SSTIs in all settings. The observed variability in antibiotic prescribing by class again points to the need for enhanced bidirectional communication between NHs and other care settings around local resistance patterns and best practice guidelines in terms of recommended first line empiric antibiotics.

This study has several important limitations that we would like to mention. First, this study was conducted using data from 5 NHs in one US state which limits generalizability. Local practice patterns vary which highlights the need for additional investigation into antibiotic prescribing appropriateness for NH residents by setting. The small number of antibiotic starts occurring in the ED and outpatient clinic setting as compared to the NHs is also a limitation. The small sample size may have reduced our ability to detect true differences in appropriateness when present. Another limitation of this study is that our reported inappropriateness rates are likely underestimates because we did not assess the appropriateness of antibiotic selection or duration. In contrast, although we reviewed all clinical records available at the NH, documentation of care provided at outside settings (ED or outpatient clinic) was not always available. Without reviewing these records directly, it is unknown if additional symptom documentation or diagnostic testing would have satisfied the criteria for antibiotic initiation. However, our approach accurately reflects appropriateness assessed from the NH perspective based on all records available to providers in that setting. The bidirectional transfer of information for NH residents treated in the ED has already been highlighted as an important area of focus to improve the quality of care in this population [43, 44]. Although this quality concern is not specific to antibiotics, the transfer of information that enables the receiving NHs to understand the rationale for initiation of antibiotics is critical to support ongoing stewardship programs and enhancing safe transitions of care.

Conclusions

In conclusion, our report represents the first comparative analysis of antibiotic use for NH residents based on setting of prescription initiation. Antibiotics initiated in the ED and outpatient clinics constitute a small but not trivial percent of all NH prescriptions and inappropriate use was high across all settings. Inappropriate antibiotic prescribing overall and by condition varied significantly by setting. Overall, outpatient clinics had significantly higher odds of inappropriate antibiotic prescribing, as compared to NHs and the ED. Antibiotic prescribing for NH residents that is initiated outside of the facility is an important area for additional investigation and must be considered in quality improvement efforts targeting antibiotic stewardship in NHs.

Funding
This project was supported by research grants from the Agency for Healthcare Research and Quality (K08HS024342, R18HS022465 & HHSA2902010000018I), the VA Health Services Research and Development (HX-16-006 & CRE-12-291), the Centers for Disease Control and Prevention (CK-15-004), the State of Wisconsin Civil Monetary Penalty Fund, the National Institutes of Health (K24AG054560), and the University of Wisconsin Institute of Clinical and Translational Research (UW ICTR) which is supported by the Clinical and Translational Science Award (CTSA) program through the NIH National Center for Advancing Translational Sciences (UL1TR000427). The content is solely the responsibility of the authors and does not necessarily represent the official views of these funding agencies. None of these funding agency played any role in the design and conduct of the study; collection, management, analysis, and interpretation of the data; and preparation, review, or approval of the manuscript.

Authors' contributions
MP and CC contributed to study conception, design, analysis and interpretation of data, and drafted the manuscript. MK, RS, ES, and MS each contributed to analysis and interpretation of the data. All authors have reviewed, provided intellectual feedback, and approved the final version of the manuscript.

Competing interests
The authors declare that they have no competing interests.

Author details
[1]BerbeeWalsh Department of Emergency Medicine, University of Wisconsin-Madison School of Medicine and Public Health, Madison, WI, USA. [2]University of Wisconsin-Madison School of Medicine and Public Health, Madison, WI, USA. [3]Department of Biostatistics and Medical Informatics, University of Wisconsin-Madison School of Medicine and Public Health, Madison, WI, USA. [4]Department of Medicine, University of Wisconsin-Madison School of Medicine and Public Health, Madison, WI, USA.

References
1. Ranji SR, Steinman MA, Shojania KG, Sundaram V, Lewis R, Arnold S, et al. Closing the quality gap: a critical analysis of quality improvement strategies (Vol. 4: antibiotic prescribing behavior). Rockville (MD): Agency for Healthcare Research and Quality (US); 2006.
2. Daneman N, Gruneir A, Newman A, Fischer HD, Bronskill SE, Rochon PA, et al. Antibiotic use in long-term care facilities. J Antimicrob Chemother. 2011;66:2856–63. https://doi.org/10.1093/jac/dkr395.
3. Rhee SM, Stone ND. Antimicrobial stewardship in long-term care facilities. Infect Dis Clin N Am. 2014;28:237–46. https://doi.org/10.1016/j.idc.2014.01.001.
4. High KP, Bradley SF, Gravenstein S, Mehr DR, Quagliarello VJ, Richards C, et al. Clinical practice guideline for the evaluation of fever and infection in older adult residents of long-term care facilities: 2008 update by the Infectious Diseases Society of America. Clin Infect Dis Off Publ Infect Dis Soc Am. 2009;48: 149–71. https://doi.org/10.1086/595683.
5. Augustine S, Bonomo RA. Taking stock of infections and antibiotic resistance in the elderly and long-term care facilities: a survey of existing and upcoming challenges. Eur J Microbiol Immunol. 2011;1:190–7. https://doi.org/10.1556/EuJMI.1.2011.3.2.
6. Crnich CJ, Duster M, Hess T, Zimmerman DR, Drinka P. Antibiotic resistance in non–major metropolitan skilled nursing facilities: prevalence and Interfacility variation. Infect Control Hosp Epidemiol. 2012;33:1172–4. https://doi.org/10.1086/668018.
7. Crnich CJ, Jump R, Trautner B, Sloane PD, Mody L. Optimizing antibiotic stewardship in nursing homes: a narrative review and recommendations for improvement. Drugs Aging. 2015;32:699–716. https://doi.org/10.1007/s40266-015-0292-7.
8. Dyar OJ, Pagani L, Pulcini C. Strategies and challenges of antimicrobial stewardship in long-term care facilities. Clin Microbiol Infect. 2015;21: 10–9. https://doi.org/10.1016/j.cmi.2014.09.005.
9. Nicolle LE. Antimicrobial stewardship in long term care facilities: what is effective? Antimicrob Resist Infect Control. 2014;3:1–7. https://doi.org/10.1186/2047-2994-3-6.
10. The Core Elements of Antibiotic Stewardship for Nursing Homes | Nursing Homes and Assisted Living (LTC) | CDC n.d. https://www.cdc.gov/longtermcare/prevention/antibiotic-stewardship.html. Accessed 16, Feb 2018.
11. Dwyer R, Gabbe B, Stoelwinder JU, Lowthian J. A systematic review of outcomes following emergency transfer to hospital for residents of aged care facilities. Age

Ageing. 2014;43:759–66. https://doi.org/10.1093/ageing/afu117.

12. Centers for Medicare & Medicaid Services. 2016–09-28. CMS Final Improv Care Saf Consum Prot Long-Term Care Facil Resid 2016. https://www.cms.gov/Newsroom/MediaReleaseDatabase/Press-releases/2016-Press-releases-items/2016-09-28.html?DLPage=1&DLEntries=10&DLSort=0&DLSortDir=descending. Accessed 20, Apr 2018.

13. Department of Health Services. Directory of Licensed Wisconsin Nursing Homes-Alphabetical By County and City 2018. https://www.dhs.wisconsin.gov/guide/nhdir.pdf. Accessed 20, Apr 2018.

14. Loeb M, Bentley DW, Bradley S, Crossley K, Garibaldi R, Gantz N, et al. Development of minimum criteria for the initiation of antibiotics in residents of long-term–care facilities: results of a consensus conference. Infect Control Hosp Epidemiol. 2001;22:120–4. https://doi.org/10.1086/501875.

15. Levy MM, Fink MP, Marshall JC, Abraham E, Angus D, Cook D, et al. 2001 SCCM/ESICM/ACCP/ATS/SIS international Sepsis definitions conference. Crit Care Med. 2003;31:1250–6. https://doi.org/10.1097/01.CCM.0000050454.01978.3B.

16. Freund Y, Lemachatti N, Krastinova E, Laer MV, Claessens Y-E, Avondo A, et al. Prognostic accuracy of Sepsis-3 criteria for in-hospital mortality among patients with suspected infection presenting to the emergency department. JAMA. 2017;317:301–8. https://doi.org/10.1001/jama.2016.20329.

17. Pulia MS, Redwood R, Sharp B. Antimicrobial stewardship in the Management of Sepsis. Emerg Med Clin North Am. 2017;35:199–217. https://doi.org/10.1016/j.emc.2016.09.007.

18. Long-term Care Facilities | NHSN | CDC n.d. http://www.cdc.gov/nhsn/ltc/. Accessed 16, Feb 2018.

19. Barlam TF, Soria-Saucedo R, Cabral HJ, Kazis LE. Unnecessary antibiotics for acute respiratory tract infections: association with care setting and patient demographics. Open Forum Infect Dis. 2016;3:1–7. https://doi.org/10.1093/ofid/ofw045.

20. Bergmark RW, Sedaghat AR. Antibiotic prescription for acute rhinosinusitis: emergency departments versus primary care providers. Laryngoscope. 2016;126:2439–44. https://doi.org/10.1002/lary.26001.

21. Jones BE, Sauer B, Jones MM, Campo J, Damal K, He T, et al. Variation in outpatient antibiotic prescribing for acute respiratory infections in the veteran population: a cross-sectional study. Ann Intern Med. 2015;163:73–80. https://doi.org/10.7326/M14-1933.

22. Caterino JM. Evaluation and management of geriatric infections in the emergency department. Emerg Med Clin North Am. 2008;26:319–43, viii. https://doi.org/10.1016/j.emc.2008.01.002.

23. Core Elements of Outpatient Antibiotic Stewardship | Community | Antibiotic Use | CDC 2017. https://www.cdc.gov/antibiotic-use/community/improving-prescribing/core-elements/core-outpatient-stewardship.html. Accessed 16 Feb 2018.

24. Caterino JM, Stevenson KB. Disagreement between emergency physician and inpatient physician diagnosis of infection in older adults admitted from the emergency department. Acad Emerg Med. 2012;19:908–15. https://doi.org/10.1111/j.1553-2712.2012.01415.x.

25. Drinka PJ, Crnich CJ. Diagnostic accuracy of criteria for urinary tract infection in a cohort of nursing home residents. J Am Geriatr Soc. 2008;56:376–7; author reply 378. https://doi.org/10.1111/j.1532-5415.2007.01533.x.

26. Juthani-Mehta M, Tinetti M, Perrelli E, Towle V, Van Ness PH, Quagliarello V. Diagnostic accuracy of criteria for urinary tract infection in a cohort of nursing home residents. J Am Geriatr Soc. 2007;55:1072–7. https://doi.org/10.1111/j.1532-5415.2007.01217.x.

27. Nace DA, Drinka PJ, Crnich CJ. Clinical uncertainties in the approach to long term care residents with possible urinary tract infection. J Am Med Dir Assoc. 2014;15:133–9. https://doi.org/10.1016/j.jamda.2013.11.009.

28. Loeb M, Brazil K, Lohfeld L, McGeer A, Simor A, Stevenson K, et al. Effect of a multifaceted intervention on number of antimicrobial prescriptions for suspected urinary tract infections in residents of nursing homes: cluster randomised controlled trial. BMJ. 2005;331:669. https://doi.org/10.1136/bmj.38602.586343.55.

29. Tomas ME, Getman D, Donskey CJ, Hecker MT. Over-diagnosis of urinary tract infection and under-diagnosis of sexually transmitted infection in adult women presenting to an emergency department. J Clin Microbiol. 2015;53:2686–92. https://doi.org/10.1128/JCM.00670-15.

30. Watson JR, Sánchez PJ, Spencer JD, Cohen DM, Hains DS. Urinary tract infection and antimicrobial stewardship in the emergency department. Pediatr Emerg Care. 2018;34:93–5. https://doi.org/10.1097/PEC.0000000000000688.

31. Yin P, Kiss A, Leis JA. Urinalysis orders among patients admitted to the general medicine service. JAMA Intern Med. 2015;175:1711–3. https://doi.org/10.1001/jamainternmed.2015.4036.

32. Sullivan W, Tintinalli J, Hoffman J, Kanzari H, Probst M. Pro/con: 'unnecessary' testing. Emergency Physicians Monthly n.d. http://epmonthly.com/article/pro-con-unnecessary-testing/. Accessed 14, May 2018.

33. Framework for Quality and Safety in the Emergency Department n.d. https://www.ifem.cc/wp-content/uploads/2016/03/Framework-for-Quality-and-Safety-in-the-Emergency-Department-2012.doc.pdf. Accessed 16 Feb 2018.

34. Fine JM, Fine MJ, Galusha D, Petrillo M, Meehan TP. Patient and hospital characteristics associated with recommended processes of care for elderly patients hospitalized with pneumonia: results from the medicare quality indicator system pneumonia module. Arch Intern Med. 2002;162:827–33.

35. Harper C, Newton P. Clinical aspects of pneumonia in the elderly veteran. J Am Geriatr Soc. 1989;37:867–72. https://doi.org/10.1111/j.1532-5415.1989.tb02268.x.

36. Marrie TJ, Haldane EV, Faulkner RS, Durant H, Kwan C. Community-acquired pneumonia requiring hospitalization. J Am Geriatr Soc. 1985;33:671–80. https://doi.org/10.1111/j.1532-5415.1985.tb01775.x.

37. Metlay JP, Schulz R, Li YH, Singer DE, Marrie TJ, Coley CM, et al. Influence of age on symptoms at presentation in patients with community-acquired pneumonia. Arch Intern Med. 1997;157:1453–9.

38. Muder RR, Brennen C, Swenson DL, Wagener M. Pneumonia in a long-term care facility. A prospective study of outcome. Arch Intern Med. 1996;156:2365–70.

39. Starczewski AR, Allen SC, Vargas E, Lye M. Clinical prognostic indices of fatality in elderly patients admitted to hospital with acute pneumonia. Age Ageing. 1988;17:181–6. https://doi.org/10.1093/ageing/17.3.181.

40. Waterer GW, Kessler LA, Wunderink RG. Delayed administration of antibiotics and atypical presentation in community-acquired pneumonia. Chest. 2006;130:11–5. https://doi.org/10.1378/chest.130.1.11.

41. Loeb M, Carusone SC, Goeree R, Walter SD, Brazil K, Krueger P, et al. Effect of a clinical pathway to reduce hospitalizations in nursing home residents with pneumonia: a randomized controlled trial. JAMA. 2006;295:2503–10. https://doi.org/10.1001/jama.295.21.2503.

42. Feldstein D, Sloane PD, Weber D, Ward K, Reed D, Zimmerman S. Current prescribing practices for skin and soft tissue infections in nursing homes. J Am Med Dir Assoc. 2017;18:265–70. https://doi.org/10.1016/j.jamda.2016.09.024.

43. Terrell KM, Hustey FM, Hwang U, Gerson LW, Wenger NS, Miller DK, et al. Quality indicators for geriatric emergency care. Acad Emerg Med. 2009;16:441–9. https://doi.org/10.1111/j.1553-2712.2009.00382.x.

44. Terrell KM, Miller DK. Challenges in transitional care between nursing homes and emergency departments. J Am Med Dir Assoc. 2006;7:499–505. https://doi.org/10.1016/j.jamda.2006.03.004.

13

Chlorhexidine is not an essential component in alcohol-based surgical hand preparation: a comparative study of two handrubs based on a modified EN 12791 test protocol

Thomas-Jörg Hennig[1][*], Sebastian Werner[2], Kathrin Naujox[2] and Andreas Arndt[1]

Abstract

Background: Surgical hand preparation is an essential part of modern surgery. Both alcohol-based and antiseptic detergent-based hand preparation are recommended practices, with a trend towards use of alcohol based handrubs. However, discussion has arisen whether chlorhexidine is a required ingredient in highly efficacious alcohol-based formulations, in view of providing sustained antimicrobial efficacy.

Methods: One alcohol-only formulation (product A), containing ethanol and n-propanol, and one formulation containing a chlorhexidine-ethanol combination (product B) were directly compared with each other using a modified test protocol based on European standard EN 12791 (2016) with 25 volunteers. The alcohol-only formulation (product A) was applied for only 90 s, the chlorhexidine-alcohol formulation (product B) for 180 s. Microbial log reduction factors were determined and statistically compared immediately after application and at 6 h under surgical gloves.

Results: The alcohol-only formulation (product A) achieved mean log reduction factors of 1.96 ± 1.06 immediately after application and 1.67 ± 0.71 after 6 h. The chlorhexidine-alcohol combination (product B) achieved mean log reduction factors of 1.42 ± 0.79 and 1.24 ± 0.90 immediately and after 6 h, respectively. The values for product A were significantly greater than those for product B at both measured time points ($p \leq 0.025$ immediately after application and $p \leq 0.01$ after 6 h).

Conclusions: An optimized alcohol-only formulation tested according to a modified EN 12791 protocol in 25 healthy volunteers outperformed a chlorhexidine-alcohol formulation both immediately after application and at 6 h under surgical gloves, despite a much shorter application time. Thus, optimized alcohol-only formulations do not require chlorhexidine to achieve potent immediate and sustained efficacy. In conclusion, chlorhexidine is not an essential component for alcohol-based surgical hand preparation.

Keywords: Surgical hand antisepsis, Surgical scrubbing, Chlorhexidine, Alcohol, Handrub evaluation

* Correspondence: thomas.hennig@bbraun.com
[1]B. Braun Medical AG, Centre of Excellence Infection Control, Seesatz 17, 6204 Sempach, Switzerland
Full list of author information is available at the end of the article

Background

Surgical hand preparation, also termed surgical hand antisepsis or surgical scrubbing, has become an essential part of modern surgery. It was introduced as part of the post-Listerian system of aseptic surgery that was widely adopted in Europe and the USA at the turn of the twentieth century [1]. The goal of surgical hand preparation is to generate a near-elimination of transient hand flora or hand contamination, and a substantial reduction of resident hand flora that would be sustained for the duration of the surgery [2]. The aim is to prevent wound contamination or infection by accidental glove leaks or glove rupture. Although the basic necessity of surgical hand preparation, as compared to no preparation, has never been tested in a randomized clinical trial (RCT), the practice is nevertheless strongly supported by the principles of microbiology, by existing models of pathogen transmission and by empirical observations. Hands are frequently contaminated with microorganisms, accidental sterile glove leaks are common and there are observations of case clusters of surgical infections when hand preparation protocols were inadequate or breached [2–5].

The two main approaches to surgical hand preparation are (a) aqueous preparation, using antiseptics such as chlorhexidine (CHG) or povidone-iodine (PVI) in a detergent base that are applied and then rinsed off with running water, and (b) preparation with alcohol-based handrubs, without rinsing with water, where the alcohol provides the bulk of the microbicidal action. The preference for either of the two approaches differs in different healthcare settings, and both aqueous and alcohol-based hand preparation have been incorporated as suitable alternatives into important major guidelines [2, 6, 7]. Alcohol-based hand preparation has four main advantages over aqueous preparation, (a) it generally achieves much greater reduction of microorganisms on hands, (b) formulations with suitable emollients are usually associated with less skin damage and dermatitis, (c) it requires shorter application times, and (d) it saves considerable amounts of running water [2, 3, 8, 9]. One large RCT of alcohol-based versus aqueous preparation found equivalence in terms of surgical site infection (SSI) rates and concluded that the alcohol-based protocol was better tolerated by the surgical teams and improved compliance with hand hygiene guidelines [10]. Modern alcohol-based handrub formulations can meet efficacy requirements within application times as short as 1.5 min, which can translate to time savings for surgeons and surgical teams [11].

The efficacy of surgical hand preparation formulations and protocols is routinely tested using standardized in vivo microbiological protocols on the hands of volunteers [2]. The European standard EN 12791 [12] compares a given formulation to a reference alcohol consisting of 60% (v/v) n-propanol on clean hands and stipulates that the microbial log reduction factors of the tested formulation must not be statistically inferior to the reference, both immediately after application and after 3 h under surgical gloves. The US standard ASTM E1115 [13], applied with the US Food and Drug Administration (FDA) criteria [14], stipulates that a given formulation on clean hands must achieve absolute microbial log reduction factors of 1.0 on the first day of application, of 2.0 on the second day, and of 3.0 on the fifth day after a total of 11 sequential applications, and must show sustained efficacy by way of microbial counts not exceeding those at baseline after 6 h under surgical gloves. Both standards require that adequately-validated neutralizers are used during testing, in order to prevent false-positive results from sustained antimicrobial activity that is exerted after the end of the planned antiseptic exposure [15].

Discussion has arisen as to whether alcohol-based surgical handrubs should contain CHG as a second agent, to ensure persistency of the antiseptic effects for the duration of the operation. A few studies [16, 17] indeed reported superiority of CHG-alcohol combination rubs over alcohol-only products at time points of up to 6 h under surgical gloves. However, concerns were subsequently raised about methodological details of these studies, such as whether initial antiseptic application and subsequent neutralization were adequate [18, 19]. In order to investigate this question further, we initiated a comparative study of an alcohol-only versus a CHG-alcohol combination handrub, based on a modified EN 12791 test protocol with an extended period of 6 h under surgical gloves.

Methods

Two commercially available alcohol-based handrubs were investigated. Product A was an alcohol-only handrub containing 45% (w/v) ethanol, 18% (w/v) n-propanol and emollients (Softa-Man®, also branded as Softalind®, B. Braun, Sempach, Switzerland). Product B was a CHG-alcohol combination handrub containing 1% (w/w) chlorhexidine gluconate, 61% (w/w) ethanol and emollients (3 M™ Avagard™ Surgical and Healthcare Personnel Hand Antiseptic with Moisturizers, 3 M Health Care, St. Paul, MN, USA).

Twenty-five healthy volunteers were included in two experimental runs in a randomized, cross-over design according to a modified EN 12791 protocol [12]. The two modifications were that instead of using 60% (v/v) n-propanol as a reference, the two products (A and B) were directly compared as part of a benchmarking exercise, and that a prolonged period of 6 h instead of 3 h under surgical gloves was used to assess sustained efficacy. Hands were prewashed for 1 min with non-antiseptic soap. Pretreatment bacterial counts (prevalues) were obtained by rubbing fingertips and thumb tips in 10 ml tryptic soy broth (TSB) for 1 min. Subsequently, each subject used either product A or product B by applying 3 portions of 3 ml of the product to the hands, in such a way as to keep the hands moist with the product for the duration of the application. Product A was applied for a shortened application time of 90 s, product B was applied for the full 3 min duration, as usually done for the reference alcohol in EN 12791. Immediate postexposure bacterial counts (first postvalues) were taken from one hand by rubbing fingertips and thumb tips in 10 ml TSB containing neutralizers, and the other hand remained gloved for 6 h. Another set of bacterial counts (second postvalues) was taken after glove removal. Validated neutralizers (a combination of 5.0% polysorbate 80 + 0.6% sodium oleate +2.0% lecithine) according to EN 13727 [20] were used in the TSB for sampling (postvalues). Samples in TSB were plated on neutralizer-free tryptic soy agar (TSA), incubated at 36+/−1 °C for 48 h, and colonies were subsequently enumerated. The differences between the $\log_{10}$ pre- and postvalues (log reduction factors) were determined for each subject, and the means of these differences were statistically compared using the Wilcoxon matched-pairs signed-ranks test.

Results

The results of the direct comparison between the alcohol-only (product A) versus the CHG-alcohol (product B) handrub are shown in Table 1. Product A achieved mean log reduction factors (± standard deviation) of 1.96 ± 1.06 immediately after application, and 1.67 ± 0.71 after 6 h. Product B achieved mean log reduction factors of 1.42 ± 0.79 and 1.24 ± 0.90 immediately and after 6 h, respectively. The mean log reduction factors obtained with use of product A were significantly greater than those of product B at both time points, immediately after application ($p \leq 0.025$) and after 6 h under surgical gloves ($p \leq 0.01$).

Discussion

Our results show that an alcohol-only handrub that contains an optimized composition of two alcohol species, ethanol and n-propanol, achieved a significantly greater initial microbial reduction after surgical hand preparation than a CHG-alcohol combination handrub when tested according to a modified EN 12791 protocol, and that a significant difference in reduction factors in favor of the alcohol-only rub was maintained for 6 h under surgical gloves. These results are consistent with findings from a previous comparative study [21], in which an 80% (w/w) ethanol-only rub passed EN 12791 requirements both immediately and at 3 h after application, while the same 1% (w/w) CHG and 61% (w/w) ethanol combination rub as was used in the present study failed at both time points. Among the three common alcohol species (ethanol, isopropanol and n-propanol) that are used for hand and skin antisepsis, n-propanol has the most potent general microbicidal activity and exerts this at relatively lower concentrations [22]. This supports its inclusion into alcohol-based handrubs and explains the potent activity exhibited by a combination of n-propanol and ethanol at an overall concentration of 63% (w/v) in product A as observed in the present study.

The results in this study were obtained despite the absence of CHG in handrub A, despite the extended test interval of 6 h under surgical gloves and despite the fact that handrub B was given a very substantial a priori advantage by having had twice the initial application time (180 s) of handrub A (90 s), with the application volume (3 × 3 ml) and other conditions being equal. These findings are consistent with earlier findings indicating that the application of alcohols, despite the absence of residual activity per se, is followed by substantially delayed regrowth of skin flora or even continued microbial killing [23, 24] and that the contribution of dedicated supplements for persistency is relatively modest or even absent when tested for durations of up to 6 h [25, 26]. This is further consistent with the concept that an initially strong and immediate microbial killing capacity

Table 1 Comparison of an alcohol-only handrub (product A) versus a chlorhexidine-alcohol combination handrub (product B) for surgical hand preparation in a modified test arrangement according to EN 12791 (2016)

| | Application time | Application volume | Prevalues ($\log_{10}$ ± SD) | Immediate effects | | 6-h effects | | |
				Mean RF ($\log_{10}$ ± SD)	p value[a]	Prevalues ($\log_{10}$ ± SD)	Mean RF ($\log_{10}$ ± SD)	p value[a]
Product A (alcohol only)	90 s	3 × 3 ml	4.68 ± 0.5	1.96 ± 1.06	≤0.025	4.79 ± 0.51	1.67 ± 0.71	≤0.01
Product B (CHG-alcohol)	180 s	3 × 3 ml	4.79 ± 0.52	1.42 ± 0.79		4.73 ± 0.50	1.24 ± 0.90	

RF reduction factor, SD standard deviation, CHG chlorhexidine
[a]Calculated using the Wilcoxon matched-pairs signed-ranks test

continues to translate into low viable microorganism numbers for several hours under surgical gloves. The extended duration of 6 h under surgical gloves was chosen for the present experiments, instead of the usual 3 h for EN 12791, in order to simulate tougher test conditions that resemble those of the US ASTM E1115 standard in this aspect. Furthermore, our results as well as those of others [11, 27] support shorter application times, as short as 1.5–2 min, when highly potent alcohol-based handrubs are used.

In addition to using an effective alcohol-based handrub, the technique of application is also considered important [28]. While EN 12791 requires coverage of only the hand surfaces for the purpose of efficacy testing, the World Health Organization hand hygiene guidelines [2] state that complete coverage of hands and forearms requires about 15 ml (about 3 × 5 ml) and emphasize that it is important to keep hands and forearms wet with alcohol for the entire duration of application. Some protocols that include very small applied volumes [29] are therefore a cause for concern, as they are likely to lead to incomplete skin surface coverage and interrupted action of the antiseptic.

In the area of skin antisepsis, CHG has been the subject of a considerable amount of incorrect assessment. What had happened was that a substantial proportion of the clinical trial-based literature on skin antisepsis had attributed favorable clinical outcomes achieved with CHG-alcohol combinations (two effective antiseptics) to CHG alone and concluded that CHG alone (instead of the combination) was the agent supported by evidence [30, 31]. This had happened despite a strong microbiological literature base that showed alcohols to be potent antiseptics. The misinterpretation of trial outcomes was carried over into prominent guidelines, led to a number of prominent recommendations for CHG alone, and created widespread but in parts unsubstantiated views of CHG as an "in" antiseptic.

Microbiological assessment of antiseptics may similarly be subject to errors. Both European and US standards stipulate that adequately validated neutralizer substances must be used at the point of sampling after antiseptic exposure [15]; this is in order to prevent continued killing due to residual bacteriostatic or bactericidal action after the end of the dedicated exposure. While this applies to the testing of all antiseptics, CHG in particular is prone to false-positive efficacy assessment in the absence of adequate neutralization, due to strong bacteriostatic activity that it exerts at concentrations far below bactericidal levels [32–34]. It has been suggested that this is a factor that likely led to a systematic skewing of the antiseptic literature [35]. Previous reports of superior performance of CHG-alcohol combination rubs for surgical hand antisepsis

[16, 17] indeed attracted letters to the editor that expressed concern about adequate neutralization [18, 19]. In the present study, adequate neutralizers were used during the entire testing process, thus creating equal sampling conditions for both comparator rubs.

Among the different hand hygiene agents, alcohol-based handrubs are generally most well tolerated on skin; true alcohol allergies have not been documented beyond reasonable doubt, and irritant contact dermatitis from alcohols is rare when handrubs are well formulated with emollients [2]. On the other hand, CHG is a known allergen and a frequent cause of irritant contact dermatitis among healthcare personnel [2, 36, 37]. It has also been the subject of a recent US FDA warning about rare but serious anaphylactic reactions [38]. Thus, there is a clear potential for a tolerability advantage from alcohol-only handrubs for surgical hand preparation, especially if their antimicrobial performance characteristics are equal to or even better than those of CHG-containing ones.

It is a limitation of our study that it was performed according to a modified EN 12791 protocol, and results from EN 12791 testing do not necessarily translate into congruent results according to the US standard ASTM E1115 [13], mainly due to the US standard's requirement for incremental increases (cumulative effects) in log reduction factors on subsequent days of testing [15, 39]. However, the clinical relevance of this requirement has been questioned, because it is not intuitive why a surgeon's hands after antisepsis should be permitted to have different microbial counts on different working days of the week [39]. In any case, EN 12791 is a very stringent standard in which only very potent handrubs tend to pass, and it has high inter-laboratory reproducibility [40].

Conclusions

In the present study, an alcohol-only handrub containing a mix of ethanol and n-propanol outperformed a CHG-alcohol handrub both immediately after application and at 6 h when applied for 1.5 min and tested according to a modified EN 12791 protocol in 25 healthy volunteers. This means that optimized and well-formulated alcohol-only handrubs can provide superior performance to CHG-alcohol combination rubs for the purpose of surgical hand preparation, even with shortened application times, and this includes sustained efficacy for an extended period of 6 h under surgical gloves. In conclusion, given that CHG has a greater potential for skin irritation than alcohols alone, CHG is not an essential or even necessary component of alcohol-based handrubs for surgical hand preparation. Further studies in routine practice are warranted.

Acknowledgements
None.

Funding
This work was funded by B. Braun Medical AG.

Authors' contributions
SW, KN, AA modified the EN 12791 test method, analyzed and interpreted the data regarding the efficacy. TH has born the idea for this investigation and was a major contributor in writing the manuscript. All authors reviewed and approved the final manuscript.

Consent for publication
Not applicable.

Competing interests
A. Arndt and T.-J. Hennig are paid employees of B. Braun Medical AG, the manufacturer of the Softa-Man® alcohol-based handrub described in this article. The authors declare that they have no competing interests.

Author details
[1]B. Braun Medical AG, Centre of Excellence Infection Control, Seesatz 17, 6204 Sempach, Switzerland. [2]HygCen Germany GmbH, Bornhövedstrasse 78, 19055 Schwerin, Germany.

References
1. Gröschel DHM, Pruett TL. Surgical antisepsis. In: Block SS, editor. Disinfection, sterilisation and preservation. 4th ed. London: Lea & Febiger; 1991. p. 642–54.
2. World Health Organization. WHO guidelines on hand hygiene in health care. Geneva: World Health Organization; 2009.
3. Widmer AF. Surgical hand hygiene: scrub or rub? J Hosp Infect. 2013;83(Suppl 1): S35–9.
4. Graves PB, Twomey CL. Surgical hand antisepsis: an evidence-based review. Periop Nurs Clin. 2006;1:235–49.
5. Tanner J. Surgical hand antisepsis: the evidence. J Perioper Pract. 2008;18(8): 330–4. 9
6. Boyce JM, Pittet D. Guideline for hand hygiene in health-care settings. Recommendations of the healthcare infection control practices advisory committee and the HICPAC/SHEA/APIC/IDSA hand hygiene task force. Society for Healthcare Epidemiology of America/Association for Professionals in infection control/Infectious Diseases Society of America. MMWR Recomm Rep. 2002;51(RR-16):1–45. quiz CE1-4
7. Association of perioperative Registered Nurses (AORN). Recommended practices for surgical hand antisepsis/hand scrubs. AORN J. 2004;79(2):416–8. 21-6, 29-31
8. Hsieh HF, Chiu HH, Lee FP. Surgical hand scrubs in relation to microbial counts: systematic literature review. J Adv Nurs. 2006;55(1):68–78.
9. Graf ME, Machado A, Mensor LL, Zampieri D, Campos R, Faham L. Surgical hands antisepsis with alcohol-based preparations: cost-effectiveness, compliance of professionals and ecological benefits in the Brazilian healthcare scenario (in Portuguese). J Bras Econ Saúde. 2014;6(2):71–80.
10. Parienti JJ, Thibon P, Heller R, et al. Hand-rubbing with an aqueous alcoholic solution vs traditional surgical hand-scrubbing and 30-day surgical site infection rates: a randomized equivalence study. JAMA. 2002;288(6):722–7.
11. Kampf G, Ostermeyer C, Heeg P. Surgical hand disinfection with a propanol-based hand rub: equivalence of shorter application times. J Hosp Infect. 2005;59(4):304–10.
12. European Committee for Standardization (CEN). EN 12791:2016. Chemical disinfectants and antiseptics. Surgical hand disinfection. Test method and requirement (phase 2/step2). Brussels: European Committee for Standardization (CEN); 2016.
13. American Society for Testing and Materials (ASTM). ASTM E1115–11. Standard test method for evaluation of surgical hand scrub formulations West Conshohocken, PA: ASTM International; 2011.
14. Food and Drug Administration_(FDA). Tentative final monograph for health-care antiseptic drug products; proposed rule. 21 CFR parts 333 and 369. Fed Regist. 1994;59(116):31402–52.
15. Heeg P, Ostermeyer C, Kampf G. Comparative review of the test design

16. Beausoleil CM, Paulson DS, Bogert A, Lewis GS. In vivo evaluation of the persistant and residual antimicrobial properties of three hand-scrub and hand-rub regimes in a simulated surgical environment. J Hosp Infect. 2012;81(4):283–7.
17. Olson LK, Morse DJ, Duley C, Savell BK. Prospective, randomized in vivo comparison of a dual-active waterless antiseptic versus two alcohol-only waterless antiseptics for surgical hand antisepsis. Am J Infect Control. 2012; 40(2):155–9.
18. Kampf G. "Persistent activity"-should the effect of chlorhexidine in the sampling fluid and nutrient broth and on agar plates really be regarded as the effect on hands? Am J Infect Control. 2012;40(6):579.
19. Kampf G. How valid are the 'persistent and residual antimicrobial properties' described by Beausoleil et al.? J Hosp Infect. 2012;82(4):301–2.
20. European Committee for Standardization (CEN). EN 13727:2012+A2:2015. Chemical disinfectants and antiseptics. Quantitative suspension test for the evaluation of bactericidal activity in the medical area. Test method and requirements (phase 2, step 1). Brussels: European Committee for Standardization (CEN); 2015.
21. Kampf G, Ostermeyer C. Efficacy of two distinct ethanol-based hand rubs for surgical hand disinfection – a controlled trial according to prEN 12791. BMC Infect Dis. 2005;5:17.
22. Rotter ML. Hand washing, hand disinfection, and skin disinfection. In: Wenzel RP, editor. Prevention and control of nosocomial infections. 3rd ed. Baltimore: Williams &Wilkins; 1997. p. 691–709.
23. Lilly HA, Lowbury EJ, Wilkins MD, Zaggy A. Delayed antimicrobial effects of skin disinfection by alcohol. J Hyg. 1979;82(3):497–500.
24. Ayliffe GA. Surgical scrub and skin disinfection. Infect Control. 1984;5(1):23–7.
25. Rotter ML, Kampf G, Suchomel M, Kundi M. Population kinetics of the skin flora on gloved hands following surgical hand disinfection with 3 propanol-based hand rubs: a prospective, randomized, double-blind trial. Infect Control Hosp Epidemiol. 2007;28(3):346–50.
26. Kampf G, Kramer A, Suchomel M. Lack of sustained efficacy for alcohol-based surgical hand rubs containing 'residual active ingredients' according to EN 12791. J Hosp Infect. 2017;95(2):163–8.
27. Weber WP, Reck S, Neff U, et al. Surgical hand antisepsis with alcohol-based hand rub: comparison of effectiveness after 1.5 And 3 minutes of application. Infect Control Hosp Epidemiol. 2009;30(5):420–6.
28. Maiwald M. Technique is important for alcohol-based surgical hand antisepsis. Healthc Infect. 2012;17(3):106–7.
29. Burch TM, Stanger B, Mizuguchi KA, Zurakowski D, Reid SD. Is alcohol-based hand disinfection equivalent to surgical scrub before placing a central venous catheter? Anesth Analg. 2012;114(3):622–5.
30. Maiwald M, Chan ES. The forgotten role of alcohol: a systematic review and meta-analysis of the clinical efficacy and perceived role of chlorhexidine in skin antisepsis. PLoS One. 2012;7(9):e44277.
31. Maiwald M, Chan ES. Pitfalls in evidence assessment: the case of chlorhexidine and alcohol in skin antisepsis. J Antimicrob Chemother. 2014;69(8):2017–21.
32. Kampf G, Shaffer M, Hunte C. Insufficient neutralization in testing a chlorhexidine-containing ethanol-based hand rub can result in a false positive efficacy assessment. BMC Infect Dis. 2005;5(1):48.
33. Kampf G. What is left to justify the use of chlorhexidine in hand hygiene? J Hosp Infect. 2008;70(Suppl 1):27–34.
34. Kampf G, Reichel M, Hollingsworth A, Bashir M. Efficacy of surgical hand scrub products based on chlorhexidine is largely overestimated without neutralizing agents in the sampling fluid. Am J Infect Control. 2013;41(1):e1–5.
35. Maiwald M, Petncy TN, Assam PN, Chan ES. Use of statistics as another factor leading to an overestimation of chlorhexidine's role in skin antisepsis. Infect Control Hosp Epidemiol. 2013;34(8):872–3.
36. Kampf G, Kramer A. Epidemiologic background of hand hygiene and evaluation of the most important agents for scrubs and rubs. Clin Microbiol Rev. 2004;17(4):863–93. table of contents
37. Stingeni L, Lapomarda V, Lisi P. Occupational hand dermatitis in hospital environments. Contact Dermatitis. 1995;33(3):172–6.
38. US Food and Drug Administration (FDA). FDA Drug Safety Communication: FDA warns about rare but serious allergic reactions with the skin antiseptic chlorhexidine gluconate. 2017. https://www.fda.gov/Drugs/DrugSafety/ucm530975.htm. Accessed 12 Sept 2017.
39. Kampf G, Ostermeyer C, Heeg P, Paulson D. Evaluation of two methods of determining the efficacies of two alcohol-based hand rubs for surgical hand antisepsis. Appl Environ Microbiol. 2006;72(6):3856–61.

14

In vitro evaluation of the susceptibility of *Acinetobacter baumannii* isolates to antiseptics and disinfectants: comparison between clinical and environmental isolates

Sanae Lanjri[*], Jean Uwingabiye, Mohammed Frikh, Lina Abdellatifi, Jalal Kasouati, Adil Maleb, Abdelouahed Bait, Abdelhay Lemnouer and Mostafa Elouennass

Abstract

Background: This study aims to assess the susceptibility of *Acinetobacter baumannii* isolates to the antiseptics and disinfectants commonly used, and to the non-approved product.

Methods: This is a prospective study carried out from February to August 2015, in the Bacteriology department of Mohammed V Military Teaching hospital of Rabat on *A.baumannii* isolates collected from colonized and/or infected patients and environmental samples. The antiseptics and disinfectants susceptibility testing was assessed using the micromethod validated in our department. The antiseptics and disinfectants studied were: 70% ethyl alcohol, chlorhexidine, povidone-iodine, didecyldimethylammonium chloride and a commercial product which was presented as a hospital disinfectant (non-registered product).

Results: Povidone-iodine, 0.5% chlorhexidine digluconate, 70% ethyl alcohol and didecyl dimethyl ammonium chloride in combination with N- (3-aminopropyl) -N-dodecylpropane-1, 3-diamine were effective against all the 81 *A.baumannii* isolates tested, and their logarithmic reduction ≥ 5 were observed in 100% of the isolates in their undiluted form. The strains isolated from patients were more resistant than environmental strains: at a dilution of ½ for 70% ethyl alcohol (37. 77% vs 11.11%, $p = 0.007$) and at a dilution of 1/10 (100% vs 69.44%, $p < 0.001$) for povidone iodine. The non-registered product was ineffective with a resistance rate of 96.29% at a dilution of 1/50, 45.67% at a dilution of 1/10 and 13.58% in its purest form.

Conclusion: Our study revealed the effectiveness of the main disinfectants and antiseptics used in Morocco; three antiseptics tested were effective in their purest form against the 81 *A.baumannii* isolates. Regarding disinfectants, our results showed an efficacy of didecyl dimethyl ammonium at the recommended use concentration and in its purest form. This study emphasizes the need for using disinfectants and antiseptics in dilutions recommended by the manufacturer because the insufficient dilutions of these products are not effective. Our findings also demonstrated an inefficiency of the non-registered product against *A.baumanii* isolates. However, the non-registered products should be prohibited.

Keywords: *Acinetobacter baumannii*, Resistance, Antiseptics, Disinfectants

* Correspondence: lanjrisanae@gmail.com
Department of Clinical Bacteriology, Mohammed V Military teaching hospital, research team of Epidemiology and Bacterial resistance, Faculty of Medicine and Pharmacy, Mohammed V University, Rabat, Morocco

Background

Acinetobacter baumannii is a Gram-negative bacillus that has emerged in recent years as one of the pathogens that poses the most problems of antibiotic resistance, morbidity and mortality in health facilities worldwide [1].

A.baumannii is a ubiquitous bacterium that can be isolated from both the environment [2] and the human's skin [3, 4]. It mainly affects debilitated patients [5] and it is responsible for a variety of life-threatening infections including bacteremia and pneumonia [1]. In an American study, 5 to 10% of nosocomial pneumonia and 1.3% of bacteremia were due to *A. baumannii* [6, 7]. In a Moroccan study published in 2016, *Acinetobacter spp.* isolates represented 6.94% of all bacterial clinical isolates and 9.6% of Gram negative rods [8].

The remarkable ability of *A.baumannii* to easily acquire resistance factors ranked it among the organisms that threaten the current therapeutic armamentarium. *A. baumannii* strain resistant to all known antibiotics has already been reported in France [9]. The Moroccan studies showed that the resistance rate to imipenem, ceftazidime, amikacin and ciprofloxacin increased from 23 to 76%, 63 to 86%, 41 to 52% and 68 to 87% respectively during the last 13 years [8, 10].

The importance of hand transmission in the spread of this bacteria and prolonged survival in the environment (>8 days) complicates the prevention and control of these infections [1]. Indeed, hand hygiene and environmental cleanliness are the keystone of the infection control measures for the prevention of the spread of *A.bauamannii*. The use of antiseptics and disinfectants is an important means in these infection control strategies. Their use allows the reduction or elimination of bacterial reservoir and prevents the transition from colonization to infection [11].

Contrary to antibiotics, studies that have been devoted to the emergence of *A. baumannii* resistant to antiseptics and disinfectants are very few. Some emphasize the increase in resistance rates to these products. A study assessing the susceptibility of 445 bacterial strains from various genera against more than 50 types of disinfectants revealed that *A. baumannii* isolates were the most resistant species. Resistance rates were higher against oxidizing agents while the lowest resistance rate was observed against quaternary ammonium compounds and amines [12].

Antiseptic resistance rates vary. One study showed that on hands artificially contaminated with *A. baumannii,* ethyl alcohol and povidone-iodine had higher removal ratio than chlorhexidine and ordinary soap [13].

The aim of our study was to assess the susceptibility of *A. baumannii* strains to the antiseptics and disinfectants commonly used, and to a non-registered product.

Methods

Type of the study

This is a prospective study performed in the Bacteriology department of Mohammed V Military Teaching hospital (HMIMV) of Rabat from February to August 2015. HMIMV has a hospital capacity of more than 700 beds and contains 2 intensive care units (medical and surgical) with 10 beds each, a center for burns treatment, surgical and medical units, and laboratory and imagery departments.

Bacterial isolates

The *A. baumannii* strains tested were isolated from colonized and/or infected patients, and environmental samples in the HMIMV.

In addition to these isolates, a reference strain was tested (*Escherichia coli* ATCC® 25922™).

Antiseptics and disinfectants tested

In our institution, the antiseptics mainly used are polividone iodine and chlorhexidine. For the bio-cleaning of floors and surfaces, the disinfectant used is didecyl dimethyl ammonium chloride.

During our study, five products were tested including three antiseptics and two disinfectants including a commercial detergent-disinfectant whose composition is unknown (Table 1).

Methods

The sensitivity of *A.baumannii* isolates to antiseptics and disinfectants was assessed using the microdilution method (micromethod), validated in our laboratory.

The validation of our method was made by comparing its results with those obtained by the tube dilution method (macromethod) for three isolates to Surfanios®, as it was described by Mama et al. (2014) [14].

Validation of a micromethod for the determination of the susceptibility to antiseptics and disinfectants

Inoculum preparation

After thawing the bacterial isolates to be tested, a brain heart broth was inoculated and incubated at 37 °C for 18 to 24 h. The broths were subsequently subcultured on blood agar and incubated at 37 °C for 18 to 24 h. The inoculum was prepared by saline suspension of isolated colonies selected from an 18 to 24 h agar plate. The turbidity of these suspensions was adjusted to. 0.5 McFarland standard.

Dilution of the initial inoculum

After calculating the different volumes to be used for the micromethod by respecting the proportions used in the macromethod, the volume of the bacterial suspension was found very low (1 µl). To increase the volume, 1/10

Table 1 The recommended dilutions, abbreviation, active ingredient and the dilutions tested for each product in our study

Product	Abbreviation	Active ingredient	Recommended dilutions	dilutions tested
Betadine scrub®	PVPI	4% povidone-iodine	Pure, 1|3	pure, 1|3, 1|10, 1|100, 1|1000
septeal®	CHX	0.5% chlorhexidine digluconate	Pure	pure, 1|10, 1|100, 1|1000
ethyl alcohol 70	AL	70% ethyl Alcohol	Pure	pure, 1|2, 1|10, 1|100, 1|1000
Surfanios®	DDA	N- (3-aminopropyl) -N-dodécylpropane-1, 3-diamine (51 mg/g) + didecyl dimethyl ammonium chloride (25 mg/g)	1|400 (0,25%)	pure, 1|10, 1|100, 1|200, 1|400, 1|1000, 1|10000, 1|1000000
Non registered product	NRP	unknown composition	1|50 (2%)	pure, 1|10, 1|50, 1|100, 1|1000

dilution of the previously standardized bacterial suspension at 0.5 McFarland was performed.

Preparation of antiseptic and disinfectant solutions

The different prepared dilutions of each product were chosen according to the concentration recommended by the manufacturer (Table 1).

Validation tests
Macromethod validation

In a sterile test tube, 4.9 ml of sterile trypticase soy broth was mixed with 5 ml of each dilution of the antimicrobial agent. To obtain a final volume of 10 ml, 0.1 ml of standardized bacterial suspension was inoculated into each tube.

Two control tubes were used; positive control tube containing only the nutrient broth and the strain to be tested, while negative controls were established as follows: nutrient broth only, nutrient broth and antimicrobial agent.

After 24 h at 37 °C, the visible signs of bacterial growth (turbidity) were not possible to detect given the macroscopic qualities of the product-broth mixture in all the tubes including the control tubes. All tubes were then subcultured on Bromocresol Purple (BCP) agar and incubated at 37 °C for 24 h. The reading of each culture plate has been validated by the absence of growth in sterility control wells and bacterial growth in fertility control wells.

Micromethod validation, and antiseptics and disinfectants susceptibility testing

The wells of a microplate were filled with appropriate volumes of increasing concentrations of antiseptic or disinfectant solution and then completed with corresponding volumes of broth and suspension of the inoculum.

In practice, each well of a sterile 96-well plate was inoculated with 50 μl of dilution of the antimicrobial agent, 40 μl of trypticase soy and 10 μl of diluted bacterial suspension.

The positive control wells were inoculated with 40 μl of nutrient broth and 10 μl of the bacterial suspension

(fertility testing), while the negative controls were inoculated with nutrient broth and the antimicrobial agent (sterility testing).

After 24 h at 37 °C, all tubes were then subcultured on BCP agar and incubated at 37 °C for 24 h. Reading of agar plates was performed as described in macromethod validation.

The macromethod was used as reference for validating the micromethod, with both methods leading to the same results.

The evaluation of the A. baumanni susceptibility to antiseptics and disinfectants was realized by using micromethod as it was described in the validation's paragraph. The number of colony-forming units was counted on each plate. The plates on which manual counting of bacterial colony-forming units was not possible, the number of colony-forming unit was considered to be above 10^7.

The rate of the log reduction of the different products was calculated. The ⩾5 log10 reduction was considered as significant reduction of growth.

Statistical analysis

Statistical analysis was performed using SPSS statistical software version 13.0 and Microsoft Office Excel 2007. Susceptibility comparisons of the isolates from the patient and environmental samples to different products were established using the chi test-square. P values less than 0.05 were considered statistically significant.

Results

During this study, 81 A.baumannii isolates were tested: 45 strains from patient samples and 36 strains from the environmental samples. The majority of clinical isolates were predominantly collected from intensive care unit's (ICUs) patients ($n = 34$, 75.5%), followed by those from medical department ($n = 8$, 17.8%) and external consultants ($n = 3$, 6.7%). Of the clinical isolates, 23 (51.1%) were colonizing isolates and 22 (48.9%) were infectious ones. The colonizing isolates were isolated from anal margin (43.5%), groin area (8.34.8%) and mouth (n21.7%), while the isolation sites of infectious isolates were: broncho-pulmonary (45.5%), urine (31.8%) and blood culture (13.6%), catheters (4.5%), joint fluid (4.5%) and cutaneous lesions (4.5%). The environmental isolates were exclusively recovered from the ICUs. The distribution of isolation sites for environmental isolates was: bed sheets (38.9%), soil (36.1%), hospital respirators (11.1%), trolleys (5.6%), gallows (2.8%), pillows (2.8%) and monitors (2.8%).

All chemical agents tested were found to be effective on the *Escherichia coli ATCC 25922* reference strain in their purest form (Table 2).

The Tables 3 and 4 represent respectively the resistance rates of *A.baumannii* strains and the logarithmic reduction ≥ 5 over the initial time zero inoculum levels of the various products tested. Povidone-iodine, 0.5% chlorhexidine digluconate, 70% ethyl alcohol and didecyl dimethyl ammonium chloride in combination with N-(3-aminopropyl) -N-dodecylpropane-1, 3-diamine were effective against all the 81 *A.baumannii* isolates tested and their logarithmic reduction ≥ 5 was observed in 100% of isolates in their undiluted form. The strains isolated from patients were more resistant than environmental strains: at a dilution of ½ for70 % ethyl alcohol (37.77% vs 11.11% and $p = 0.007$) and at a dilution of 1/10 (100% vs 69.44%, $p < 0.001$) for povidone iodine. The

Table 2 Efficacy of antiseptics and disinfectants tested on *Escherichia coli ATCC® 25922™* reference strain

Product	Dilution	Bacterial growth
PVPI	PURE	-
	1|3	-
	1|10	+
	1|100, 1|1000	+
CHX	PURE	-
	1|10	-
	1|100	-
	1|1000	+
AL	PURE	-
	1|2	+
	1|10	+
	1|100, 1|1000	+
DDA	PURE, 1|10, 1|100, 1|400	-
	1|1000	-
	10–4	+
	10–5, 10–6	+
NRP	PURE	-
	1|10	+
	1|50	+
	1|100, 1|1000	+

PVPI povidone-iodine, *CHX* chlorhexidine digluconate, *AL* ethyl Alcohol, *DDA* N-(3-aminopropyl)-N-dodécylpropane-1,3-diamine + didecyl dimethyl ammonium chloride, *NRP* non registered product, *(+)* Growth, *(-)* No growth

non-registered product was ineffective with resistant rate of 96.29% at a dilution of 1/50, 45.67% at a dilution of 1/10 and 13.58% in its purest form.

Discussion

Our study was focused on three commonly used antiseptics: 70% ethyl alcohol, chlorhexidine and povidone-iodine, on a disinfectant (didecyldimethylammonium chloride) and on a commercial product which was presented as a hospital disinfectant.

The 70% ethyl alcohol is used for antisepsis of small superficial wounds and skin before an injection. It's a component of several hand sanitizers. Other alcohols, such as propanol and isopropanol, are also used as hand sanitizers [11]. In our study, pure ethyl alcohol (70%) was effective against all *A.baumannii* isolates. At a dilution of 1/2, the resistance rate was 25.92%. The strains isolated from patients were more resistant than environmental strains (37.77% vs 11, 11%, $p = 0.007$). The ≥ 5 $\log_{10}$ reduction was obtained in 100% of isolates at undiluted state, in 74% at dilution of ½ and in 12.34% at dilution of 1/10. Wisplinghoff et al. [15] used 60% propanol and found the results similar to ours while the contact time was 15 s, 30s, 60s and 120 s.

The 0.5% chlorhexidine digluconate is recommended in antisepsis of surgical wounds, common skin infections, and antisepsis of healthy skin prior to minor surgery. It is applied to the skin without rinsing [11]. In our study, chlorhexidine at its undiluted state has shown its effectiveness against all 81 isolates tested. The logarithmic reduction ≥ 5 was observed in 100% of isolates in its undiluted state and in 92.59% of isolates at a dilution of 1/10. The difference in resistance rates between isolates from the patient and the environmental samples was not significant. Comparing these rates with those of 70% ethyl alcohol, the chlorhexidine is more effective. Our results agree with Wisplinghoff et al's study [15]. Another study showed that daily bathing with chlorhexidine 2% in the ICU reduced the rate of acquisition of *A.baumannii* isolates resistant to carbapenems by 51.8% [16].

The povidone iodine is a foam solution composed of iodine and is used for scrubbing, antisepsis of healthy skin, preoperative shower; for which, it should be used in its purest form. For the cleansing of contaminated wounds, it is recommended that one-third be diluted with water [11]. In our study, all isolates were sensitive to pure povidone-iodine. While at the dilution of 1/3(dilution recommended for cleansing of wounds), 18.51% isolates were resistant. In Povidone Iodine's purest form and at a dilution of 1/3, the difference in resistance rates between isolates from patients and the environmental isolates was not significant. Clinical strains were more resistant than the environmental strains at a dilution of 1/10(100% vs 69.44%, $p < 0.05$). The logarithmic reduction ≥ 5 was observed in 100% in its

Table 3 Comparison of resistance rates between *A.baumannii* strains isolated from patients and from environmental samples to different products tested

Products	Dilution	Origin of the strains		Total ($n = 81$)	P
		Patients ($n = 45$)	Environment ($n = 36$)		
PVPI	PURE	0% (0)	0% (0)	0% (0)	-
	1|3	24.44% (11)	11.11% (4)	18.51% (15)	0.125
	1|10	100% (45)	69.44% (25)	86.41%(70)	<0.001
	1|100, 1|1000	100% (45)	100% (36)	100% (81)	-
CHX	PURE	0% (0)	0% (0)	0% (0)	-
	1|10	13.33% (6)	0% (0)	7.40% (6)	0.31
	1|100	51.11% (23)	66.66% (24)	58.02 (47)	0.159
	1|1000	100% (45)	100% (36)	100% (81)	-
AL	PURE	0% (0)	0% (0)	0% (0)	-
	1|2	37.77% (17)	11.11% (4)	25.92% (21)	0.007
	1|10	93.33% (42)	80.55% (29)	87.65% (71)	0.100
	1|100, 1|1000	100%(45)	100% (36)	100% (81)	-
DDA	PURE, 1|10,1|100, 1|400	0% (0)	0% (0)	0% (0)	-
	1|1000	24.44% (11)	8.33% (3)	17.28% (14)	0.057
	10–4	86.66% (39)	69.44% (25)	79.01% (64)	0.059
	10–5, 10–6	100% (45)	100% (36)	100%(81)	-
NRP	PURE	24.44% (11)	0% (0)	13.58% (11)	0.001
	1|10	66.66% (30)	19.44% (7)	45.67% (37)	<0.001
	1|50	97.77% (44)	94.44%(34)	96.29% (78)	0.582
	1|100, 1|1000	100% (45)	100% (36)	100% (81)	-

PVPI povidone-iodine, *CHX* chlorhexidine digluconate, *AL* ethyl Alcohol, *DDA* N-(3-aminopropyl)-N-dodécylpropane-1,3-diamine + didecyl dimethyl ammonium chloride, *NRP* non registered
- : *p* value not calculated

purest form, in 81.48% at the dilution of 1/3 and in 13.58% at a dilution of 1/10. In the study conducted by Wisplinghoff et al [15], pure povidone iodine was active against all *Acinetobacter* isolates tested.

Environmental hygiene plays an important role in cross-transmission of *A. baumannii*. Prolonged survival of *A.baumannii* in a dry environment has been correlated with ongoing epidemics in ICUs [17]. During an *A. baumannii* outbreak which occurred over a period of 14 months in a neurosurgery ICU in the United Kingdom, a significant correlation was observed between the number of infected or colonized patients and the number of environmental isolates ($p = 0.004$) [18]. The majority of detergent-disinfectants for floors and surfaces are composed of quaternary ammonium compounds only [19] or associated with other substances (Biguanide derivatives, aldehydes, isopropanol, alkylamine, amino acid, hydrogen peroxide, ethanol …). Some studies reported acquired resistance to quaternary ammonium compounds, and that these products have a higher effectiveness against Gram-positive bacteria than against Gram-negative bacteria [11, 20]. Didecyldimethylammonium chloride in association with the amino acid

hydrochloride (Surfanios®) is used in the hospital, diluted to 0.25%(1/400) according to the manufacturer's recommendations, for the biocleaning of floors and surfaces. In our study, Surfanios® was effective against all isolates at the recommended dilution (1/400). Resistance was observed at a dilution of 1/1000 with a rate of 17.28%. There was no significant difference in resistance between the clinical and environmental isolates. In the study of Reichel et al [21], three Quaternary ammonium compound products were effective against three *A. baumannii* strains.

Another product tested in this study, is presented as a hospital-level disinfectant and its composition is unknown (non-registered product). The concentration recommended by the manufacturer is 2% (1/50). This product was ineffective with resistance rate of 96.29% at a dilution of 1/50, 45.67% at a dilution of 1/10 and 13.58% in its purest form. Our results show the ineffectiveness of this product and emphasize the advantage of using the products inscribed on the positive lists published by learned societies. The right choice of antiseptics and disinfectants plays a crucial role in preventing the development of resistance.

Table 4 The rate of isolates presenting logarithmic reduction ≥ 5 from initial inoculum

Product	Dilution	The rate of isolates presenting logarithmic ≥ 5 Log_{10} reduction
PVPI	PURE	100%
	1|3	81.48%
	1|10	13.58%
	1|100, 1|1000	0%
CHX	PURE	100%
	1|10	92.59%
	1|100	41.97%
	1|1000	0%
AL	PURE	100%
	1|2	74.07%
	1|10	12.34%
	1|100, 1|1000	0%
DDA	PURE, 1|10, 1|100, 1|400	100%
	1|1000	82.71%
	10–4	20.98%
	10–5, 10–6	0%
NRP	PURE	86.4%
	1|10	54.32%
	1|50	3.70%
	1|100, 1|1000	0%

PVPI povidone-iodine, *CHX* chlorhexidine digluconate, *AL* ethyl Alcohol, *DDA* N-(3-aminopropyl)-N-dodécylpropane-1,3-diamine + didecyl dimethyl ammonium chloride, *NRP* non registered product

Globally, the clinical isolates were more resistant to the antiseptics and disinfectants in their diluted state than the environmental ones. This shows that the minimum inhibitory concentrations of clinical and those of environmental isolates to biocides are not the same. The colonizing and infecting *A.baumannii* isolates were the most resistant to the antiseptics and disinfectants. This can probably be explained by the selection pressure exerted by the use of antiseptics and sometimes facilitated by the sub-inhibitory concentrations [22].

Conclusion

Our study revealed the effectiveness of the main disinfectants and antiseptics used in Morocco: three antiseptics tested were effective in their purest form against the 81 *A.baumannii* isolates. However, with povidone iodine diluted at one third, 18.51% of isolates were resistant. Regarding disinfectants, our results showed an efficacy of Didecyldimethylammonium at the recommended concentration. This study emphasizes the need for using disinfectants and antiseptics in dilutions recommended by the manufacturer because the insufficient concentrations of these products are ineffective. Our findings also demonstrated an inefficiency of the non-registered product against Acinetobacter isolates. The market for these products is constantly increasing but it is potentially associated with risks. Therefore, a regulatory framework for the use of these products must be implemented both for hospital and community use.

Abbreviations
A.baumannii: *Acinetobacter baumannii*; AL: Ethyl alcohol; BCP: Bromocresol purple; CHX: Chlorhexidine digluconate; DDA: N-(3-aminopropyl)-N-dodécylpropane-1,3-diamine + didecyl dimethyl ammonium chloride; HMIMV: *Mohammed V military teaching hospital of Rabat*; ICUs: Intensive care units; NRP: Non registered; PVPI: Povidone-iodine

Acknowledgements
Not applicable.

Funding
No external funding was received for this study.

Authors' contributions
SL, UJ and ME designed the study, collected data and wrote the manuscript. MF, AL and LA were involved in the review of literature, AB and AM provided critical revision of the manuscript. JK participated in statistical analysis. All authors contributed to the interpretation of the results, the revision of the draft manuscript and approval of the final version.

Competing interests
The authors declare that they have no competing interests.

Consent for publication
Not applicable.

References
1. Peleg AY, Seifert H, Paterson DL. *Acinetobacter baumannii*: emergence of a successful pathogen. Clin Microbiol Rev. 2008;21(3):538.
2. Fournier PE, Richet H. The epidemiology and control of *Acinetobacter baumannii* in health care facilities. Clin Infect Dis. 2006;42(5):692–9.
3. Seifert H, Dijkshoorn L, Gerner-Smidt P, Pelzer N, Tjernberg I, Vaneechoutte M. Distribution of Acinetobacter species on human skin: comparison of phenotypic and genotypic identification methods. J Clin Microbiol. 1997;35:2819–25.
4. Berlau J, Aucken H, Malnick H, Pitt T. Distribution of *Acinetobacter* species on skin of healthy humans. Eur J Clin Microbiol Infect Dis. 1999;18(3):179–83.
5. Bergogne-Bérézin E, Towner KJ. *Acinetobacter spp.* as nosocomial pathogens: microbiological, clinical, and epidemiological features. Clin Microbiol Rev. 1996;9(2):148–65.
6. Gaynes R, Edwards JR, National Nosocomial Infections Surveillance System. Overview of nosocomial infections caused by gram-negative bacilli. Clin Infect Dis. 2005;41:848–54.
7. Wisplinghoff H, Bischoff T, Tallent SM, Seifert H, Wenzel RP, Edmond MB. Nosocomial bloodstream infections in US hospitals: analysis of 24,179 cases from a prospective nationwide surveillance study. Clin Infect Dis. 2004;39:309–17.
8. Uwingabiye J, Frikh M, Lemnouer A, Bssaibis F, Belefquih B, Maleb A, Dahraoui S, Belyamani L, Bait A, Haimeur C, Louzi L, Ibrahimi A, Elouennass M. Acinetobacter infections prevalence and frequency of the antibiotics resistance: comparative study of intensive care units versus other hospital units. Pan Afr Med J. 2016;23:191.
9. Rolain JM, Roch A, Castanier M, Papazian L, Raoult D. Acinetobacter baumannii resistant to colistin with impaired virulence: a case report from France. J Infect Dis. 2011;204:1146–7.
10. Elouennass M, Bajou T, Lemnouer AH, Foissaud V, Hervé V, Baaj AJ. Acinetobacter baumannii : étude de la sensibilité des souches isolées à l'hôpital militaire d'instruction Mohammed V, Rabat. Maroc Med Mal Infect. 2003;33:361–4.
11. Boyce JM, Pittet D, Healthcare Infection Control Practices Advisory Committee, HICPAC/SHEA/APIC/IDSA Hand Hygiene Task Force. Guideline for hand hygiene in health-care settings. Recommendations of the Healthcare Infection Control Practices Advisory Committee and the HICPAC/SHEA/APIC/IDSA Hand Hygiene Task Force. Society for Healthcare Epidemiology of America/Association for Professionals in Infection Control/Infectious Diseases Society of America. MMWR Recomm Rep. 2002;51(RR-16):1–45.
12. Saperkin N, Kovalishena O, Blagonravova A. P089: surveillance of bacterial resistance to disinfectants. Antimicrob Resist Infect Control. 2013;2 Suppl 1:89.
13. Cardoso CL, Pereira HH, Zequim JC, Guilhermetti M. Effectiveness of hand-cleansing agents for removing Acinetobacter baumannii strain from contaminated hands. Am J Infect Control. 1999;27:327–31.
14. Mama M, Abdissa A, Sewunet T. Antimicrobial susceptibility pattern of bacterial isolates from wound infection and their sensitivity to alternative topical agents at Jimma University specialized hospital, South-West Ethiopia. Ann Clin Microbiol Antimicrob. 2014;13:14.
15. Wisplinghoff H, Schmitt R, Wöhrmann A, Stefanik D, Seifert H. Resistance to disinfectants in epidemiologically defined clinical isolates of *Acinetobacter baumannii*. J Hosp Infect. 2007;66(2):174–81.
16. Chung YK, Kim JS, Lee SS, Lee JA, Kim HS, Shin KS, Park EY, Kang BS, Lee HJ, Kang HJ. Effect of daily chlorhexidine bathing on acquisition of carbapenem-resistant *Acinetobacter baumannii* (CRAB) in the medical intensive care unit with CRAB endemicity. Am J Infect Control. 2015;43(11):1171–7.
17. Catalano M, Quelle LS, Jeric PE, Di Martino A, Maimone SM. Survival of *Acinetobacter baumannii* on bed rails during an outbreak and during sporadic cases. J Hosp Infect. 1999;42:27–35.
18. Denton M, Wilcox MH, Parnell P, Green D, Keer V, Hawkey PM, Evans I, Murphy P. Role of environmental cleaning in controlling an outbreak of *Acinetobacter baumannii* on a neurosurgical intensive care unit. J Hosp Infect. 2004;56:106–10.
19. Smith K, Gemmell CG, Hunter IS. The association between biocide tolerance and the presence or absence of qac genes among hospital-acquired and community-acquired MRSA isolates. J Antimicrob Chemother. 2008;61(1):78–84.
20. Block BB. Peroxygen compounds. In: Block SS, editor. Disinfection, sterilization, and preservation. 4th ed. Philadelphia, Pa, USA: Lea & Febiger; 1991. p. 167.
21. Reichel M, Schlicht A, Ostermeyer C, Kampf G. Efficacy of surface disinfectant cleaners against emerging highly resistant gram-negative bacteria. BMC Infect Dis. 2014;14:292.
22. Gilbert P, McBain AJ. Potential impact of increased use of biocides in consumer products on prevalence of antibiotic resistance. Clin Microbiol Rev. 2003;16(2):189–208.

15

Alcohol-based hand rub and incidence of healthcare associated infections in a rural regional referral and teaching hospital in Uganda ('WardGel' study)

Hiroki Saito[1]* ⓘ, Kyoko Inoue[2], James Ditai[3], Benon Wanume[4], Julian Abeso[4], Jaffer Balyejussa[4] and Andrew Weeks[5]

Abstract

Background: Good hand hygiene (HH) practice is crucial to reducing healthcare associated infections (HAIs). Use of alcohol-based hand rub (ABHR) at health facilities is strongly recommended but it is limited in Uganda. Data on the practice of HH and the incidence of HAIs is sparse in resource-limited settings. We conducted a quasi-experimental study to evaluate HH practices of health care providers (HCPs) utilizing locally made ABHR and the incidence of HAIs.

Methods: HH compliance among HCPs and the incidence of HAIs were assessed at Mbale Regional Referral Hospital, a teaching hospital in rural Uganda. Inpatients from the obstetrics/gynecology (OBGYN), pediatric and surgical departments were enrolled on their day of admission and followed up during their hospital stay. The baseline (pre-intervention) phase of 12-weeks was followed by a 12-week intervention phase where training for HH practice was provided to all HCPs present on the target wards and ABHR was supplied on the wards. Incidence of HAIs and or Systemic Inflammatory Response Syndrome (SIRS) was measured and compared between the baseline and intervention phases. Multivariate survival analysis was performed to identify associated variables with HAIs/SIRS.

Results: A total of 3335 patients (26.3%) were enrolled into the study from a total of 12,665 admissions on the study wards over a 24-week period. HH compliance rate significantly improved from 9.2% at baseline to 56.4% during the intervention phase ($p < 0.001$). The incidence of HAIs/SIRS was not significantly changed between the baseline and intervention phases (incidence rate ratio (IRR) 1.07, 95% CI: 0.79 – 1.44). However, subgroup analyses showed significant reduction in HAIs/SIRS on the pediatric and surgical departments (IRR 0.21 (95% CI: 0.10 – 0.47) and IRR 0.39 (95% CI: 0.16 – 0.92), respectively) while a significant increase in HAIs/SIRS was found on the OBGYN department (IRR 2.99 (95% CI: 1.92 – 4.66)). Multivariate survival analysis showed a significant reduction in HAIs/SIRS with ABHR use on pediatric and surgical departments (adjusted hazard ratio 0.26 (95% CI: 0.15 – 0.45)).

Conclusions: To our knowledge, this study is one of the largest studies that address HAIs in Africa. During the 24-week study period, significant improvement in HH compliance was observed by providing training and ABHR. The intervention was associated with a significant reduction in HAIs/SIRS on the pediatric and surgical departments. Further research is warranted to integrate HAIs surveillance into routine practice and to identify measures to further prevent HAIs in resource limited settings.

Keywords: Healthcare epidemiology, Infection prevention and control, Alcohol-based hand rub

* Correspondence: saitohrk@bu.edu
1 Japan Ministry of Health, Labour and Welfare, Health Bureau, Tokyo, Japan
Full list of author information is available at the end of the article

Background

Hand hygiene (HH) is a basic yet critical practice to prevent healthcare associated infections (HAIs) [1]. However, studies have been conducted mostly in high-income countries and little is known about HH practice and HAIs in the resource limited settings [2]. Alcohol-based hand rub (ABHR) has been recommended over hand washing with soap and water by the World Health Organization (WHO) because of its wide microbiological spectrum, time efficiency, availability at the point of care, and improved skin tolerance [2]. Local production of ABHR has been shown to be feasible globally, even in low- and middle-income countries (LMICs) [3]. However, multiple other behavioral, cultural and religious factors also need to be considered in HH improvement programs.

The current high disease burden of HAIs and their preventability have led to a global emphasis on HAI prevention in the face of antimicrobial resistance as described in Global Health Security Agenda and WHO global action plan on antimicrobial resistance [4, 5]. In the USA, for example, HAI prevention has been included as one of the national health objectives [6]. However, the studies on HAIs from LMICs are limited, variable, and often of poor quality, and mainly focused on a single disease entity such as surgical site infection (SSI) [7–9]. Moreover, the association between HH improvement, especially with use of ABHR, and HAIs reduction has been rarely described in the resource limited setting. We therefore carried out a clinical study with the following aims in Uganda:

1. To assess the baseline HH practice among health care providers (HCPs) and the impact of ABHR and training in its use on the HH practice improvement
2. To determine the incidence of HAIs and the effectiveness of ABHR on the reduction of HAIs

Methods

Study design and setting

We conducted a quasi-experimental study (named as the 'WardGel' study) in which HH compliance and HAI rates were compared before and after the introduction of ABHR on 3 clinical departments in Mbale Regional Referral Hospital (MRRH), a government hospital in eastern Uganda. MRRH is one of the 14 governmental regional referral hospitals in Uganda, and serves over four million people in its catchment area of 15 local districts and beyond. The hospital has 12 wards with 550 beds. It also functions as a teaching hospital where there are 40 physicians (including interns), 170 nurses and students including medical students and nursing students. Before this study, ABHR was only used by a small number of senior HCPs such as nursing supervisors who carried portable ABHR bottles. This was mainly because

of financial constraints that prevented its purchase by the hospital. As such, ABHR use was almost non-existent prior to this study. Typically, only one or no functional sinks/taps were available in each ward. Portable water bottles and basins were an alternative for hand washing. Gloves, even non-sterile ones, were rarely available. A ward was usually a single, open space without isolation rooms. The hospital followed a standard operating procedure for general environmental cleaning, which was unchanged during the study period.

We selected five wards across three departments as the study sites, namely; the acute and general pediatric wards (pediatric department), the gynecology and post-natal wards (obstetrics/gynecology (OBGYN) department), and the general surgical ward (surgical department). The two pediatric wards were selected because evidence of the impact of ABHR on HAIs among pediatric patients has been particularly scarce in resource limited settings [7]. The latter three were selected because there were relatively few cases of infection on admission on those wards, and it was thought that HAIs would be more accurately observed than at other wards where febrile illnesses such as malaria were more common on admission. Overall, the study was designed so that a wide variety of the patients were observed for multiple types of HAIs to enhance generalisability of the study.

The study was conducted over 24 weeks between October 2014 and April 2015, with the first 12 weeks of the baseline (pre-intervention) phase followed by 12 weeks of the intervention phase. There was a 4-week study interruption between December 2014 and January 2015 (after week 8) due to the holiday seasons in Uganda when the number of inpatients and HCPs were low. Inclusion criteria for the study were all the patients who were admitted on the above selected wards during the study period (hospital day 1 = day of admission).

During the baseline phase, the HH compliance rate among HCPs was assessed by direct observations performed by the trained research assistants on the wards, based on the WHO hand hygiene technical reference manual and the WHO five moments for HH, i.e. before touching a patient, before clean/aseptic procedure, after body fluid exposure risk, after touching a patient, and after touching patient surroundings [2]. Each trained research assistant on each ward observed HCPs during the day-times only for targeted ward activities including busy times such as ward rounds by physicians. The research assistants conducted observations openly, without interfering with the ongoing clinical work, but kept the identity of the HCP confidential, observing up to a maximum of three HCPs simultaneously provided there were no missing opportunities. One observation session lasted for 10-30 min; and only prolonged the sessions in situations of observing a care sequence to its end.

The HH compliance was calculated by the number of observed HH actions (using either ABHR or hand washing with soap and water) upon an opportunity divided by the total number of opportunities for HH actions. The amount of ABHR consumption from non-portable bottles was assessed as a supplemental indication for HH compliance through ABHR. The incidence of HAIs was also measured during the baseline phase through prospective follow-up of patients by research assistants (see below).

During the intervention phase, in addition to the study activities performed during the baseline phase, the one-litre ABHR bottles fitted in a locally-made metallic holder were mounted on the walls of the wards where the access to ABHR was thought to be convenient. Mobile bottles were also placed on the trolleys for ward rounds, on the reception area, and on the treatment area. Portable 40 ml hand-sized bottles were also provided to HCPs and kept available throughout the intervention phase. The ABHR used in the study was Alsoft V, ABHR locally made from sugar cane in Uganda by Saraya East Africa Co. Ltd. It manufactured locally, but according to international standards (Good Manufacturing Practice), and contained the recommended concentration of ethanol (76.9 to 81.4 vol%) [2, 10, 11]. An introductory training session on ABHR use was provided to all the HCPs on the target wards by the research team in week 12 with the help of staff trainers from Saraya East Africa Co. Ltd. In order to maintain the HH compliance, the introductory training was followed by the distribution of educational posters on HH in week 17 and follow-up training in week 18. Additional training was also conducted as required when new medical students and nursing students came to the wards. As the first training session was provided in the last week of the baseline phase, patients who were hospitalized in week 12 and week 13 were excluded from the final analysis of the incidence of HAIs to minimize study contamination between the baseline and the intervention phases.

For the assessments, a paper-based surveillance form was created to record demographics, patient interventions (e.g. surgical interventions), vital signs, clinical findings, antibiotic use and patient's outcomes. SSIs, urinary tract infections (UTIs), pneumonia, central nervous system (CNS) infections, gastroenteritis and episiotomy infections were selected as the HAIs measured in this study. Each definition of HAIs was modified from the 2014 version of United States Center for Disease Control and Prevention's National Healthcare Safety Network (CDC/NHSN) surveillance definitions of HAIs, considering locally available resources [12]. Research assistants (mainly registered nurses but

with one physician) were trained to fill out the surveillance form, to measure vital signs, to identify relevant clinical signs from patients' medical records, and to record laboratory and imaging findings. After enrollment into the study, the patients were prospectively followed on a daily basis until discharge. Post-discharge follow-up calls were also attempted for all the patients around 1 month after their discharge. Individual patients' data collected from patients' medical records and vital signs measured by the research assistants were also reviewed by research supervisor for quality assurance of the data. All the data collected on the paper-based forms were entered into an Epi Info® database installed onto computers at the Sanyu Africa Research Institute (SAfRI). The only exception was the HH compliance data that was entered into the WHO-produced Microsoft Word® data collection sheet for analysis [13].

Outcomes

The primary outcomes were the HH compliance rates among HCPs and the incidence rates of HAIs before and after the intervention. The secondary outcomes included antibiotic usage, length of hospital stay and hospital mortality of the study participants.

During the run-in period, it was noted that medical documentation by physicians and clinical officers was not always sufficient to make a diagnosis of an HAI as defined for this study. Direct questioning of the physicians and clinical officers involved with the patient management was also difficult due to their busy schedule and difficulty in recall given the large volume of patients seen per physician. There was therefore a post-hoc change in the primary outcome from HAIs only to the composite outcome of HAIs and or criteria for systemic inflammatory response syndrome (SIRS) occurring on hospital day 3 or after (SIRS/HAI) (c.f. SIRS criteria for adult patients, two or more of: 1. temperature > 38 °C or <36 °C, 2. heart rate > 90/min, 3. respiratory rate > 20/min or $Paco_2$ < 32 mmHg, 4. white blood cell (WBC) count >12,000/mm^3 or <4000/mm^3 or >10% immature bands. SIRS criteria for pediatric patients, two or more of the same four items with variable thresholds for age, at least one of which must be temperature or WBC) [14, 15]. Those with SIRS on hospital day 1 or 2 of their hospital stay were excluded from the composite primary outcome. $Paco_2$ and WBC were rarely performed at MRRH, therefore vital signs measured by research staff were mostly used to determine whether SIRS criteria was met or not.

Statistical analysis

Means, standard deviations (SD) with t-tests, and proportions with chi-squared tests were calculated for continuous and categorical variables in bivariate analyses, respectively, in order to describe demographics and clinical variables of the study participants. Poisson regression analysis was used to compare HH compliance rates before and after the intervention. Linear regression analysis was used to compare HH compliance rate and ABHR consumption during the intervention. Relative risks and incidence rate ratios of SIRS/HAI were also calculated to compare risks and incidence rates before and after the intervention, respectively. Survival analyses with the cox proportional hazard model were performed to calculate hazard ratios (HRs) in order to describe the associated variables for SIRS/HAI. Multivariate survival analysis with backward selection and plausible causal interpretation was used to calculate adjusted HRs. Statistical significance was defined as a p value of <0.05 and 95% confidence intervals (CIs) were reported. All statistical analysis was conducted using Statistical Analysis System (SAS®) version 9.3 (SAS Institute, Cary, NC, USA).

There was no formal HAI rate reported in Uganda that we could use for the sample size calculation. We therefore used the WHO data for developing countries to estimate that 10% of the hospitalized patients would develop any type of HAI [16]. We estimated a 3% reduction in HAIs after the intervention. With the level of significance defined as α = 0.05, and statistical power as β = 0.80, we estimated 1356 patients each would be required before and after the intervention.

Role of the funding source

The study was conducted with funding provided by Saraya East Africa Co. Ltd., who also provided the ABHR made at their local factory in Uganda. Their staff helped the research team conduct HH training on the wards. Otherwise, the funder was not involved in the study design, data collection, data analysis, data interpretation, or manuscript writing.

The study was approved by the Mbale Regional Hospital Institutional Review Committee (MRHIRC)(REIRC IN – COM 098/2014) and registered to ClinicalTrials.gov (NCT02435719).

Results

Hand hygiene compliance

In total, 7102 HH opportunities were observed (3770 and 3332 opportunities in baseline and intervention phases, respectively). HH compliance rate remained very low for most of the baseline weeks (Fig. 1). The overall compliance rate from week 1 to week 9 was 4.6%. During week 10, a neonatal unit was opened in one section of the pediatric wards. As part of that initiative, the pediatricians provided HH education (without ABHR provision). All staff on the unit were requested to wash their hands with soap and water before entering the neonatal unit and touching the patients. In addition, educational posters were placed at the entrance and the patient registration area of the unit. As a result, the HH compliance rate rose on the pediatric wards, starting with an increased rate in week 10. There is evidence that there was higher compliance elsewhere in the hospital with the surgical department also showing higher rates starting in week 10. During week 12, when the introductory HH training was provided along with portable ABHR bottles for HCPs by our study group, the HH

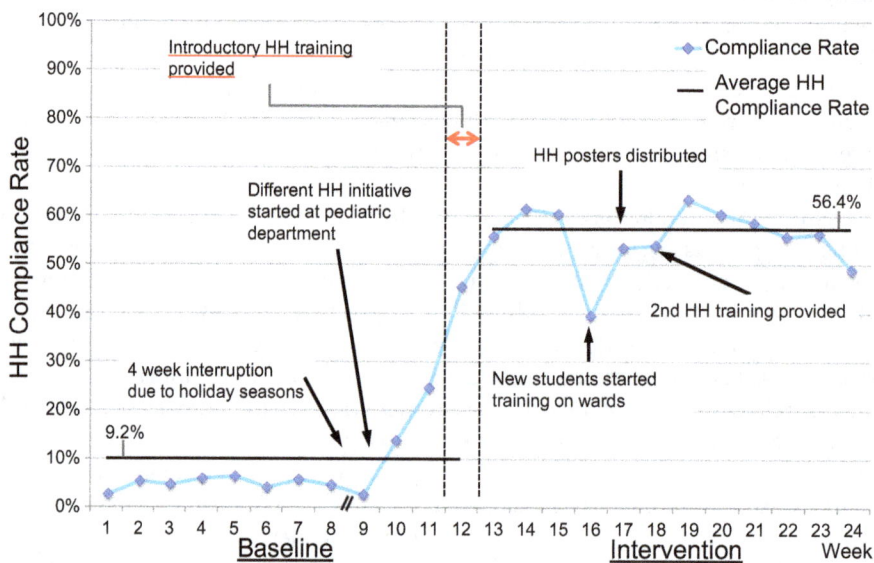

Fig. 1 Overall Hand Hygiene (HH) Compliance Before and After Intervention. x-axis: study week (Week 1-12: Baseline, Week 13-24: Intervention). y-axis: HH compliance rate (%). light blue line: HH compliance rate

compliance rate continued to rise steadily. The average HH compliance rate during the intervention phase (week 13 through 24) was significantly higher compared with that during the baseline (56.4% vs. 9.2%, rate difference 47.2, 95% CI 44.5-50.0, $p < 0.001$ (Poisson regression)). During the intervention phase, the HH compliance rate dropped once in week 16 when a large group of new medical students and nursing students started clinical rotations on the wards. The effect was seen amongst the new students, but also seen in other cadres of staff during that week. However, the rate increased after the posters for HH promotion and second HH training were provided during week 17 and 18, respectively, and remained at the similar level thereafter. The HH compliance rates by department during the intervention phase were 75.9% at the pediatric department, 54.4% at the surgical department, and 44.1% at the OBGYN department, respectively ($p < 0.001$ (chi-square)), and the HH compliance rate during the intervention phase was significantly lower at the OBGYN department than the other departments (44.1% vs. 67.6%, rate difference 23.5%, 95% CI 20.3-26.8, $p < 0.001$ (chi-square)) (Fig. 2). The HH compliance rates by profession during the intervention phase were 66.0% among nurses, 61.0% among physicians, 51.5% among midwives, 50.6% among students, and 46.9% among nurse assistants, respectively (p < 0.001 (chi-square); Fig. 3). During the intervention phase, the amount of ABHR consumption from non-portable bottles attached on the wards was measured. There was no significant linear correlation between HH compliance rate and

ABHR consumption ($r = -0.27$, $p = 0.39$ (Pearson correlation)).

Baseline characteristics of the study participants

There were 12,665 admissions across the selected five wards during the entire study period. From these, a total of 3335 patients (26.3%) were enrolled into the study, excluding those who were hospitalized in study weeks 12 and 13 from the analyses. Enrollment of patients into the study was limited by the availability of research staff who only attended the wards once a day to collect data. Those patients who were admitted and discharged between their visits were therefore missed by the data collectors. The 1723 (51.7%) adult patients had a mean age of 29.7 years whilst the 1612 (48.3%) pediatric patient had a mean age of 3.9 years (Table 1). Patients in the OBGYN department composed 47.8% of the study patients with the post-natal ward being the largest of the five wards studied. During their hospitalization 2286 (68.6%), 573 (17.3%), and 873 patients (26.3%) received antibiotic therapy, urinary catheter placement, and surgery respectively. Two hundred ten patients (6.3%) required mechanical ventilation, but virtually all of these (208; 99.0%) required it peri-operatively on the day of surgery only. Although there were relatively few pediatric patients and an excess of surgical patients enrolled into the study during the intervention phase, the rest of the patient characteristics were comparable between the baseline and intervention phases (Table 1).

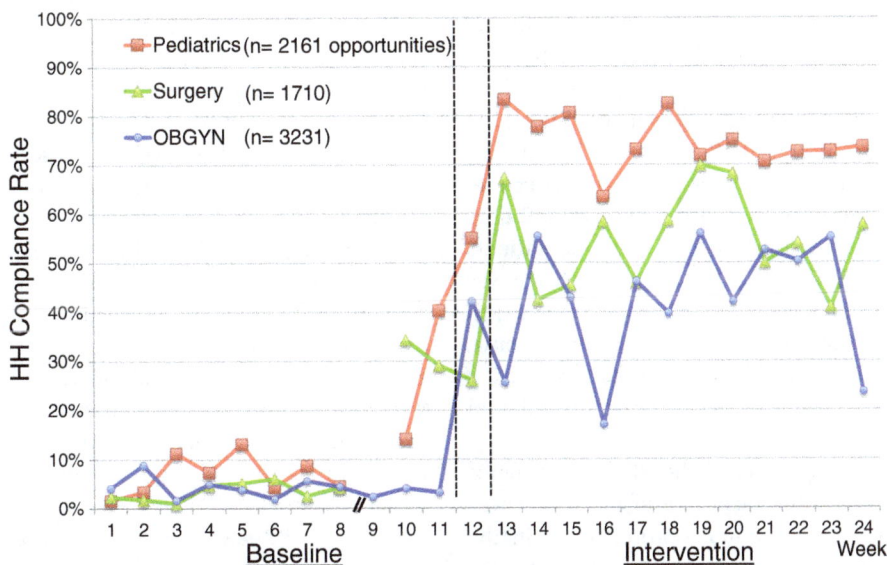

Fig. 2 Hand Hygiene (HH) Compliance by Department. x-axis: study week (Week 1-12: Baseline, Week 13-24: Intervention). y-axis: HH compliance rate (%). red line: Pediatrics. green line: Surgery. blue line: OBGYN

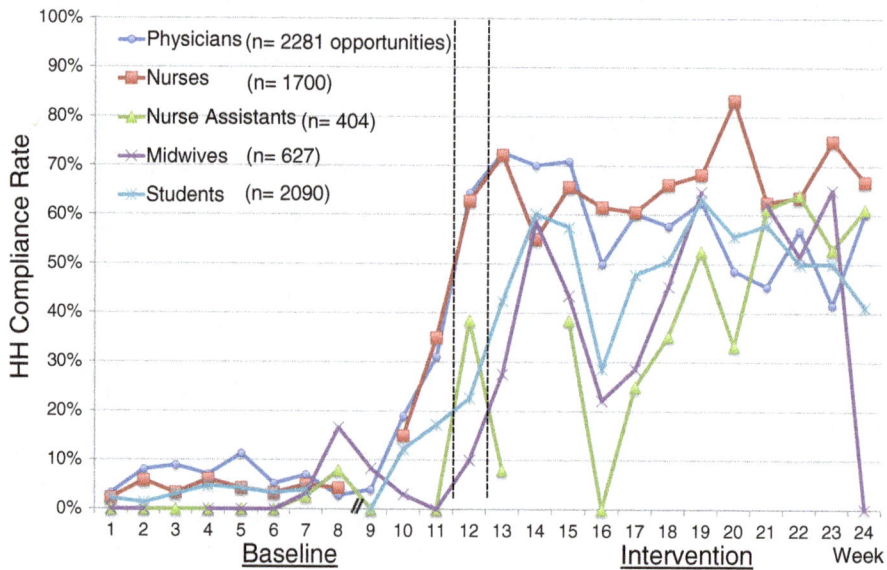

Fig. 3 Hand Hygiene (HH) Compliance by Profession. x-axis: study week (Week 1-12: Baseline, Week 13-24: Intervention). y-axis: HH compliance rate (%). blue line: Physicians. red line: Nurses. green line: Nurse Assistants. purple line: Midwives. light blue line: Students

Healthcare associated infections

There were 95 (5.1%) and 87 (5.9%) patients who were diagnosed as having HAIs and or met the SIRS criteria during the baseline and intervention phases, respectively (relative risk (RR) of 1.14, 95% CL 0.86-1.51, $p = 0.37$; Table 2). Among the total 182 patients with SIRS/HAI during the whole study period, 178 patients (97.8%) met SIRS criteria whilst 20 patients (11.0%) were diagnosed with at least one of HAIs. Only 4 had a diagnosis of HAIs without meeting the SIRS criteria. The most commonly diagnosed HAI was SSI (12 patients, 0.4%), followed by pneumonia (8 patients, 0.2%), gastroenteritis (1 patient) and episiotomy infection (1 patient). UTI and CNS infections were not diagnosed. The median hospital day of SIRS/HAI incidence was day 3 (range 3-17) whilst the median post-operative day (POD) of SIRS/HAI incidence was day 2 (range 0-12, $n = 100$). For the 87 patients who had a urinary catheter placed and later met the SIRS criteria, SIRS was identified a median of 2 days after catheter placement (range 0-11). Fifty-one patients (58.6%) had a urinary catheter in place when SIRS was identified. For 33 patients who received mechanical ventilation and later developed SIRS and or pneumonia, the incidence of SIRS and or pneumonia occurred a median of 2 days after the start of mechanical ventilation (range 1-9).

When stratified by departments, the RR and incidence rate ratio (IRR) showed the incidence of SIRS/HAI was significantly lower during the intervention phase in the pediatric and surgical departments whilst the incidence rose significantly in the OBGYN department (Table 2). The incidence of SIRS/HAI per surgery was also lower

in the surgical department during the intervention phase (RR 0.38, 95% CI 0.12-1.18, $p = 0.10$) while it was increased in the OBGYN department (RR 3.14, 95% CI 2.05-4.82, $p < 0.01$). On the other hand, the incidence of SIRS in those with a urinary catheter and the incidence of SIRS and or pneumonia in those who had mechanical ventilation were both significantly higher during the intervention in the OBGYN department (RR for SIRS in those with a urinary catheter 3.18, 95% CI 2.02-5.00, $p < 0.01$; and RR for SIRS and or pneumonia in those receiving mechanical ventilation 3.30, 95% CI 1.35-8.08, $p < 0.01$, respectively) while those at the surgical department were not significantly changed (RR for SIRS per urinary catheter use 2.11, 95% CI 0.35-12.67, $p = 0.30$; and RR for SIRS and or pneumonia per mechanical ventilation 0.28, 95% CI 0.05-1.61, $p = 0.16$, respectively).

Bivariate survival analysis to describe the associated variables for SIRS/HAI showed no overall statistical association between the intervention and the SIRS/HAI incidence (HR 1.10, 95% CI 0.83-1.48, $p = 0.50$; Table 3), but multivariate analysis stratified by department showed the intervention was significantly associated with the lower SIRS/HAI incidence at the pediatric and surgical departments (adjusted HR 0.26, 95% CI 0.15-0.45, $p < 0.01$), after adjusting for gender and occurrence of surgery. Conversely, the intervention was significantly associated with increased SIRS/HAI incidence at OBGYN department (adjusted HR 3.10, 95% CI 1.98-4.84, $p < 0.01$), after adjusting for occurrence of surgery, prior antibiotic use (including antibiotic prophylaxis for those who received surgery) and mechanical ventilation, the latter two of

Table 1 Characteristics of enrolled patients

	All n (%)	Baseline n (%)	Intervention n (%)	p value
Number of patients enrolled	3335	1848 (55.4)	1487 (44.6)	
Adult	1723 (51.7)	898 (48.6)	825 (55.5)	<0.01
Female	2369 (71.0)	1290 (69.8)	1079 (72.6)	0.08
Mean age among adult patients, (SD), y	29.7 (12.6)	29.4 (11.9)	30.1 (13.3)	0.21
Mean age among pediatric patients, (SD), y	3.9 (5.0)	3.8 (5.0)	4.1 (4.9)	0.24
Department				
OBGYN	1595 (47.8)	854 (46.2)	741 (49.8)	<0.01
Pediatrics	1336 (40.1)	814 (44.1)	522 (35.1)	
Surgery	404 (12.1)	180 (9.7)	224 (15.1)	
Ward				
Post-natal	1139 (34.1)	621 (33.6)	518 (34.8)	<0.01
Gynecology	456 (13.7)	233 (12.6)	223 (15.0)	
General pediatrics	669 (20.1)	359 (19.4)	310 (20.8)	
Acute pediatric unit	667 (20.0)	455 (24.6)	212 (14.3)	
Surgery	404 (12.1)	180 (9.8)	224 (15.1)	
Living in rural region	2634 (79.0)	1455 (78.8)	1179 (79.3)	0.74
Education (adult patients only)				
None	786 (45.7)	401 (44.8)	385 (46.7)	0.28
Primary	605 (35.1)	313 (34.9)	292 (35.4)	
Secondary	255 (14.8)	135 (15.1)	120 (14.5)	
Tertiary	75 (4.4)	47 (5.2)	28 (3.4)	
Antibiotic use	2286 (68.6)	1290 (69.8)	996 (67.0)	0.08
Mean length of antibiotic use (SD), d	2.4 (2.6)	2.2 (2.1)	2.7 (3.1)	<0.01
Urinary catheter use	573 (17.3)	323 (17.6)	250 (16.9)	0.58
Mean length of urinary catheter use, (SD), d	2.3 (3.8)	1.3 (1.4)	3.5 (5.2)	<0.01
Mechanical ventilation Use	210 (6.3)	78 (4.3)	132 (8.9)	<0.01
Mean length of mechanical ventilation use, (SD), d	0.0 (0.1)	0.0 (0.2)	0.0 (0.0)	0.07
Surgery performed	873 (26.3)	491 (26.8)	382 (25.7)	0.51
Major surgery	611 (70.0)	339 (69.0)	272 (71.2)	0.49
General anesthesia	324 (37.3)	159 (32.7)	165 (43.3)	<0.01
Prophylaxis antibiotic use	800 (91.6)	443 (90.2)	357 (93.5)	0.09

which were considered confounders for occurrence of surgery.

The incidence of SIRS/HAI was significantly associated with higher hospital mortality (RR11.55, 95% CI 4.78-27.93, p < 0.01), longer length of hospital stay (mean difference 3.8 days, 95% CI 3.4-4.2, p < 0.01), and longer duration of antibiotic use (mean difference 2.3 days, 95% CI 1.9-2.7, p < 0.01)(Table 4).

During the entire study period, there were only 14 blood cultures sent (0.4% of the total 3335 enrolled patients), 12 swab wound cultures sent (0.3%), and one X-ray performed. Other relevant laboratory and imaging tests such as urine cultures and gram stain of cerebrospinal fluid were never performed.

Discussion

HAIs are a serious but often overlooked problem in many LMICs. Introduction of locally made ABHR with HH education significantly improved HH practice at this regional teaching hospital in rural Uganda, leading to a significant reduction in the incidence of HAIs and or SIRS on the pediatric and surgical services. In contrast, however, there was an increase in SIRS/HAI on the OBGYN wards. The incidence of SIRS/HAI was found to be associated with adverse clinical outcomes such as higher hospital mortality, longer length of hospital stay and longer length of antibiotic use. We believe therefore that ABHR use with improved HH practice can have a significant impact both at the individual level for

Table 2 Incidence of systemic inflammatory response syndrome (SIRS) and healthcare associated infections (HAIs)

	All n (%) (N = 3335)	Baseline n (%) (N = 1848)	Intervention n (%) (N = 1487)	Relative risk (RR) or incidence rate ratio (IRR) (95% CI, p value)
SIRS incidence since hospital day 3 and/or HAIs diagnosed	182 (5.5)	95 (5.1)	87 (5.9)	1.14 (0.86-1.51, 0.37)
OBGYN	99 (6.2)	27 (3.2)	72 (9.7)	3.07 (2.00-4.73, <0.01)
Pediatrics	58 (4.3)	51 (6.3)	7 (1.3)	0.21 (0.10-0.47, <0.01)
Surgery	25 (6.2)	17 (9.4)	8 (3.6)	0.38 (0.17-0.86, 0.01)
SIRS criteria met	178 (5.4)	91 (5.0)	87 (5.8)	1.18 (0.89-1.57, 0.25)
Diagnoses of HAIs made	20 (0.6)	13 (0.7)	7 (0.5)	0.67 (0.27-1.67, 0.39)
Surgical site infection[a]	12 (0.4)	6 (0.3)	6 (0.4)	1.24 (0.40-3.84, 0.71)
Pneumonia[a]	8 (0.2)	8 (0.4)	0 (0.0)	0 (, 0.01)
Gastroenteritis[a]	1 (0.03)	1 (0.05)	0 (0.0)	0 (, 0.55)
Episiotomy infection[a]	1 (0.03)	1 (0.05)	0 (0.0)	0 (, 0.55)
Incidence rate of SIRS/HAI (cases/1000 patient-days)	18.0	17.4	18.6	1.07 (0.79–1.44, 0.66)
OBGYN	25.6	13.4	40.1	2.99 (1.92–4.66, <0.01)
Pediatrics	15.0	21.7	4.6	0.21 (0.10–0.47, <0.01)
Surgery	10.2	15.8	6.2	0.39 (0.16–0.92, 0.02)
SIRS/HAI incidence per 100 surgeries (n = 873)	11.5	7.5	16.5	2.19 (1.49-3.21, <0.01)
OBGYN (n = 639)	13.5	7.2	22.5	3.14 (2.05-4.82, <0.01)
Surgery (n = 234)	6.0	8.8	3.3	0.38 (0.12-1.18, 0.10)
SIRS incidence per 100 urinary catheter use (n = 573)	14.8	7.7	24.0	3.10 (2.00-4.80, <0.01)
OBGYN (n = 545)	14.9	7.6	24.1	3.18 (2.02-5.00, <0.01)
Surgery (n = 28)	14.3	10.5	22.2	2.11 (0.35-12.67, 0.30)
SIRS/pneumonia incidence per 100 mechanical ventilation (n = 210)[b]	15.7	11.5	18.2	1.58 (0.77-3.22, 0.20)
OBGYN (n = 112)	24.1	10.4	34.4	3.30 (1.35-8.08, <0.01)
Surgery (n = 97)	5.2	10.3	2.9	0.28 (0.05-1.61, 0.16)

[a] Multiple diagnoses are possible for each individual
[b] Includes one case each who had mechanical ventilation without surgery at pediatric and OGBYN departments

patients' health and at the hospital level in resource limited settings where hospitals are commonly overcrowded and drug supplies are limited and unstable.

Our study showed the baseline HH compliance was only 9.2%, lower than previous studies that reported 16.5%, 12%, and 34.1% in the hospital setting in Ethiopia, Ghana and Rwanda, respectively, though there were some differences in the methods used to measure HH compliance rate [17–19]. Before the start of the neonatal unit on the pediatric wards, the HH compliance was as low as 4.6%, implying the HH practice was almost nonexistent at worst. However, the ABHR provision and HH education significantly improved the HH compliance to 56.4%, peaking at 75.9% in the pediatric department. A cross-sectional study conducted in Ethiopia showed that the knowledge of HH and availability of ABHR on the ward were associated with better HH practice [17]. Our study confirmed their findings in a quasi-experimental model and showed that impressive improvements in HH are possible through ABHR provision and HH education: we found a 6-fold increase in the HH compliance

rate from under 10%. The different HH initiative that started at the pediatric department during our baseline phase accidentally provided an interesting insight: that HH education alone, without ABHR provision, also improved the HH compliance in all departments. In our study, ABHR use was not differentiated from hand washing with soap and water when the compliance rate was measured. Interestingly, the chief surgeon and nurse in the surgical department started using the water basin during inpatient rounds after the hospital infection-prevention committee suggested it, as follow-up from the pediatric initiative. It was also observed that once HCPs began to use ABHR properly on the wards, they remarked that the smell on the wards improved and the number of flies flying around admitted patients on the bed reduced. This led to HCPs encouraging one another to HH practice, and provided the senior nurses with further motivation to promote HH in the ward areas. Thus, the presence of the right champions along with effective HH education can influence the culture and behavior of HCPs beyond the intervention area.

Table 3 Patient characteristics associated with systemic inflammatory response syndrome (SIRS) and healthcare associated infections (HAIs)

	Hazard ratio (HR) of SIRS/HAI (95% CI, p value)	Adjusted HR (95% CI, p value)	
		Pediatrics or Surgery (n = 1740)	OBGYN (n = 1595)
Alcohol based hand gel provision and hand hygiene promotion (intervention)	1.10 (0.83-1.48, 0.50)	0.26 (0.15-0.45, <0.01)	3.10 (1.98-4.84, <0.01)
Adult	1.64 (1.22-2.20, <0.01)		a
Female	2.11 (1.49-3.00, <0.01)	1.43 (0.93-2.20, 0.11)	a
Age among adult patients, y	0.99 (0.98-1.01, 0.24)		
Age among pediatric patients, y	1.02 (0.97-1.06, 0.47)		
Pediatrics/Surgery (vs. OBGYN)	0.40 (0.30-0.54, <0.01)	a	a
Living in rural region	1.01 (0.70–1.46, 0.94)		
Education – none (adult patients only)	0.93 (0.63-1.35, 0.69)		
Surgery performed prior to SIRS/HAI	1.80 (1.34-2.41, <0.01)	0.57 (0.31-1.04, 0.07)	1.42 (0.75-3.00, 0.28)
Antibiotic used prior to SIRS/HAI	1.85 (1.05–3.25, 0.03)		4.99 (1.47-16.98, 0.01)
Urinary catheter used prior to SIRS/HAI	2.63 (1.96-3.53, <0.01)		
Mechanical ventilation used prior to SIRS/HAI	1.59 (1.09-2.34, 0.02)		1.53 (0.97-2.42, 0.07)

[a]Variables were not used because they were completely discrete in the models

Furthermore our study showed the HH compliance rate was improved more among nurses and physicians, and this finding was favorable given that those clinical staff, who are recognized as a senior, can have a powerful influence on the rest of the HCPs [20]. The final extent of the education-only improvements is not known as the ABHR provision started shortly afterwards and resulted in further improved HH across the wards.

The ABHR was widely distributed around the wards according to the HCPs' wishes. This included placing it in dispensers on the walls and on the trolleys for ward rounds. Even though the amount of ABHR consumption from non-portable bottles was not associated with compliance rate during the intervention, it is possible that the portable bottles provided to each member of the clinical staff were more convenient and more often used than the static bottles as the biggest increase in HH compliance was observed in week 12 when the portable bottles were provided. The HH compliance rate was the highest at the pediatric department where our informal follow-up interviews suggested better ABHR "buy-in" from the staff. On the other hand, the HH compliance rate dropped regardless of profession on week 16 when new students started clinical rotations. It was observed that many HCPs were much busier teaching and supervising the new students, giving lower priority to the HH practice. Therefore, in this setting, it appears to be easy to compromise HH practice early in the implementation when it has yet to become established practice. During the intervention, it was noted that the improved HH practice was mostly due to ABHR use. This suggests that knowledge and attitude alone may be insufficient, and that it is critical to have good access to a product for HH such as ABHR bottles. This is particularly important in resource limited settings where water, soap or clean towels to dry hands may not be available on wards.

With the improvements in HH practice through ABHR provision and HH education, a lower incidence of HAIs and or SIRS was observed in the pediatric and surgical departments. Even though the incidence of this composite outcome was mainly explained by SIRS rather than HAIs, the incidence was significantly associated with critical clinical outcomes such as higher hospital mortality, implying that the obtainment of accurate vital signs by trained

Table 4 Clinical outcomes associated with systemic inflammatory response syndrome (SIRS) and healthcare associated infections (HAIs)

	All n (%) (N = 3335)	SIRS/HAI n (%) (N = 182)	No SIRS/HAI n (%) (N = 3153)	Relative risk (RR) (95% CI, p value) or p value of t-test
Hospital mortality	20 (0.6)	8 (4.4)	12 (0.4)	11.55 (4.78-27.93, <0.01)
Left against medical advice	395 (11.8)	17 (9.3)	378 (12.0)	0.78 (0.49-1.24, 0.28)
Mean length of stay, (SD), d	2.7 (3.0)	6.3 (6.7)	2.5 (2.5)	<0.01
Mean length of antibiotic use, (SD), d (n = 2286)	2.4 (2.6)	4.5 (5.6)	2.2 (2.1)	<0.01

staff and identifying SIRS correctly could serve as an intermediate variable when a formal surveillance system of HAIs is not established or reliable.

Surprisingly, our study found that the incidence of HAIs and or SIRS was increased in the OBGYN department following the intervention. There are several possible explanations for this finding. First, construction/partitioning work for the neonatal unit establishment started on part of the post-natal ward on week 13, leading to a higher patient throughput in the rest of the ward. This led to many mothers having to sleep on the floor or in the corridors in the overcrowded environment, which could have potentially exposed many of these mothers to infections. Second, the new interns started clinical rotations in the OBGYN department on week 13, and started learning basic OBGYN skills such as cesarean section. Our intervention didn't cover labor room where vaginal deliveries are performed, or the OBGYN operating room. Therefore, other important preventative measures, such as good aseptic technique during deliveries or surgery might have been suboptimal and may be areas for improvement in the future. Third, HH compliance in the OBGYN department was significantly lower than in the other two departments, and this could account for the lack of positive effect. Sick leave in several of the head midwives during this period resulted in a lack of overall leadership and support, and this is likely to have contributed to the low compliance rate. These factors clearly demonstrate how the ward provision of ABHR and HH education is not enough on its own to prevent all infections. It needs to be provided alongside clinical leadership, good personal hygiene in the operating and labor rooms, as well as good overall hospital space, facilities and cleanliness to reduce the overall infection risk.

Even though this large study provides further insights into ABHR use and HAIs in the resource limited setting, there are several study limitations. First, this study was conducted at a single location with a simple before-and-after design, mainly due to the financial constraints. However, MRRH has a large catchment area as a referral hospital, and the studied population is considered to be representative of the population of eastern Uganda. Longer monitoring of HH compliance, even after the intervention was stopped, could have provided further insight. Second, the HH compliance rate was measured through direct observation by the research staff. This is likely to have caused spontaneous improvements in practice, also known as the Hawthorne effect [21]. This is a bias resulting from a change in behavior of observed study participants leading to improved outcomes. However, direct observation is still considered the gold standard for monitoring HH practice [2]. The lack of a significant association between ABHR consumption

from non-portable bottles and observed HH compliance suggests that measuring product consumption may not be an effective way to measure HH compliance. Third, our composite outcome mostly relied on the incidence of SIRS. There was no standardized surveillance system for HAIs at MRRH, and physicians' and clinical officers' documentation was often of insufficient quality to make an accurate diagnosis of HAIs. Our research assistants were capable of measuring accurate vital signs to identify SIRS incidence after training, but for them to assess additional clinical findings would have required further training and would have been impractical given the large patient volume. Patients with HAIs may not always develop abnormal vital signs to meet SIRS, and the SIRS incidence on hospital day 3 may not necessarily result from HAIs. However, our study revealed a clear association between SIRS/HAI and more clinically important clinical outcomes such as mortality and length of hospital stay. We therefore consider the composite outcome to be a practical and realistic measure of HAI in resource-limited settings. An impact of a recent change in the definition of sepsis by Third International Consensus Definitions Task Force (Sepsis-3) including utility of quick Sequential [Sepsis-related] Organ Failure Assessment (qSOFA) score for non-intensive care unit patients on diagnosis and treatment of HAIs in the resource limited setting would merit further research as the study, which was conducted in USA, showed qSOFA was a superior predictor of mortality to SIRS [22–24]. Fourth, the study was further compromised by the low use of laboratory and imaging studies for the accurate diagnosis of HAIs. A study in the USA showed that empiric antibiotic therapy was common even when there were no clinical signs of infections, and that obtaining cultures and imaging were associated with narrowing or discontinuation of antibiotics [25]. This requires increased funding into laboratory services, as well as a change in culture of clinical staff. However, it is critical if the world-wide problem of antimicrobial resistance is to be overcome [5, 25]. Fifth, it was very difficult to conduct follow-up of patients post-discharge given the large catchment area and the limited financial resources for the patients. As a re-visit to the hospital for follow-up was logistically difficult for most, we attempted telephone follow-up. However, some phone contacts were not available and in some, the calls went through to family members who were away from the individual patient. The limited successful follow-up calls suggested that some post-operative patients might have developed SSI after discharge, but the other HAIs were difficult to assess by phone alone. This, and the multiple other sources of community infection, led us to focus on the more immediate outcomes that occurred around the time of hospitalization. This was thought to be a more reliable way to assess the impact of our study intervention. Sixth, we did not provide feedback to HCPs, or involve patients and or family members in HH promotion. These interventions could potentially have further improved HH practice among HCPs [26–28]. In addition, HH among patients' family members may play a role in HAI incidence, particularly in the setting where they are more involved in patients' care at health facilities. Lastly, we did not incorporate formal qualitative research into our study. This would have helped to explain some of the facilitators and barriers to ABHR use that affected the success of the intervention. We relied instead on field notes collected by the research staff.

Conclusion

Our study showed that improved HH practice is feasible in resource limited settings and that provision of locally made ABHR and HH education can result in reduced rates of HAIs, especially if there is effective clinical leadership. However, it needs to be seen within a broad context and is unlikely to be effective unless preventive measures are taken within operating and labor rooms, and the problem of hospital hygiene and overcrowding is addressed.

Abbreviations

ABHR: Alcohol-based hand rub; CDC/NHSN: United States Center for Disease Control and Prevention's National Healthcare Safety Network; CI: Confidence interval; CNS: Central nervous system; HAI: Healthcare associated infection; HCP: Health care provider; HH: Hand hygiene; HR: Hazard ratio; IRR: Incidence rate ratio; LMICs: Low- and middle- income countries; MRRH: Mbale Regional Referral Hospital; OBGYN: Obstetrics/gynecology; POD: Post-operative day; qSOFA: quick sequential [Sepsis-related] organ failure assessment; RR: Relative risk; SAfRI: Sanyu Africa Research Institute; SIRS: Systemic inflammatory response syndrome; SSI: Surgical site infection; UTI: Urinary tract infection; WBC: White blood cell; WHO: World Health Organization

Acknowledgements

We acknowledge the following data clerks (Macreen Mudoola, Emily Nasiyo, Rose Wataka and Grace Abongo), research assistants (Winfred Mutaki, Takali Sylvia, Christine Limio, Ekido Lossira, Rosemary Lunyolo, Proscovia Auma, Florence Ouchi, Bumba Ebyesali and Michael Maweda) who ensured smooth data collection.
The views presented here belong to the author HS and do not reflect the views of the organization.

Funding

The study was conducted with funding provided by Saraya East Africa Co. Ltd., who also provided the ABHR made at their local factory in Uganda. Their staff helped the research team conduct HH training on the wards. Otherwise, the funder was not involved in the study design, data collection, data analysis, data interpretation, or manuscript writing.

Authors' contributions

HS was closely involved in protocol design and data cleaning, and played a lead role in the analysis and the manuscript writing. AW and JD conceived the idea. JD wrote the original protocol for this study. KI and JD were involved in protocol design, data collection, data input, and manuscript writing. KI was involved in data cleaning. BW, JB and JA were involved in data collection and data input. AW was the principal investigator and actively involved at every stage of the manuscript, from protocol design to manuscript writing. All authors were involved in the write up of the manuscript and in the review of drafts. All authors read and approved the final manuscript.

Consent for publication

Not applicable

Competing interests

The authors declare that they have no competing interests.

Author details

[1]Japan Ministry of Health, Labour and Welfare, Health Bureau, Tokyo, Japan. [2]Institute of Tropical Medicine, Nagasaki University, Nagasaki, Japan. [3]Sanyu Africa Research Institute, Mbale, Uganda. [4]Mbale Regional Referral Hospital, Departments of Community Medicine, Paediatrics and Surgery, Mbale, Uganda. [5]University of Liverpool, Sanyu Research Unit, Liverpool, UK.

References

1. Allegranzi B, Pittet D. Role of hand hygiene in healthcare-associated infection prevention. J Hosp Infect. 2009;73(4):305–15.
2. World Health Organization. WHO guidelines on hand hygiene in health care: first global patient safety challenge: clean care is safer care. Geneva: World Health Organization; 2009.
3. Bauer-Savage J, Pittet D, Kim E, Allegranzi B. Local production of WHO-recommended alcohol-based handrubs: feasibility, advantages, barriers and costs. Bull World Health Organ. 2013;91(12):963–9.
4. Global Health Security Agenda. Global Health Security Agenda: Action Packages. 2014. https://www.cdc.gov/nhsn/PDFs/pscManual/validation/pcsManual-2014-valid.pdf. Accessed 11 Mar 2017.
5. World Health Organization. Global Action Plan on Antimicrobial Resistance. World Health Organization; 2015. http://www.who.int/iris/handle/10665/193736. Accessed 19 Aug 2017.
6. U.S. Department of Health and Human Services, Office of Disease Prevention and Health Promotion. Healthy People 2020: Healthcare-Associated Infections. ODPHP; 2010. https://www.healthypeople.gov/sites/default/files/HP2020_brochure_with_LHI_508_FNL.pdf. Accessed 21 Mar 2017.
7. Allegranzi B, Nejad SB, Combescure C, et al. Burden of endemic health-care-associated infection in developing countries: systematic review and meta-analysis. Lancet. 2011;377(9761):228–41.
8. Nthumba PM, Stepita-Poenaru E, Poenaru D, et al. Cluster-randomized, crossover trial of the efficacy of plain soap and water versus alcohol-based rub for surgical hand preparation in a rural hospital in Kenya. Br J Surg. 2010;97(11):1621–8.
9. Aiken AM, Karuri DM, Wanyoro AK, Macleod J. Interventional studies for preventing surgical site infections in sub-Saharan Africa - a systematic review. Int J Surg. 2012;10(5):242–9.
10. Japan Ministry of Health, Labour and Welfare. Japanese Pharmacopoeia Seventeenth Edition: Official Monographs D to K. 2016. http://jpdb.nihs.go.jp/jp17e/000217653.pdf. Accessed 14 Mar 2017.
11. Suchomel M, Kundi M, Pittet D, Weinlich M, Rotter ML. Testing of the World Health Organization recommended formulations in their application as hygienic hand rubs and proposals for increased efficacy. Am J Infect Control. 2012;40(4):328–31.
12. Center for Disease Control and Prevention. CDC/NHSN surveillance definitions for specific types of infections 2014. 2014.
13. World Health Organization. HH - Observation Tool. 2009. http://www.who.int/entity/gpsc/5may/Observation_Form.doc?ua=1. Accessed 21 Mar 2017.
14. Levy MM, Fink MP, Marshall JC, et al. 2001 SCCM/ESICM/ACCP/ATS/SIS international sepsis definitions conference. Intensive Care Med. 2003;29(4):530–8.
15. Goldstein B, Giroir B, Randolph A. International consensus conference on Pediatric sepsis. International pediatric sepsis consensus conference: definitions for sepsis and organ dysfunction in pediatrics. Pediatr Crit Care Med J Soc Crit Care Med World Fed Pediatr Intensive Crit Care Soc. 2005; 6(1):2–8.
16. World Health Organization. Health care-associated infections: Fact Sheet. http://www.who.int/gpsc/country_work/gpsc_ccisc_fact_sheet_en.pdf .

Accessed 24 Aug 2016.

17. Abdella NM, Tefera MA, Eredie AE, Landers TF, Malefia YD, Alene KA. Hand hygiene compliance and associated factors among health care providers in Gondar University hospital, Gondar, North West Ethiopia. BMC Public Health. 2014;14(1):1–7.

18. Owusu-Ofori A, Jennings R, Burgess J, Prasad PA, Acheampong F, Coffin SE. Assessing hand hygiene resources and practices at a large African teaching hospital. Infect Control Hosp Epidemiol. 2010;31(8):802–8.

19. Holmen IC, Seneza C, Nyiranzayisaba B, Nyiringabo V, Bienfait M, Safdar N. Improving hand hygiene practices in a rural Hospital in sub-Saharan Africa. Infect Control Hosp Epidemiol. 2016;37(7):834–9.

20. Lankford MG, Zembower TR, Trick WE, Hacek DM, Noskin GA, Peterson LR. Influence of role models and hospital design on the hand hygiene of health-care workers. Emerg Infect Dis. 2003;9(2):217–23.

21. Gillespie R. Manufacturing knowledge: a history of the Hawthorne experiments. New York: Cambridge University Press; 1993. http://www.tandfonline.com/doi/abs/10.1080/03612759.1993.9948526.

22. Singer M, Deutschman CS, Seymour C, et al. The third international consensus definitions for sepsis and septic shock (Sepsis-3). JAMA. 2016;315(8):801–10.

23. Seymour CW, Liu VX, Iwashyna TJ, et al. Assessment of clinical criteria for sepsis: for the third international consensus definitions for sepsis and septic shock (Sepsis-3). JAMA. 2016;315(8):762–74.

24. Govindan S, Iwashyna TJ. Inpatient notes: Sepsis-3 for hospitalists—sepsis without SIRS. Ann Intern Med. 2016;165(4):HO2.

25. Braykov NP, Morgan DJ, Schweizer ML, et al. Assessment of empirical antibiotic therapy optimisation in six hospitals: an observational cohort study. Lancet Infect Dis. 2014;14(12):1220–7.

26. Stewardson AJ, Sax H, Gayet-Ageron A, et al. Enhanced performance feedback and patient participation to improve hand hygiene compliance of health-care workers in the setting of established multimodal promotion: a single-centre, cluster randomised controlled trial. Lancet Infect Dis. 2016;16(12):1345–55.

27. Pittet D, Panesar SS, Wilson K, et al. Involving the patient to ask about hospital hand hygiene: a National Patient Safety Agency feasibility study. J Hosp Infect. 2011;77(4):299–303.

28. Longtin Y, Sax H, Leape LL, Sheridan SE, Donaldson L, Pittet D. Patient participation: current knowledge and applicability to patient safety. Mayo Clin Proc. 2010;85(1):53–62.

16

Weekly screening supports terminating nosocomial transmissions of vancomycin-resistant enterococci on an oncologic ward

Stefanie Kampmeier[1*], Dennis Knaack[2], Annelene Kossow[1], Stefanie Willems[1,4], Christoph Schliemann[3], Wolfgang E. Berdel[3], Frank Kipp[1,4] and Alexander Mellmann[1]

Abstract

Background: To investigate the impact of weekly screening within the bundle of infection control measures to terminate vancomycin-resistant enterococci (VRE) transmissions on an oncologic ward.

Methods: A cluster of 12 VRE colonisation and five infections was detected on an oncologic ward between January and April 2015. Subsequently, the VRE point prevalence was detected and, as part of a the bundle of infection control strategies to terminate the VRE cluster, we isolated affected patients, performed hand hygiene training among staff on ward, increased observations by infection control specialists, intensified surface disinfection, used personal protective equipment and initiated an admission screening in May 2015. After a further nosocomial VRE infection in August 2015, a weekly screening strategy of all oncology patients on the respective ward was established while admission screening was continued. Whole genome sequencing (WGS)-based typing was applied to determine the clonal relationship of isolated strains.

Results: Initially, 12 of 29 patients were VRE colonised; of these 10 were hospital-acquired. During May to August, on average 7 of 40 patients were detected to be VRE colonised per week during the admission screening, showing no significant decline compared to the initial situation. WGS-based typing revealed five different clusters of which three were due to *vanB*- and two *vanA*-positive enterococci. After an additional weekly screening was established, the number of colonised patients significantly declined to 1/53 and no further nosocomial cases were detected.

Conclusions: Weekly screening helped to differentiate between nosocomial and community-acquired VRE cases resulting in earlier infection control strategies on epidemic situations for a successful termination of nosocomial VRE transmissions.

Keywords: Vancomycin-resistant enterococci, *E. faecium*, Screening, Infection control bundle strategies, Outbreak, Whole genome sequencing

* Correspondence: Stefanie.Kampmeier@ukmuenster.de
[1]Institute of Hygiene, University Hospital Münster, Robert-Koch-Strasse 41, 48149 Münster, Germany
Full list of author information is available at the end of the article

Background

Vancomycin-resistant enterococci (VRE) are important causes of healthcare associated infections [1, 2]. Acquisition of VRE has been associated with prolonged hospital stay and duration of previous hospitalization, neutropenia, antibiotic treatment, exposure to high-dose corticosteroids and immunosuppression [3–6]. Patients with hematologic malignancies have many of these predisposing factors and are at high-risk for VRE colonisation and infection.

Recent studies report an increase in VRE outbreaks on wards, hosting immunocompromised patients [7–9]. Mathematical modelling estimated a basic reproductive number R_0 of 1.32, underlining the epidemic potential of VRE [10]. Via shedding VRE, colonised patients serve as potential sources for transmission on other patients, healthcare workers or surfaces [4]. Limiting the spread of VRE requires infection control bundle strategies such as antibiotic stewardship, patient isolation, enhanced hand hygiene, surface disinfection, and increased active surveillance [11, 12].

Screening to detect VRE carriage in risk patients is usually used to identify previously unrecognized cases on a ward in order to prevent further nosocomial spread and subsequent infections of VRE. Distinguishing community-acquired VRE cases from cases transmitted in the hospital is often difficult. Appropriate screening strategies can help to differentiate among these cases and to detect clusters of VRE. International recommendations prefer active rather than passive screening methods in hospitals [13] but due to imprecise definitions, currently performed screening strategies diverge, depending on the respective hospital. In current studies, VRE screening is mainly considered within the context of preventive activities [14]. Here, we investigate the impact of weekly VRE screening within the bundle of infection control measures to terminate VRE outbreaks on an oncologic ward.

Methods

Outbreak detection, screening and infection control measures

In the 1500-bed University Hospital Muenster, routine surveillance, i.e. regular review of patients' charts and microbiological test results, detected five VRE infections on the hematologic/oncologic ward between January and April 2015. In addition 12 VRE colonisations could be detected coincidentally in anal swabs or stool samples in epidemiologically linked patients. As these rates exceeded the baseline of two infections and three incidentally detected colonisations every 12 months, an outbreak investigation was initiated. Subsequently, VRE point prevalence among all patients on ward was determined and environmental samples were taken. A VRE infection control strategy (hereafter called "VRE bundle strategy") was established including the following measures:

Patients were screened upon admission and contact precautions were implemented. Patients with positive VRE testing were isolated. Isolation of more than one patient in one room was performed if patients were colonized or infected with enterococci harbouring identical *vanA/B* resistance genes. Separation of toilets, showers, and water supplies was performed and previously shared bathing rooms were closed for colonised patients from this moment on. Staff was instructed to wear personal protective equipment in case of entering a patient room, consisting of gloves, surgical masks and gowns. Surface disinfection was performed initially in every room, including washrooms, patient rooms, nurses' room, storage rooms, and staff rest rooms once a day using Perform® (Schülke & Mayr GmbH, Norderstedt, Germany). Hand hygiene training was performed among nurses, physicians, cleaning personnel, and kitchen staff. Implementation of hygienic measures was observed by infection control staff every day. A time line was compiled, documenting every patient's VRE status on the ward. Patients with known VRE colonisations, detected during previous hospital stays, were immediately isolated in a single patient room. De-isolation was only performed in case of three negative swab samples collected in three consecutive weeks without application of any antibiotics within this period.

After an additional VRE infection (sepsis) in August 2015, a weekly screening was added to the VRE bundle strategy in order to clearly identify hospital-acquired colonisations and infections. Transmissions were classified as nosocomial colonisations or infections if they occurred >48 h after hospitalization and the initial screening was negative or not performed.

VRE screening, culture and PCR testing methods

VRE screening was performed obtaining rectal (5 cm *ab ano*) swabs (Transwab ® m40 compliant, mwe, Corsham, Wiltshire, UK) that were applied to blood agar (Columbia sheep blood agar, Oxoid, Wesel, Germany) and a chromogenic selective agar (VRESelect™, Biorad, Hercules, California, USA) and incubated for up to 48 h at 37 °C. Bacterial species of suspected colonies were confirmed by MALDI-TOF-MS (Bruker Corporation, Bremen, Germany) and antibiotic susceptibility testing was performed and verified using VITEK®2 system (BioMérieux, Nürtingen, Germany) in accordance with the EUCAST standards for clinical breakpoints. In case of vancomycin resistance, the GenoType Enterococcus system (Hain Lifescience, Nehren, Germany) was used to differentiate vancomycin resistance genes *vanA*, *vanB*, *vanC1* and *vanC2/C3*.

Environmental sampling and testing methods

Two series of environmental sampling were performed: first during the initial phase after transmission detection in May 2015, second after cleaning of hand contact surfaces in June 2015. Polywipes (mwe, Corsham, Wiltshire, UK) were applied on surfaces and incubated in Tryptic Soy Broth + LT (Merck Millipore, Eppelheim, Germany) for 24 h at 37 °C. Following, 10 μL of broth were applied to blood agar and VRE selective agar and incubated for 24 h at 37 °C. Suspected colonies were subcultured on blood agar and species identification was performed with the help of MALDI-TOF-MS (Bruker Corporation). Susceptibility testing for vancomycin was performed using Etest® (Bestbion GmbH, Liofilchem, Italy) and evaluated in accordance with the EUCAST standards for clinical breakpoints.

Whole genome sequence-based typing

To determine the clonal relationship of isolated VRE strains, the isolates were subjected to whole genome sequencing (WGS) using the Illumina MiSeq platform (Illumina Inc., San Diego, USA) as described previously [15]. After sequencing, quality-trimming and de novo assembly were performed, coding regions were compared in a gene-by-gene approach (core genome Multilocus SequenceTyping, cgMLST) [16] using the SeqSphere+ software version 2.0 beta (Ridom GmbH, Muenster, Germany). The clonal relationship was displayed in a minimum-spanning tree that was generated using the same software. For backwards compatibility with classical molecular typing, i. e. MLST, the MLST sequence types (ST) were extracted from the WGS data in silico.

Statistical analysis

All data are expressed as absolute numbers or percentage, if not stated otherwise. Statistical analyses were performed using the Fisher's exact test for categorical data. Statistical significance was declared at $p < 0.05$.

Results

Between January and April 2015 five VRE isolates from clinically relevant specimens (two blood cultures, three urines) were detected in patients on the haematology/oncology ward. Point prevalence determination of patients on the ward revealed 12 of 29 patients positive for VRE, of which 10 were per definition hospital-acquired, since admission screening was not performed or negative. After establishing the VRE bundle strategy, on average 7 of 40 (17.5%) patients were detected to be VRE colonised in in admission screenings, showing no significant decline compared to the initial situation. In total 30% of investigated outbreak strains harboured vanA, 68.3% vanB and 1.6% both resistance genes. MLST ST 192 (41.7%) and ST 203 (18.3%) were most prevalent (Table 1). cgMLST revealed five different VRE clusters in parallel comprising patients and environmental isolates; of these clusters three exhibited a vanB and two a vanA resistance genotype (Fig. 1).

To evaluate effectiveness of weekly screening in addition to the VRE bundle strategy, percentages of screened, colonised, hospital-acquired and isolated patients were analysed: After implementation of admission screening in May 2015 the percentage of screened patients was 76%. With establishing weekly screening in the end of August 2015 on average 91% of all patients on ward were screened (see also Fig. 2). The number of colonised patients in January 2016 declined to 1 of 53 (~2%, $p = 0.00001$) and no further nosocomial cases were detected ($p = 0.00001$) (Fig. 3). Closely connected to this situation, the number of weekly isolated patients due to a positive VRE status declined significantly from 21 of 55 patients in May 2015 to 6 of 59 patients in January 2016 ($p = 0.00007$) (Fig. 3a). While the number of community-acquired VRE did not change remarkably comparing May 2015 to January 2016, the number of total VRE colonisations decreased significantly due to a decline in hospital-acquired VRE colonisations (Fig. 3).

Discussion

Within the here presented study, spread of VRE on the oncologic ward was suspected, in particular after the initial point prevalence of VRE colonisations was determined 41.3%. During the following months (May–August) VRE colonisation rate on admission was 17.5%, which clearly exceeds admission prevalence published elsewhere [12]. This might be due to the fact, that a high number of patients, including VRE colonised patients, was repeatedly admitted in two- or three-week- intervals for chemotherapeutic treatment. Data of detected MLST ST and vangenotypes, both comparable to published investigations on clinical E. faecium isolates [17], provided a first hint, that different VRE clones were circulating on this ward. Of note, we found MLST ST 192 and ST 203, which are the most causative STs of German VRE outbreaks [17–19], to be most prevalent on this ward. Interestingly, MLST ST 117 or ST 80, as e.g. found during VRE outbreaks in German neighbouring countries (Denmark, the Netherlands) [16], did not play a major role in our setting. cgMLST, which can be used to precisely monitor transmission rates [15], helped to illustrate, that spread of different VRE clones had taken place.. This spread was ended after establishment of weekly screening in addition to common infection control bundle strategies. Published studies mostly evaluate screening within non-outbreak settings. Here, active screening on high-risk wards was shown to reduce the incidence of VRE bacteraemia and colonisations compared to wards also hosting high-risk patients but not performing active screening [20]. The results of the present study indicate that even in situations of VRE spread, weekly screening supports reduction of VRE colonisations and infections. The combination of VRE bundle strategies plus weekly screening turned out to

Table 1 Collection dates, *van*-genotypes, MLST sequence types (all isolates) and antimicrobial resistance expression (only patient isolates) of VRE strains

Isolate no.	Collection date	van-genotype	MLST-ST	AMP	SAM	AX	AMC	PRL	TPZ	IPM	CIP	LEV	TEC	QD	TGC	LNZ	F	SXT	CN-HLR	S-HLR
P1	2015-03-01	vanA	203	r	r	r	r	r	r	r	r	r	r	s	s	s	r	r	+	+
P2	2015-03-18	vanB	192	r	r	r	r	r	r	r	r	r	s	s	s	s	s	r	+	−
P3	2015-04-16	vanB	192	r	r	r	r	r	r	r	r	r	s	s	s	s	s	r	+	−
P4	2015-04-26	vanA	117	r	r	r	r	r	r	r	r	r	r	s	s	s	s	r	+	−
P5	2015-05-01	vanB	80	r	r	r	r	r	r	r	r	r	s	s	s	s	s	r	−	−
P6	2015-05-22	vanA	769	r	r	r	r	r	r	r	r	r	s	s	s	s	s	r	−	+
P7	2015-05-22	vanB	192	r	r	r	r	r	r	r	r	r	r	s	s	s	s	r	+	−
P8	2015-05-23	vanA	769	r	r	r	r	r	r	r	r	r	r	s	s	s	s	r	−	+
P9	2015-05-23	vanB	117	r	r	r	r	r	r	r	r	r	s	s	s	s	r	r	+	+
P10	2015-05-23	vanA + vanB	17	r	r	r	r	r	r	r	r	r	s	s	s	s	r	r	+	+
P11	2015-05-23	vanB	N/A	r	r	r	r	r	r	r	r	r	s	s	s	s	s	r	−	+
P12	2015-05-23	vanB	192	r	r	r	r	r	r	r	r	r	s	s	s	s	s	r	−	−
P13	2015-05-24	vanB	N/A	r	r	r	r	r	r	r	r	r	s	s	s	s	s	r	−	−
P14	2015-05-25	vanA	769	r	r	r	r	r	r	r	r	r	r	s	s	s	s	r	+	+
P15	2015-05-28	vanA	203	r	r	r	r	r	r	r	r	r	s	s	s	r	r	r	+	−
P16	2015-06-02	vanB	192	r	r	r	r	r	r	r	r	r	s	s	s	s	s	r	+	−
P17	2015-06-02	vanA	769	r	r	r	r	r	r	r	r	r	s	s	s	s	s	r	+	+
P18	2015-06-02	vanB	192	r	r	r	r	r	r	r	r	r	r	s	s	s	s	r	+	−
P19	2015-06-07	vanA	769	r	r	r	r	r	r	r	r	r	s	s	s	s	s	r	+	+
P20	2015-06-08	vanB	192	r	r	r	r	r	r	r	r	r	r	s	s	s	s	r	+	−
P21	2015-06-09	vanA	203	r	r	r	r	r	r	r	r	r	r	s	r	s	s	r	−	+
P22	2015-06-09	vanA	203	r	r	r	r	r	r	r	r	r	r	s	r	s	r	r	−	+
P23	2015-06-09	vanB	192	r	r	r	r	r	r	r	r	r	s	s	s	s	s	r	−	−
P24	2015-06-09	vanB	192	r	r	r	r	r	r	r	r	r	r	s	s	s	s	r	−	−
P25	2015-06-16	vanB	192	r	r	r	r	r	r	r	r	r	s	s	s	s	s	r	+	+
P26	2015-06-16	vanB	N/A	r	r	r	r	r	r	r	r	r	s	s	s	s	s	r	−	−
P27	2015-06-17	vanA	203	r	r	r	r	r	r	r	r	r	s	s	s	s	r	r	−	+
P28	2015-06-19	vanB	192	r	r	r	r	r	r	r	r	r	s	s	s	s	s	r	+	−

Table 1 Collection dates, *van*-genotypes, MLST sequence types (all isolates) and antimicrobial resistance expression (only patient isolates) of VRE strains (*Continued*)

	Collection date	van-genotype	MLST ST																	
P29	2015-06-23	vanB	192	r	r	r	r	r	r	r	r	s	s	s	s	s	r	s	+	−
P30	2015-06-23	vanB	N/A	r	r	r	r	r	r	r	r	s	s	s	s	s	r	s	−	+
P31	2015-07-01	vanA	192	r	r	r	r	r	r	r	s	r	s	s	s	r	r	r	+	+
P32	2015-07-02	vanB	17	r	r	r	r	r	r	r	r	s	s	s	s	s	r	s	−	+
P33	2015-07-02	vanB	80	r	r	r	r	r	r	r	r	s	s	s	s	s	r	s	+	−
P34	2015-07-07	vanB	192	r	r	r	r	r	r	r	r	s	s	s	s	s	r	s	+	−
P35	2015-07-07	vanA	203	r	r	r	r	r	r	r	s	r	s	s	s	r	r	r	+	+
P36	2015-07-12	vanB	N/A	r	r	r	r	r	r	r	r	s	s	s	s	s	r	s	−	+
P37	2015-07-16	vanB	192	r	r	r	r	r	r	r	r	s	s	s	s	s	r	s	+	−
P38	2015-07-21	vanB	N/A	r	r	r	r	r	r	r	r	s	s	s	s	s	r	s	−	+
P39	2015-07-21	vanB	N/A	r	r	r	r	r	r	r	r	s	s	s	s	s	r	s	−	+
P40	2015-07-21	vanB	N/A	r	r	r	r	r	r	r	r	s	s	s	s	s	r	s	−	+
P41	2015-07-21	vanB	192	r	r	r	r	r	r	r	r	s	s	s	s	s	r	s	+	+
P42	2015-07-21	vanA	203	r	r	r	r	r	r	r	s	r	s	s	s	r	r	r	+	+
P43	2015-07-30	vanB	N/A	r	r	r	r	r	r	r	r	s	s	s	s	s	r	s	+	−
P44	2015-07-30	vanB	N/A	r	r	r	r	r	r	r	r	s	s	s	s	s	r	s	+	+
P45	2015-07-30	vanA	203	r	r	r	r	r	r	r	s	r	s	s	s	r	r	r	−	+
P46	2015-08-06	van3	N/A	r	r	r	r	r	r	r	r	s	s	s	s	s	r	s	+	−
P47	2015-08-06	van3	192	r	r	r	r	r	r	r	r	s	s	s	s	s	r	s	+	−
P48	2015-08-13	van3	N/A	r	r	r	r	r	r	r	r	s	s	s	s	s	r	s	+	+
P49	2015-08-20	vanB	N/A	r	r	r	r	r	r	r	r	s	s	s	s	s	r	s	−	+
P50	2015-08-31	vanB	N/A	r	r	r	r	r	r	r	r	s	s	s	s	s	r	s	−	+
P51	2015-09-02	vanB	80	r	r	r	r	r	r	r	r	s	s	i	s	s	r	s	+	+
P52	2015-09-07	vanB	N/A	r	r	r	r	r	r	r	r	s	s	s	s	s	r	s	+	+
P53	2015-10-08	vanB	80	r	r	r	r	r	r	r	r	s	s	s	s	s	r	s	+	+
P54	2015-10-19	vanB	80	r	r	r	r	r	r	r	r	s	s	s	s	s	r	s	+	+
P55	2015-10-19	vanB	N/A	r	r	r	r	r	r	r	r	s	s	s	s	s	r	s	−	+
P56	2015-10-26	vanB	80	r	r	r	r	r	r	r	r	s	s	s	s	s	r	s	+	−

Table 1 Collection dates, *van*-genotypes, MLST sequence types (all isolates) and antimicrobial resistance expression (only patient isolates) of VRE strains (*Continued*)

ID	Date	van-genotype	MLST	AMP	SAM	AX	AMC	PRL	TPZ	IPM	CIP	LEV	TEC	QD	TGC	LNZ	F	SXT	CN-HLR	S-HLR
P57	2015–11–25	vanB	N/A	r	r	r	r	r	r	r	r	r	s	s	s	s	r	r	–	+
P58	2015–11–30	vanA	203	r	r	r	r	r	r	r	r	r	s	s	s	s	r	r	–	–
P59	2015–12–21	vanA	203	r	r	r	r	r	r	r	r	r	s	s	s	s	r	r	+	+
P60	2015–12–21	vanA	203	r	r	r	r	r	r	r	r	r	s	s	s	s	r	r	+	+
P$_{ref}$	2015–05–15	vanA	192	r	r	r	r	r	r	r	r	r	s	s	s	s	r	r	+	+
E1	2015–05–11	vanB	192																	
E2	2015–05–11	vanB	192																	
E3	2015–05–11	vanB	192																	
E4	2015–05–11	vanB	192																	
E5	2015–05–11	vanB	769																	
E6	2015–05–11	vanA	192																	
E7	2015–05–19	vanB	192																	
E8	2015–06–02	vanB	80																	
E9	2015–06–02	vanB	192																	
E10	2015–06–02	vanB	80																	
E11	2015–06–02	vanB	N/A																	

AMP ampicillin, *SAM* ampicillin/sulbactam, *AX* amoxicillin, *AMC* amoxicillin/clavulanic acid, *PRL* piperacillin, *TPZ* piperacillin/tazobactam, *IPM* imipenem, *CIP* ciprofloxacin, *LEV* levofloxacin, *CN-HLR* gentamicin-high level resistance, *S-HLR* streptomycin-high level resistance, *TEC* teicoplanin, *QD* quinopristin/dalfopristin, *TGC* tigecyclin, *LNZ* linezolid, *F* nitrofurantoin, *SXT* trimetoprim/sulfamethoxazole, *MLST* Multi Locus Sequence Typing, *VRE* Vancomycin resistant enterococci

r resistant, *s* susceptible

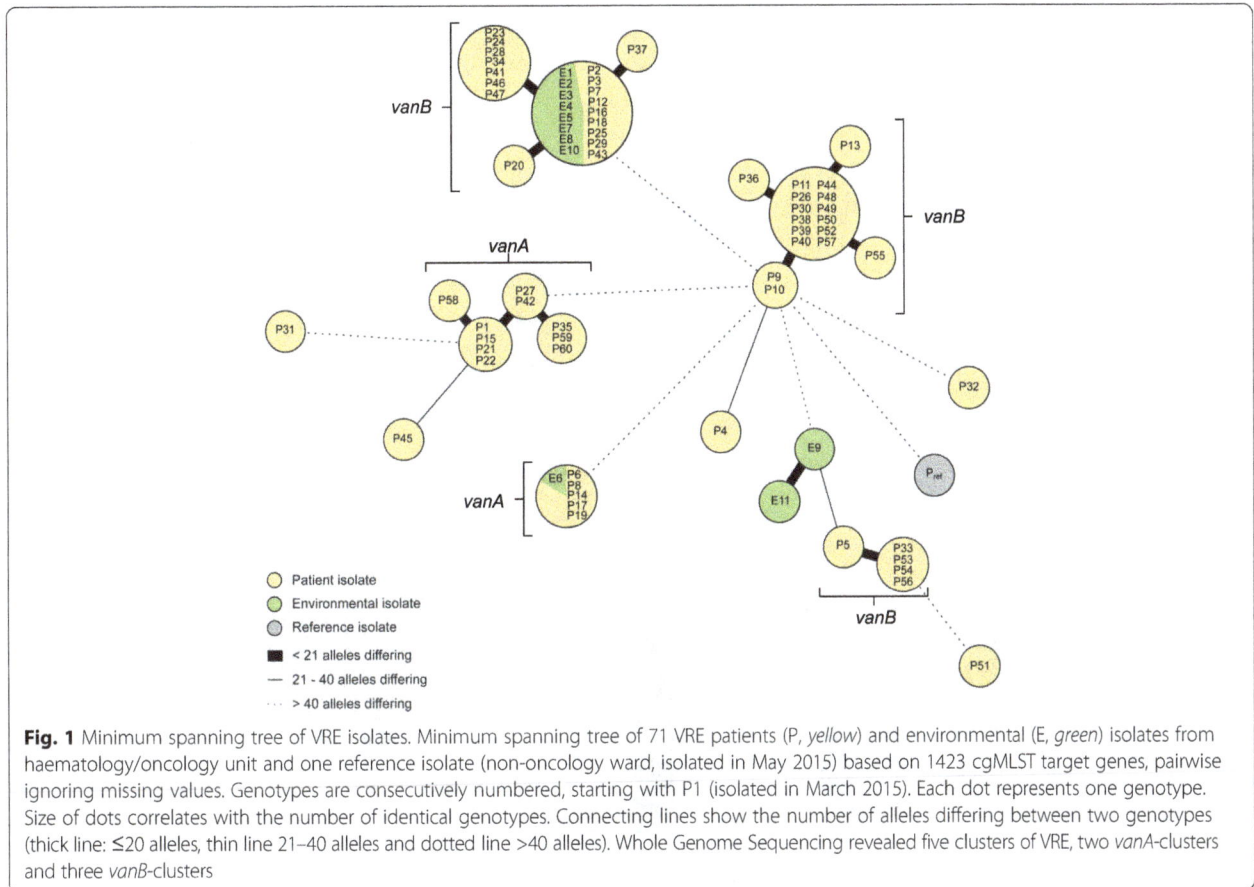

Fig. 1 Minimum spanning tree of VRE isolates. Minimum spanning tree of 71 VRE patients (P, *yellow*) and environmental (E, *green*) isolates from haematology/oncology unit and one reference isolate (non-oncology ward, isolated in May 2015) based on 1423 cgMLST target genes, pairwise ignoring missing values. Genotypes are consecutively numbered, starting with P1 (isolated in March 2015). Each dot represents one genotype. Size of dots correlates with the number of identical genotypes. Connecting lines show the number of alleles differing between two genotypes (thick line: ≤20 alleles, thin line 21–40 alleles and dotted line >40 alleles). Whole Genome Sequencing revealed five clusters of VRE, two *vanA*-clusters and three *vanB*-clusters

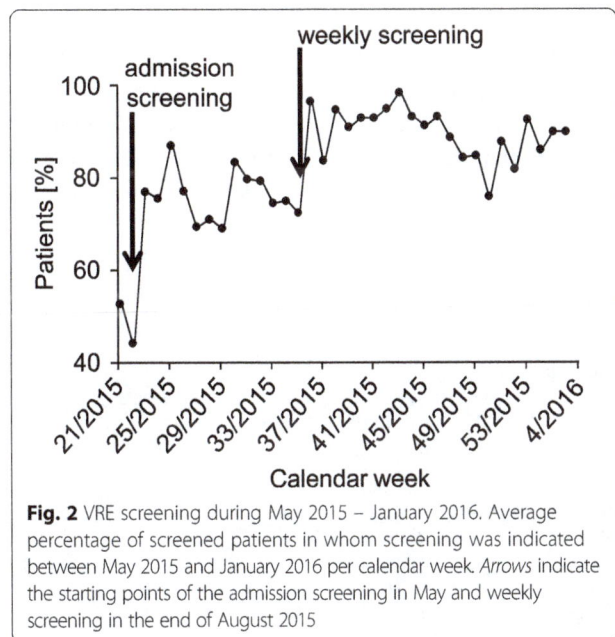

Fig. 2 VRE screening during May 2015 – January 2016. Average percentage of screened patients in whom screening was indicated between May 2015 and January 2016 per calendar week. *Arrows* indicate the starting points of the admission screening in May and weekly screening in the end of August 2015

be most effective. These findings surprise, as weekly screening *per se* does not reduce transmission rates [21]. Screening approaches alone can help uncover undetected VRE colonisations and identify potential patient reservoirs early in order to prevent transmission of VRE within a bundle of infection control strategies, while the application of infection control measures as hand hygiene and contact precautions has more significant effect on terminating VRE transmissions [13, 22]. A possible explanation why weekly screening has a direct influence in terminating spread of VRE might be that personnel's awareness is increased, if patients are weekly monitored and detected. In addition, since VRE cannot only be transmitted via direct or indirect contact but can also be selected due to the use of antibiotic agents, weekly screening serves the possibility of a colonisation follow up. Standard and extended hygienic measures can than concentrated and expanded when appropriate and VRE colonisation dynamics among patients on ward is more apparent.

Our study has limitations. First, we did not perform a case-control study. Hence, other interventions on the ward could have been responsible for decreased VRE colonisations. However, since all other

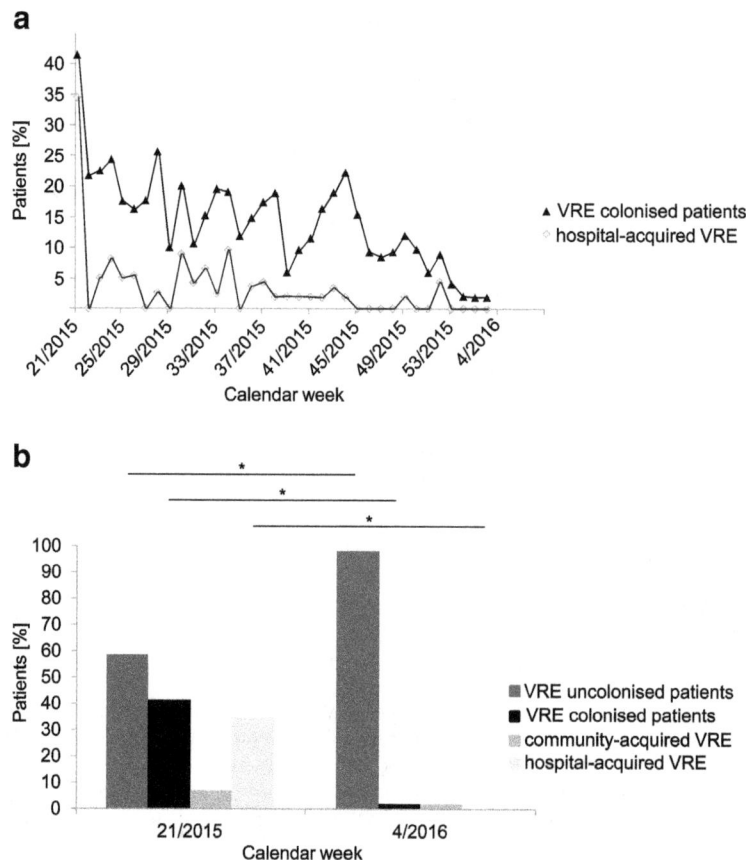

Fig. 3 Colonised, community- and hospital-acquired VRE patients between May 2015 and January 2016. **a** Average percentage of colonised and hospital- acquired VRE patients between May 2015 and January 2016 per calendar week. **b** Statistical comparison of uncolonised patients, colonised patients, community-acquired and hospital-acquired VRE patients before (May 2015) and at the end (January 2016) of performing VRE bundle strategies plus additional weekly screening

measures of our VRE bundle were already implemented when transmission began and were not changed during the intervention period, this fact has a presumably small influence on the presented results. Second, we used different methods for susceptibility testing of either clinical or environmental samples. Routinely clinical samples are tested via VITEK 2 in order to have other therapeutic possibilities for patient's treatment. In contrast, environmental samples, that are collected to clarify the distribution of VRE on surfaces, are tested for vancomycin resistance via Etest® since no therapeutic interventions are derived from these findings. Nevertheless, susceptibility evaluation was done in accordance with the latest EUCAST criteria, thereby creating comparable results. Third, we investigated the clonal spread of VRE only using cgMLST, therefore, we could not exclude whether *vanA* or *vanB* were passed via horizontal gene transfer from one strain to another as investigated elsewhere [18, 23].

Conclusion
Our study support the hypothesis, that active screening reduces the incidence of VRE infections and colonisations in high-risk patients by the early uncovering of nosocomial transmissions prior their appearance in clinical samples. Therefore, a weekly screening should be considered as part of a bundle strategy for the successful termination of VRE outbreak situations.

Abbreviations
cgMLST: Core genome multilocus sequence typing; VRE: Vancomycin-resistant enterococci; WGS: Whole genome sequencing

Acknowledgements
None.

Funding
None.

Authors' contributions

SK, DK, AK, SW and CS were responsible for all data collection. All authors were involved in data analysis and interpretation. All authors contributed to and approved the final draft of manuscript.

Competing interests

The authors declare that they have no competing interests.

Consent for publication

Not applicable.

Author details

[1]Institute of Hygiene, University Hospital Münster, Robert-Koch-Strasse 41, 48149 Münster, Germany. [2]Institute of Medical Microbiology, University Hospital Münster, Domagkstrasse 10, 48149 Münster, Germany. [3]Department of Medicine A, Haematology and Oncology, University Hospital Münster, Albert-Schweitzer-Campus 1, 48149 Münster, Germany. [4]Present address: Institute of Hygiene, DRK Kliniken Berlin, Drontheimer Str. 39–40, 13359 Berlin, Germany.

References

1. Cetinkaya Y, Falk P, Mayhall CG. Vancomycin-resistant enterococci. Clin Microbiol Rev. 2000;13:686–707.
2. O'Driscoll T, Crank CW. Vancomycin-resistant enterococcal infections: epidemiology, clinical manifestations, and optimal management. Infect Drug Resist. 2015;8:217–30.
3. Papadimitriou-Olivgeris M, Drougka E, Fligou F, et al. Risk factors for enterococcal infection and colonization by vancomycin-resistant enterococci in critically ill patients. Infection. 2014;42:1013–22.
4. Ford CD, Lopansri BK, Haydoura S, et al. Frequency, risk factors, and outcomes of vancomycin-resistant Enterococcus colonization and infection in patients with newly diagnosed acute leukemia: different patterns in patients with acute myelogenous and acute lymphoblastic leukemia. Infect Control Hosp Epidemiol. 2015;36:47–53.
5. Popiel KY, Miller MA. Evaluation of vancomycin-resistant enterococci (VRE)-associated morbidity following relaxation of VRE screening and isolation precautions in a tertiary care hospital. Infect Control Hosp Epidemiol. 2014;35:818–25.
6. Adams DJ, Eberly MD, Goudie A, et al. Rising Vancomycin-Resistant Enterococcus Infections in Hospitalized Children in the United States. Hosp Pediatr. 2016;6:404–11.
7. Schmidt-Hieber M, Blau IW, Schwartz S, et al. Intensified strategies to control vancomycin-resistant enterococci in immunocompromised patients. Int J Hematol. 2007;86:158–62.
8. Fossi Djembi L, Hodille E, Chomat-Jaboulay S, et al. Factors associated with Vancomycin-resistant Enterococcus acquisition during a large outbreak. J Infect Public Health. 2017;10:185–90.
9. Lewis JD, Enfield KB, Cox HL, et al. A single-center experience with infections due to daptomycin-nonsusceptible Enterococcus faecium in liver transplant recipients. Transpl Infect Dis. 2016;18:341–53.
10. Satilmis L, Vanhems P, Bénet T. Outbreaks of Vancomycin-Resistant Enterococci in Hospital Settings: A Systematic Review and Calculation of the Basic Reproductive Number. Infect Control Hosp Epidemiol. 2016;37:289–94.
11. De Angelis G, Cataldo MA, De Waure C, et al. Infection control and prevention measures to reduce the spread of vancomycin-resistant enterococci in hospitalized patients. a systematic review and meta-analysis. J Antimicrob Chemother. 2014;69:1185–92.
12. Mutters NT, Mersch-Sundermann V, Mutters R, et al. Control of the spread of vancomycin-resistant enterococci in hospitals: epidemiology and clinical relevance. Dtsch Arztebl Int. 2013;110:725–31.
13. Faron ML, Ledeboer NA, Buchan BW. Resistance Mechanisms, Epidemiology, and Approaches to Screening for Vancomycin-Resistant Enterococcus in the Health Care Setting. J Clin Microbiol. 2016;54:2436–47.
14. Trubiano JA, Worth LJ, Thursky KA, et al. The prevention and management of infections due to multidrug resistant organisms in haematology patients. Br J Clin Pharmacol. 2015;79:195–207.
15. Mellmann A, Bletz S, Boking T, et al. Real-Time Genome Sequencing of Resistant Bacteria Provides Precision Infection Control in an Institutional Setting. J Clin Microbiol. 2016;54:2874–81.
16. de Been M, Pinholt M, Top J, et al. Core Genome Multilocus Sequence Typing Scheme for High- Resolution Typing of Enterococcus faecium. J Clin Microbiol. 2015;53:3788–97.
17. Werner G, Fleige C, Neumann B, et al. Evaluation of DiversiLab(R), MLST and PFGE typing for discriminating clinical Enterococcus faecium isolates. J Microbiol Methods. 2015;118:81–4.
18. Bender JK, Kalmbach A, Fleige C, et al. Population structure and acquisition of the vanB resistance determinant in German clinical isolates of Enterococcus faecium ST192. Sci Rep. 2016;6:21847.
19. Werner G, Klare I, Fleige C, et al. Vancomycin-resistant vanB-type Enterococcus faecium isolates expressing varying levels of vancomycin resistance and being highly prevalent among neonatal patients in a single ICU. Antimicrob Resist Infect Control. 2012;1:21.
20. Price CS, Paule S, Noskin GA, et al. Active surveillance reduces the incidence of vancomycin-resistant enterococcal bacteremia. Clin Infect Dis. 2003;37:921–8.
21. Derde LP, Cooper BS, Goossens H, et al. Interventions to reduce colonisation and transmission of antimicrobial-resistant bacteria in intensive care units: an interrupted time series study and cluster randomised trial. Lancet Infect Dis. 2014;14:31–9.
22. Knoll M, Daeschlein G, Okpara-Hofmann J, et al. Outbreak of vancomycin-resistant enterococci (VRE) in a hematological oncology ward and hygienic preventive measures. A long-term study. Onkologie. 2005;28:187–92.
23. Raven KE, Reuter S, Reynolds R, et al. A decade of genomic history for healthcare-associated Enterococcus faecium in the United Kingdom and Ireland. Genome Res. 2016;26:1388–96.

17

Association between antibiotic consumption and the rate of carbapenem-resistant Gram-negative bacteria from China based on 153 tertiary hospitals data in 2014

Ping Yang[1], Yunbo Chen[2], Saiping Jiang[1], Ping Shen[2], Xiaoyang Lu[1] and Yonghong Xiao[2*]

Abstract

Background: This study aimed to investigate the relationship between the rate of carbapenem-resistant Gram-negative bacteria and antibiotic consumption intensity in 153 tertiary hospitals from China in 2014.

Methods: A retrospective study using national surveillance data from 2014 was conducted. Data on the annual consumption of each antibiotic, as well as the rate of carbapenem-resistant Gram-negative bacteria, were collected from each participating hospital, and the correlation between antibiotic consumption and carbapenem- resistant rate was analyzed.

Results: The overall antibiotic consumption intensity among the hospitals varied between 23.93 and 86.80 defined daily dosages (DDDs) per 100 patient-days (median, 46.30 DDDs per 100 patient-days). Cephalosporins were the most commonly used antibiotic, followed by quinolones, penicillins, and carbapenems, and the rate of carbapenem-resistant Gram-negative bacteria from each hospital varied. The correlations between carbapenem consumption intensity and rate of carbapenem resistance revealed correlation factors of 0.271 for *Escherichia coli* ($p < 0.01$), 0.427 for *Klebsiella pneumoniae* ($p < 0.01$), 0.463 for *Pseudomonas aeruginosa* ($p < 0.01$), and 0.331 for *Acinetobacter baumannii* ($p < 0.01$).

Conclusions: A significant relationship existed between the carbapenem consumption and the rates of carbapenem-resistant gram negative bacilli. Rational use of carbapenems should be implemented to address the issue of carbapenem resistance in hospitals.

Keywords: Carbapenem-resistance, *Escherichia coli*, *Klebsiella pneumoniae*, *Pseudomonas aeruginosa*, *Acinetobacter baumannii*, Carbapenem antibiotic consumption

Background

Carbapenem is a beta-lactam antibiotic with a broad antimicrobial spectrum and effective antibacterial activity. It is generally administered as a last resort for treating drug-resistant Gram-negative bacterial infections. However, in recent years, the rate of carbapenem-resistant bacteria has steadily increased [1, 2]. Antibiotic resistance greatly limits therapeutic options, consequently resulting in higher patient morbidity, mortality and considerable economic burden [3].

According to a CHINET surveillance in 2016, *Escherichia coli*, *Klebsiella* spp., *Acinetobacter* spp., and *Pseudomonas aeruginosa* were the top 4 Gram-negative bacterial species found in all clinical samples obtained from Chinese hospitals. These bacterial species are the leading cause of nosocomial infections. The overall prevalence of carbapenem-resistant strains was 1.8% in *E. coli*, 17.9% in *K. pneumoniae*, 28.7% in *P. aeruginosa*, and 70.8% in *A. baumannii* [4]. Mortality from carbapenem-resistant Enterobacteriaceae (CRE) infection was reported by the China CRE Network to be as high as 33.5%, and most cases were determined to be caused by carbapenem-resistant *E. coli* (CREC) and *K. pneumoniae*

* Correspondence: xiao-yonghong@163.com
[2]State Key Laboratory for Diagnosis and Treatment of Infectious Diseases, the First Affiliated Hospital of Medicine School, Zhejiang University, 79 Qingchun Road, Hangzhou, China
Full list of author information is available at the end of the article

(CRKP) [5]. A meta-analysis demonstrated a > 2-fold increased risk of mortality with multidrug-resistant *P. aeruginosa* infection compared to susceptible *P. aeruginosa* [6]. In yet another study, the mortality of patients with carbapenem-resistant *A. baumannii* (CRAB) infection was as high as 16–76% [7].

The irrational use of antibiotics can increase selective pressure of bacterial resistance, which is one of the important factors responsible for antimicrobial resistance (AMR). Increasing evidence indicates that antimicrobial drug consumption is associated with AMR [8–11]. Unfortunately, most related studies involve a single hospital, and relatively few researchers have sought to analyze findings from multiple hospitals or a region. In addition, whether antibiotic consumption intensity contributes to AMR has not been widely evaluated, especially multicenter researches in China.

To determine the association between antibiotic consumption intensity and AMR, we collected data on antibiotic consumption and noted the resistances of four Gram-negative bacterial species from 153 tertiary hospitals in China. We then evaluated the correlation between rate of carbapenem resistance and antibiotic consumption intensity.

Methods

Study design

A total of 153 hospitals voluntarily participated in this cross-sectional study. Antibiotic consumption and the rate of carbapenem resistance of *E. coli*, *K. pneumoniae*, *P. aeruginosa*, and *A. baumannii* from 153 Chinese tertiary hospitals in 2014 were collected. The correlation between antibiotic consumption and resistance rate was then statistically analyzed.

Data collection

Data on antibiotic consumption were obtained from the national antibacterial drug clinical consumption survey network. Hospitals are required to report bacterial resistance data to the China AMR surveillance system, and those participating in this study were asked to report data for the whole year of 2014.

For each participating hospital, administrative data, including hospital type, administrative region, number of beds, admissions, and patient-days, were recorded.

Measurement of antibiotic consumption

The pharmacists of each hospital are required to report the annual consumption of each antibiotic to the national antibacterial drug clinical consumption survey network. Antibiotics were categorized according to the Anatomic Therapeutic Chemical (ATC) classification system [12]. Antibiotic consumption was characterized by antibiotic consumption intensity, which is the number of defined daily dosages (DDDs) per 100 patient-days. According to the World Health Organization ATC/DDD classification, DDD is the assumed average maintenance dose per day for a drug used for its main indication in adults. Patient-days were defined as number of discharged patients during the same period multiplied by the average length of stay of hospitalized patients in the same period. Then, data on the main classes of antibiotic consumption were analyzed.

Antibiotic resistance

Each participating hospital was asked to collect data on four major Gram-negative bacterial species causing infections (i.e., *E. coli*, *K. pneumoniae*, *P. aeruginosa*, and *A. baumannii*) from all sample sources (e.g., bloodstream, respiratory tract, urinary tract, wound pus, other sterile body fluids, cerebrospinal fluid, faeces, genital tract and others). The isolates were nonduplicate samples, as several isolates of each species from each patient who recovered within 7 days were considered one isolate. Data included information on the number of carbapenem-resistant isolates and the total number of bacterial strains isolated from clinical specimens. Carbapenem resistance was defined as a strain resistant to imipenem or meropenem. If the resistance rates were different, the higher resistance rate was selected as the resistance rate of the strain to carbapenems. Rate of resistance was calculated as the number of carbapenem-resistant isolates divided by the total number of isolates of the same species tested multiplied by 100. Antibiotic susceptibility tests are performed as a routine laboratory method in each hospital, and all hospitals must adhere to the Clinical and Laboratory Standards Institute 2014 guidelines. The consistency and standardized assessment of the AMR data are ensured through quality control in each laboratory. The antibiotic resistance data were processed using WHONET 5.6 software, and the quality control bacterial strains were *E. coli* ATCC25922, *K. pneumoniae* ATCC700603, *P. aeruginosa* ATCC27853, and *A. baumannii* ATCC19606. Hospital data with less than 50 isolates per year in total were excluded from the study.

Statistical analysis

Pearson's correlation analysis was performed to investigate the association between annual antibiotic consumption and rate of carbapenem resistance in 153 hospitals of China. Specifically, the relationship between the rate of carbapenem resistance and the consumption intensity of overall antibiotic, beta-lactam antibiotics, penicillins, cephalosporins, carbapenems, and fluoroquinolones were analyzed individually. Differences with $p < 0.05$ were considered to indicate statistical significance, and all analyses were conducted using Microsoft Excel 2013 and STATA 20.0 (StataCorp LLC, Texas, USA).

Results

Participating hospitals

A total of 153 hospitals voluntarily participated in this study; of these hospitals, 149 were first-class tertiary hospitals, which are described as the highest-quality hospitals in China. A total of 29 hospitals were from North China, 29 hospitals were from East China, 22 hospitals were from Central China, 26 hospitals were from Southern China, 14 hospitals were from Southwest China, 16 hospitals were from Northwest China, and 17 hospitals were from Northeast China. These hospitals had a median of 2356 beds (range, 720–8475 beds) and a median of 90,000 inpatients per year (range, 10,000–410,000). As shown in Additional file 1.

Antibiotic consumption

During the study period, the overall antibiotic consumption intensity of the hospitals varied between 23.93–86.80 DDDs per 100 patient-days (median, 46.30 DDDs per 100 patient-days). Cephalosporins were the most commonly used antibiotics, followed by fluoroquinolones, penicillins, and carbapenems. The antibiotic consumption intensities for the main antibiotic classes are presented in Table 1.

Isolated strains

A total of 159,199 E. coli, 112,135 K. pneumoniae,112,792 P. aeruginosa and 105,869 A. baumannii were analyzed. Among the 489,995 isolated strains, the most frequently isolated specimen was sputum (47.53%), then was urine (24.79%), blood (7.39%), pus (3.02%) and so on, as shown in Fig. 1.

Correlation between antibiotic consumption intensity and carbapenem-resistant gram-negative bacteria

The relationships between the rate of CREC, CRKP, Carbapenem-resistant P. aeruginosa (CRPA) and CRAB, and the consumption of various antibiotics are shown in Table 2. As shown in Table 2, carbapenem consumption intensity and the carbapenem-resistant rate of the four Gram-negative bacterial strains positively correlated.

Correlation between carbapenem consumption intensity and CREC

A total of 115 hospitals were studied to determine the relationship between carbapenem consumption intensity and CREC. A total of 132,974 strains of E. coli were isolated, 1510 strains of which were CREC. The percentage of CREC isolates in each hospital was 0.1–5.7% (median, 0.9%), and was significantly positively correlated with carbapenem antibiotic consumption ($r = 0.271$, $p < 0.01$), as demonstrated in Fig. 2a.

Correlation between carbapenem consumption intensity and CRKP

A total of 130 hospitals were studied to determine the relationship between carbapenem consumption intensity and CRKP. A total of 97,910 strains of K. pneumoniae were isolated, 11,610 of which were CRKP. The percentage of CRKP isolates in each hospital was 0.1–55.6% (median, 3.38%), and was significantly positively correlated with carbapenem antibiotic consumption ($r = 0.427$, $p < 0.01$), as exhibited in Fig. 2b.

Correlation between carbapenem consumption intensity and CRPA

A total of 136 hospitals were studied to determine the relationship between carbapenem consumption intensity and CRPA. A total of 102,739 strains of P. aeruginosa were isolated, 35,370 of which were CRPA. The percentage of CRPA isolates in each hospital was 4.3–65% (median, 31.60%), and was significantly positively correlated with carbapenem antibiotic consumption ($r = 0.463$, $p < 0.01$), as depicted in Fig. 2c.

Correlation between carbapenem consumption intensity and CRAB

A total of 120 hospitals were studied to determine the relationship between carbapenem consumption intensity and CRAB. A total of 85,692 strains of A. baumannii were isolated, 66,047 of which were CRAB. The percentage of CRAB isolates in each hospital was 39.2–92.55% (median, 75.92%), and was significantly positively correlated with

Table 1 Antibiotics consumption intensity for the main classes of antibiotics in 153 hospitals

Class (ATC category)	Antibiotics consumption intensity, median value (range, DDDs per 100 patient-days)
All antibiotics(J01)	46.30 (23.93–86.80)
β-Lactams(J01C + J01D)	33.21 (19.35–67.05)
Penicillins(J01C)	5.52 (0.61–16.89)
Cephalosporins(J01DB + J01 DC + J01DD + J01DE)	24.93 (10.81–52.52)
The third generation cephalosporin(J01DD)	11.16 (2.57–38.98)
The fourth generation cephalosporin(J01DE)	0.27 (0–5.98)
Carbapenems(J01DH)	1.96 (0.17–10.06)
Fluoroquinolones(J01MA)	5.71 (1.58–13.90)

Sites of the isolated strains

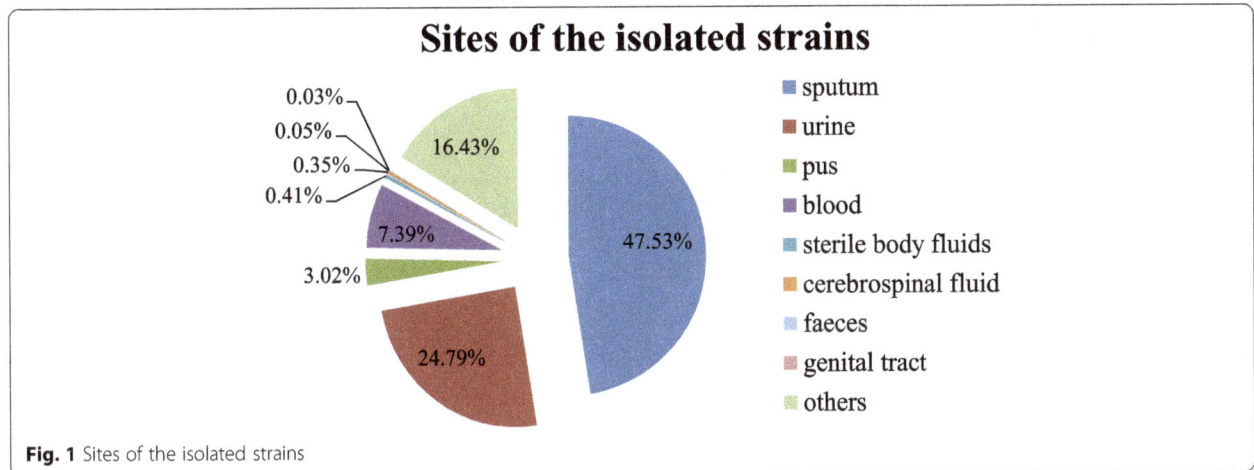

Fig. 1 Sites of the isolated strains

carbapenem antibiotic consumption ($r = 0.331$, $p < 0.01$), as shown in Fig. 2d.

Discussion

This research is the first domestic study to determine the correlations between major carbapenem-resistant Gram-negative bacteria and antibiotic consumption intensity on the basis of the national surveillance data reported by 153 voluntarily participating hospitals. During the study period, cephalosporins were found to be the most commonly used antibiotics, followed by quinolones, penicillins, and carbapenems. The percentage of carbapenem-resistant Gram-negative bacteria from each hospital varied, and correlations between carbapenem consumption intensity and rate of carbapenem-resistant *E. coli*, *K. pneumoniae*, *P. aeruginosa*, and *A. baumannii* were noted.

In our study, cephalosporins were the most common antibiotic class prescribed. This finding is consistent with previous studies conducted in China [13, 14]. Unlike doctors in our country, physicians in Europe and like doctors in our country, physicians in Europe and the United States appear to prefer penicillins. This contradiction between countries may be explained by the fact that a skin test for penicillin is required prior to the administration of the antibiotic in China. Considering the time required to conduct the test, Chinese physicians prefer to prescribe cephalosporins and quinolones instead. The clinical application of carbapenem, as a specially used antibiotic, is subject to more restrictions during its prescription.

The correlation between increased carbapenem use and increased CREC found in this study is similar to that in a previous study [15]. However, in a large survey conducted in the United States, fluoroquinolone consumption was significantly correlated with the carbapenem resistance of *E. coli* [16]. Some resistant genes could spread across strains through plasmids and integrons, leading to the emergence and widespread transmission of multidrug-resistant bacteria. A multicenter study conducted in Italy detected a significantly positive correlation between the carbapenem resistance of *E. coli* and third-generation cephalosporin and penicillin consumption [17]. The use of penicillin and

Table 2 Correlations between main classes of antibiotics consumption intensity and the rate of carbapenem-resistant in *Escherichia coli*, *Klebsiella pneumoniae*, *Pseudomonas aeruginosa* and *Acinetobacter baumannii*

Classes (ATC category)	Correlation							
	E. coli		*K. pneumoniae*		*P. aeruginosa*		*A. baumannii*	
	r [a]	p*	r	p	r	p	r	p
All antibiotics (J01)	0.093	0.324	−0.005	0.954	0.061	0.484	0.075	0.416
β-Lactams (J01C + J01D)	0.138	0.141	0.018	0.839	0.021	0.811	0.104	0.260
Penicillins (J01C)	0.121	0.198	−0.041	0.639	−0.044	0.608	−0.104	0.256
Cephalosporins (J01DB + J01 DC + J01DD + J01DE)	0.039	0.676	−0.037	0.678	−0.070	0.417	0.154	0.093
The third generation cephalosporin (J01DD)	0.024	0.803	0.004	0.961	0.000	0.996	0.132	0.151
The fourth generation cephalosporin (J01DE)	−0.080	0.393	0.064	0.471	0.143	0.097	−0.049	0.596
Carbapenems (J01DH)	0.271*	0.003	0.427*	<0.01	0.463*	<0.01	0.331*	<0.01
Fluoroquinolones (J01MA)	−0.004	0.966	0.046	0.600	0.129	0.134	0.073	0.431

[a] r denotes pearson's correlation coefficient; *statistically significant association ($p < 0.05$)

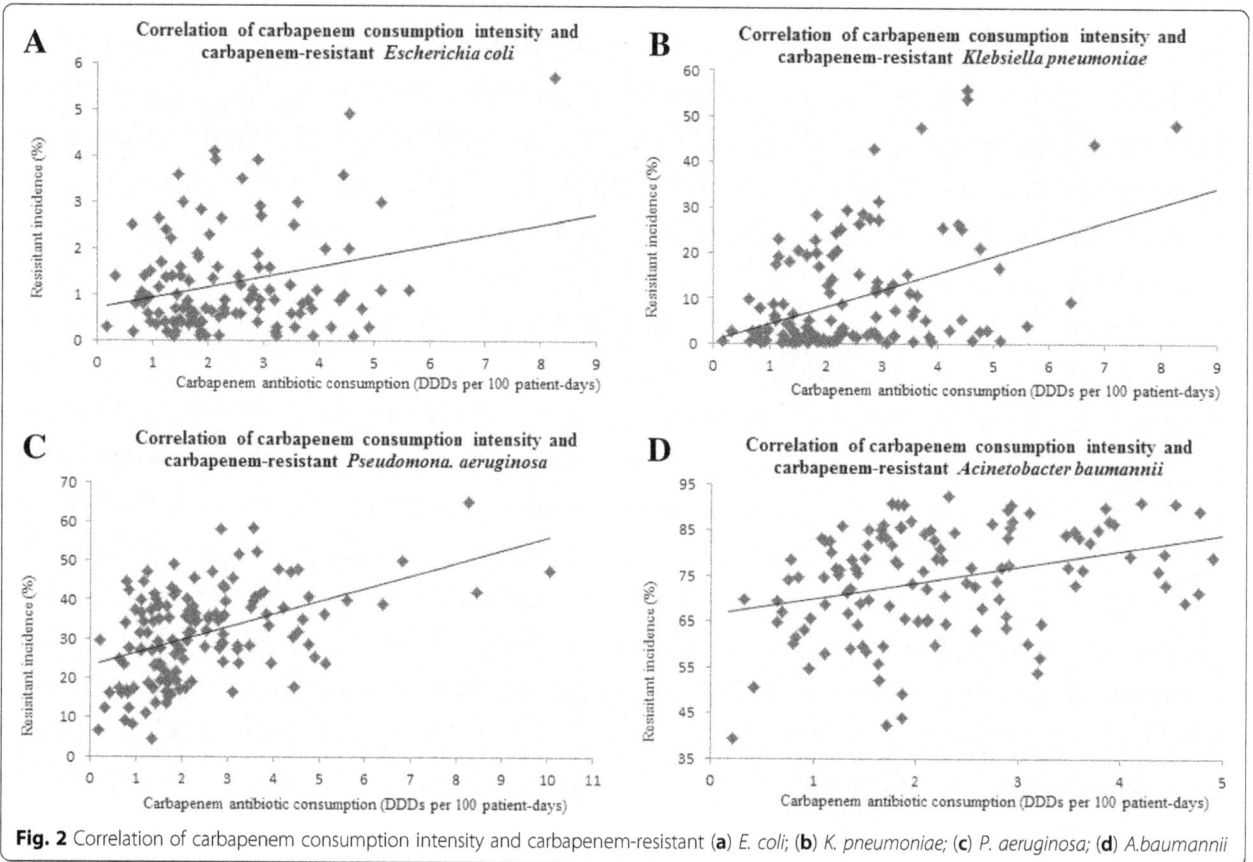

Fig. 2 Correlation of carbapenem consumption intensity and carbapenem-resistant (**a**) *E. coli*; (**b**) *K. pneumoniae*; (**c**) *P. aeruginosa*; (**d**) *A.baumannii*

third-generation cephalosporins has led to the appearance of extended-spectrum beta-lactamase (ESBL), the prevalence of which could lead to increased consumption of carbapenem antibiotics and, in turn, higher proportions of CREC.

Increased use of meropenem has been associated with the rate of CRKP [15, 18]. Our study found a positive correlation between carbapenem consumption and increases in proportion of CRKP. Increased carbapenem usage prompts the production of carbapenemases, such as *K. pneumoniae* carbapenemases (KPC) and New Delhi metallo-β-lactamase-1, which could increase the proportion of CRKP [19].

Restricting carbapenems even for a short duration has been suggested to effectively manage the problem of CRPA [20]. Our study indicated that carbapenem consumption is correlated with the rate of CRPA, similar to the conclusion of a previous study in China [14]. Such a correlation may be explained by the combination of chromosomal AmpC production and porin change. AmpC enzyme overproduction, together with reduced outer membrane porin permeability and/or efflux pump overexpression, contributes to high-level carbapenem resistance [19]. Moreover, *P. aeruginosa* harbors ESBLs, including other antibiotic-resistant enzymes, such as KPC, Verona integrin-encoded metallo-β-lactamase, and imipenem metallo- -lactamases (IMP). The combination of these enzymes could lead to a higher rate of CRPA isolates.

Research in China has revealed that quinolone consumption, besides carbapenem consumption, is substantially correlated with CRPA [14]. Another study has suggested that the CRPA rate is correlated with carbapenem plus fluoroquinolone use [21]. Quinolones and carbapenems are substrates of the same efflux pump, so the overuse of fluoroquinolones may induce the high expression of the efflux pump and lead to CRPA production [22]. Control of the usage of fluoroquinolones and carbapenems can slow down the production of multidrug-resistant *P. aeruginosa*.

A correlation between carbapenem antibiotic use and the prevalence of CRAB has been described in many previous studies [23–25]. Prior use of carbapenems is a risk factor for multidrug-resistant, extensively drug-resistant even pan drug-resistant *A. baumannii* infection [26]. This phenomenon may be attributed to selective pressure from carbapenem exposure. Excessive carbapenem use encourages the emergence of carbapenemase-producing *A. baumannii* strains, such as IMP and oxacilinase serine β-lactamases. A previous study conducted in a medical center of southern Taiwan demonstrated that carbapenem and fluoroquinolone consumption is positively correlated with increased rate of imipenem-resistant *A. baumannii*. In this particular study, fluoroquinolones were the most commonly used antibiotics [27]. The expanded use of fluoroquinolones may up-regulate the efflux pump of

AdeABC. Up-regulation of efflux transcripts has been associated with a multidrug-resistant phenotype, possibly leading to CRAB production [28].

The root causes of the rapid emergence and dissemination of drug-resistant bacteria in hospitals are multifactorial, including high selective pressure resulting from improper and widespread antibiotic usage and cross-transmission from patient to patient owing to inappropriate infection control measures or interhospital transfer of resistance [29–33]. Increasing resistance may drive the increased consumption of several so-called "last-line" antibiotics and further explain why carbapenem-resistant Gram-negative bacteria are correlated with carbapenem consumption.

Despite its important findings, this study presents some limitations. First, the design of the study is retrospective, and the effects of potential confounders, such as change in the length of hospital stay, infection control practices, and hospital scale, could not be evaluated. Second, we only considered consecutive cultures, including those isolated within 48 h after hospital admission. Consequently, community-acquired isolates were not excluded from our analysis. Finally, we researched the relationship between antibiotic usage and carbapenem resistance of four common Gram-negative bacteria in the same year but did not consider the lag of the change in bacterial resistance rate. Notwithstanding these limitations, we believe that the major strength of our study is its size. We believe that, thus far, this study is the most comprehensive investigation on the topic reported domestically.

Conclusions

In conclusion, this study highlights the positive correlation between carbapenem consumption and the rate of carbapenem resistance of four major Gram-negative bacteria. We believe that this study is a useful tool for directing antimicrobial stewardship policies. Our results also make a strong case for rationalizing the use of antibiotics to delay the occurrence of bacterial resistance. Further research on this topic may be considered in future work.

Abbreviations
A.baumannii: *Acinetobacter baumannii*; AMR: Antimicrobial resistance; ATC: Anatomic Therapeutic Chemical; CRAB: Carbapenem-resistant *A. baumannii*; CRE: Carbapenem-resistant Enterobacteriaceae; CREC: Carbapenem-resistant *E. coli*; CRKP: Carbapenem-resistant *K. pneumoniae*; CRPA: Carbapenem-resistant *P. aeruginosa*; DDDs: Defined daily dosages; *E. coli*: *Escherichia coli*; ESBLs: Extended-spectrum beta-lactamase; IMP: Imipenem metallo- -lactamases; *K. pneumoniae*: *Klebsiella pneumoniae*; KPC: *K. pneumoniae* carbapenemases; *P. aeruginosa*: *Pseudomonas aeruginosa*

Acknowledgements
Not applicable

Funding
This study was sponsored by National Natural Science Foundation of China (81361138021, 81711530049), Key Research and Development Program of Zhejiang Province (2015C03032).

Authors' contributions
PY conducted the correlation analysis and prepared the initial drafts of the manuscript. YC and PS were responsible for the bacterial resistance data analysis. SJ contributed in antibiotic consumption analysis. XL was responsible for the results interpretation and manuscript review. YX as a principal investigator designed the study, collected the data and revised the manuscript. All authors contributed to the final version of the manuscript. All authors read and approved the final manuscript.

Consent for publication
Not applicable

Competing interests
The authors declare that they have no competing interests.

Author details
[1]Department of Pharmacy, the First Affiliated Hospital of Medicine School, Zhejiang University, Hangzhou, China. [2]State Key Laboratory for Diagnosis and Treatment of Infectious Diseases, the First Affiliated Hospital of Medicine School, Zhejiang University, 79 Qingchun Road, Hangzhou, China.

References
1. Guidelines for the Prevention and Control of Carbapenem-Resistant Enterobacteriaceae, Acinetobacter baumannii and Pseudomonas aeruginosa in Health Care Facilities,Geneva: World Health Organization; 2017.
2. Fupin HU, Yan GUO, Demei ZHU. Resistance trends among clinical isolates in China reported from CHINET surveillance of bacterial resistance, 2005–2014. Chin J Infect Chemother. 2017;17:93–9.
3. Chandy SJ, Naik GS, Balaji V, et al. High cost burden and health consequences of antibiotic resistance: the price to pay. J Infect Dev Ctries. 2014;8:1096–102.
4. Fupin HU, Yan GUO, Demei ZHU, et al. CHINET surveillance of bacterial resistance across China: report of the results in 2016. Chin J Infect Chemother. 2017;17:481–91.
5. Zhang Y, Wang Q, Yin Y, et al. Epidemiology of Carbapenem-resistant Enterobacteriaceae infections: report from the China CRE network. Antimicrob Agents Chemother. 2018;62:e01882–17.
6. Nathwani D, Raman G, Sulham K, et al. Clinical and economic consequences of hospital-acquired resistant and multidrug-resistant Pseudomonas aeruginosa infections: a systematic review and meta-analysis. Antimicrob Resist Infect Control. 2014;3:32.
7. Lemos EV, de la Hoz FP, Einarson TR, et al. Carbapenem resistance and mortality in patients with Acinetobacter baumannii infection: systematic review and meta-analysis. Clin Microbiol Infect. 2014;20:416–23.
8. Arepyeva MA, Kolbin AS, Sidorenko SV, et al. A mathematical model for predicting the development of bacterial resistance based on the relationship between the level of antimicrobial resistance and the volume of antibiotic consumption. J Glob Antimicrob Resist. 2017;8:148–56.
9. Stapleton PJ, Lundon DJ, McWade R, et al. Antibiotic resistance patterns of Escherichia coli urinary isolates and comparison with antibiotic consumption data over 10 years, 2005-2014. Ir J Med Sci. 2017;186:733–41.
10. Tammer I, Geginat G, Lange S, et al. Antibiotic consumption and the development of antibiotic resistance in surgical units. Zentralbl Chir. 2016; 141:53–61.
11. Bell BG, Schellevis F, Stobberingh E, et al. A systematic review and meta-analysis of the effects of antibiotic consumption on antibiotic resistance. BMC Infect Dis. 2014;14:13.
12. de Kraker ME, Wolkewitz M, Davey PG, et al. Burden of antimicrobial resistance in European hospitals: excess mortality and length of hospital stay associated with bloodstream infections due to Escherichia coli resistant to third-generation cephalosporins. J Antimicrob Chemother. 2011;66:398–407.
13. Wushouer H, Tian Y, Guan XD, et al. Trends and patterns of antibiotic consumption in China's tertiary hospitals: based on a 5 year surveillance with sales records, 2011-2015. PLoS One. 2017;12:e0190314.
14. Wushouer H, Zhang ZX, Wang JH, et al. Trends and relationship between antimicrobial resistance and antibiotic use in Xinjiang Uyghur autonomous

region, China: based on a 3 year surveillance data, 2014-2016. J Infect Public Health. 2018;11:339–46.

15. Joseph NM, Bhanupriya B, Shewade DG, et al. Relationship between antimicrobial consumption and the incidence of antimicrobial resistance in Escherichia coli and Klebsiella pneumoniae isolates. J Clin Diagn Res. 2015;9: DC08–12.

16. Lesho EP, Clifford RJ, Chukwuma U, et al. Carbapenem-resistant Enterobacteriaceae and the correlation between carbapenem and fluoroquinolone usage and resistance in the US military health system. Diagn Microbiol Infect Dis. 2015;81:119–25.

17. Agodi A, Auxilia F, Barchitta M, et al. Antibiotic consumption and resistance: results of the SPIN-UTI project of the GISIO-SItI. Epidemiol Prev. 2015;39:94–8.

18. Zhang GB, Mao XH, Wu ZHQ, et al. Correlation between the resistant rate of *Klebsiella pneumoniae* and antibiotics use density. Chin J Nosocomiol. 2017; 27:2427–52.

19. Santajit S, Indrawattana N. Mechanisms of antimicrobial resistance in ESKAPE pathogens. Biomed Res Int. 2016;2016:2475067.

20. Abdallah M, Badawi M, Amirah MF, et al. Impact of carbapenem restriction on the antimicrobial susceptibility pattern of Pseudomonas aeruginosa isolates in the ICU. J Antimicrob Chemother. 2017;72:3187–90.

21. Székely E, Bucur G, Vass L, et al. Antimicrobial use and its correlations with the frequency of carbapenem-resistant Pseudomonas aeruginosa strains in a hospital setting. Bacteriol Virusol Parazitol Epidemiol. 2010;55:179–86.

22. Terzi HA, Kulah C, Ciftci IH. The effects of active efflux pumps on antibiotic resistance in Pseudomonas aeruginosa. World J Microbiol Biotechnol. 2014; 30:2681–7.

23. Lai CC, Shi ZY, Chen YH, et al. Effects of various antimicrobial stewardship programs on antimicrobial usage and resistance among common gram-negative bacilli causing health care-associated infections: a multicenter comparison. J Microbiol Immunol Infect. 2016;49:74–82.

24. Cao J, Song W, Gu B, et al. Correlation between carbapenem consumption and antimicrobial resistance rates of Acinetobacter baumannii in a university-affiliated hospital in China. J Clin Pharmacol. 2013;53:96–102.

25. Mascarello M, Simonetti O, Knezevich A, et al. Correlation between antibiotic consumption and resistance of bloodstream bacteria in a University Hospital in North Eastern Italy, 2008-2014. Infection. 2017;45:459–67.

26. Inchai J, Liwsrisakun C, Theerakittikul T, et al. Risk factors of multidrug-resistant, extensively drug-resistant and pandrug-resistant Acinetobacter baumannii ventilator-associated pneumonia in a medical intensive care unit of University Hospital in Thailand. J Infect Chemother. 2015;21:570–4.

27. Tan CK, Tang HJ, Lai CC, et al. Correlation between antibiotic consumption and carbapenem-resistant Acinetobacter baumannii causing health care-associated infections at a hospital from 2005 to 2010. J Microbiol Immunol Infect. 2015;48:540–4.

28. Higgins PG, Wisplinghoff H, Stefanik D, et al. Selection of topoisomerase mutations and overexpression of adeB mRNA transcripts during an outbreak of Acinetobacter baumannii. J Antimicrob Chemother. 2004;54:821–3.

29. Voor In 't Holt AF, Severin JA, Lesaffre EM, et al. A systematic review and meta-analyses show that carbapenem use and medical devices are the leading risk factors for carbapenem-resistant Pseudomonas aeruginosa. Antimicrob Agents Chemother. 2014;58:2626–37.

30. Tuon FF, Gortz LW, Rocha JL. Risk factors for pan-resistant Pseudomonas aeruginosa bacteremia and the adequacy of antibiotic therapy. Braz J Infect Dis. 2012;16:351–6.

31. Lee CH, Su TY, Ye JJ, et al. Risk factors and clinical significance of bacteremia caused by Pseudomonas aeruginosa resistant only to carbapenems. J Microbiol Immunol Infect. 2017;50:677–83.

32. Liu P, Li X, Luo M, et al. Risk factors for Carbapenem-resistant Klebsiella pneumoniae infection: a meta-analysis. Microb Drug Resist. 2018;24:190–8.

33. Hsueh PR, Chen WH, Luh KT. Relationships between antimicrobial use and antimicrobial resistance in gram-negative bacteria causing nosocomial infections from 1991–2003 at a university hospital in Taiwan. Int J Antimicrob Agents. 2005;26:463–72.

18

Chlorhexidine-coated surgical gloves influence the bacterial flora of hands over a period of 3 hours

Miranda Suchomel[1][*] [ID], Markus Brillmann[1], Ojan Assadian[2,3], Karen J. Ousey[3] and Elisabeth Presterl[2]

Abstract

Background: The risk of SSI increases in the presence of foreign materials and may be caused by organisms with low pathogenicity, such as skin flora derived from hands of surgical team members in the event of a glove breach. Previously, we were able to demonstrate that a novel antimicrobial surgical glove coated chlorhexidine-digluconate as the active ingredient on its inner surface was able to suppress surgeons' hand flora during operative procedures by a magnitude of 1.7 $\log_{10}$ cfu/mL. Because of the clinical design of that study, we were not able to measure the full magnitude of the possible antibacterial suppression effect of antimicrobial gloves over a full 3 h period.

Methods: The experimental procedure followed the method for assessment of the 3-h effects of a surgical hand rub's efficacy to reduce the release of hand flora as described in the European Norm EN 12791. Healthy volunteers tested either an antimicrobial surgical glove or non-antimicrobial surgical latex gloves in a standardized laboratory-based experiment over a wear time of 3 h.

Results: Wearing antimicrobial surgical glove after a surgical hand rub with 60% (v/v) n-propanol resulted in the highest 3-h reduction factor of 2.67 $\log_{10}$. Non-antimicrobial surgical gloves demonstrated significantly lower ($p \leq 0.01$) 3-h reduction factors at 1.96 $\log_{10}$ and 1.68 $\log_{10}$, respectively. Antibacterial surgical gloves are able to maintain a sustainable bacterial reduction on finger tips in a magnitude of almost 3 $\log_{10}$ ($\log_{10}$ 2.67 cfu) over 3 h wear time.

Conclusion: It was demonstrated that wear of an antibacterial surgical glove coated with chlorhexidine-digluconate is able to suppress resident hand flora significantly over a period of 3-h.

Keywords: Surgical glove, Perforation, Bacterial migration, Antimicrobial efficacy, Surgical site infection, Bacterial skin flora, Antimicrobial glove, Chlorhexidine, Antiseptic

Background

Surgical site infections (SSIs) constitute a large proportion of all Healthcare Associated Infections (HAI). Overall, at least one of every 20 patients undergoing open surgery will develop an SSI [1, 2]. SSIs are associated with one third of post-operative related deaths [3], but more frequently they may cause cosmetically unacceptable scars, pain, prolonged duration of hospitalization, and emotional stress to patients, relatives, and care givers [4, 5].

SSI rates are influenced by multiple clinical risk factors. However, to cause any SSI, microorganisms will need to contaminate the sterile surgical site. Bacteria involved in SSIs include patients' own endogenous flora, and those that may be introduced from the environment including the microbial flora of the operating surgical team members [6, 7]. The risk of SSI increases in the presence of foreign materials and may even be caused by organisms with low pathogenicity, such as skin flora derived from hands of surgical team members in the event of a glove breach [8].

Breach of glove integrity may cause bacterial migration from the surgeon's hand to the surgical site [9]. Therefore, various tactics have been developed to reduce the risk of surgical site contamination with bacteria originating from the surgical team's hands. The most important measure is preoperative surgical hand antisepsis using

* Correspondence: miranda.suchomel@meduniwien.ac.at
[1]Institute for Hygiene and Applied Immunology, Medical University of Vienna, Kinderspitalgasse 15, 1090 Vienna, Austria
Full list of author information is available at the end of the article

an antimicrobial soap (surgical scrub) or an alcohol-based hand rub (surgical rub), which is regarded as standard practice to decrease the microbial bio-burden on surgeons' hands [10]. However, preoperative surgical hand antisepsis can reduce, but not eradicate the resident flora on the surgeon's hands [11, 12], and re-grown skin flora therefore still may enter the surgical site in the event of a glove breach [13].

In a previous randomized clinical trial [14] we were able to demonstrate that after vascular surgical procedures involving carotid endarterectomy, peripheral bypass surgery, or revascularization of the common femoral and profunda femoris arteries the frequency of glove perforation was 14% at the end of the interventions. Furthermore, we could demonstrate that the mean number of bacterial colony forming units (cfu) retrieved from the inner layer of intact surgical gloves was 299 cfu/mL after a mean operating time of 112 min. Finally, we could show that a novel antimicrobial surgical glove coated with a complex formulation of 14 ingredients, including chlorhexidine-digluconate (CHG) as the active ingredient on its inner surface was able to suppress surgeons' hand flora during operative procedures by a magnitude of 1.7 $\log_{10}$ cfu/mL.

However, because of the design of that study, we were not able to measure the full magnitude of the possible antibacterial suppression effect of antimicrobial gloves over a full 3 h period. Therefore, the aim of this laboratory-based standardized experimental study following the European Norm (EN) 12,791 [15], the in vivo laboratory assay for testing the bactericidal efficacy of pre-surgical hand preparations, was to close this gap.

Methods

The experimental procedure followed the method for assessment of the 3-h effect of a surgical hand rub's efficacy to reduce the release of hand flora as described in the European Norm EN 12791 [15]. The study was conducted at the Institute for Hygiene and Applied Immunology, Medical University, Vienna, Austria. The laboratory was accredited according to EN ISO/IEC 17025:2005 [16] and recognized by the national accreditation body "Akkreditierung Austria". All areas of testing were approved and reported to the Federal Ministry of Science, Research and Economy, Austria. Approval for this laboratory based experimental work was obtained together with a previously published randomized controlled trial (RCT; ISRCTN 71391952) from the ethics committee of the municipality of Vienna (EK 11–201-1111), and written informed consent was obtained from all participating volunteers.

Twenty-one healthy volunteers tested either an antimicrobial surgical glove (Glove A; Gammex PF with AMT; Ansell Ltd., Richmond, Australia) made of latex or one of the following non-antimicrobial surgical latex glove types: Sempermed Supreme (Glove B; Semperit, Ternitz, Austria) or Gammex PF (Glove C; Gammex PF; Ansell Ltd., Richmond, Australia) randomly allocated to their dominant and non-dominant hand.

The proof of a non-existent antimicrobial property of the uncoated control gloves B and C was carried out in accordance with Annex B of the European Norm EN 12791 [15].

A Latin-square design was used with 3 test groups (glove A and B; glove B and C; glove C and A), each of 7 randomly allotted participants. In each test run all 3 test groups were tested concurrently. At the end of the whole test series each volunteer had used each glove combination (A/B; B/C; C/A) once. Each test run was performed strictly on a Monday in order to allow re-growth of the normal skin flora before the next test run. Hence, after 3 weeks, a total of 42 results were available for each type of glove.

Before each test, every participant washed hands in a standardized manner with non-medicated soap (APOCA; Vienna, Austria) for 1 min as described in EN 12791 [15]. Hands were dried with clean hand towels. Thereafter, fingertips were rubbed and kneaded for 1 min at the base of a petri dish (Ø 9 cm) containing 10 mL tryptic soy broth (TSB; Caso broth°, Merck) for measurement of bacterial pre-values. Subsequently, hand antisepsis was performed using minimum 3 mL reference alcohol 60% (v/v) n-propanol (pro analysi, Merck) for 3 min [15]. The bactericidal efficacy of this reference alcohol recommended by the European Norm EN 12791 was demonstrated before [17]. After the alcohol had evaporated, the volunteer donned two different sterile surgical gloves on both hands (A and B, B and C or C and A). Instead of the conditions of the EN 12791 which requires comparing the reduction factor of a test hand rub against a reference product immediately and after 3 h in pre-trained volunteers, the viable $\log_{10}$ cfu/mL means of the post-values obtained from the participants' finger tips [15] of the three groups were compared against each other only after 3 h. During the 3-h phase the participants followed the standard procedure according to the used EN 12791, which states that they shall use their gloved hands as usually simulating a surgery. In case of glove perforation the participant has to be excluded.

After 3 h gloves were donned by a second person without contamination and finger tips of both hands were massaged in petri dishes - one for each hand - filled with 10 mL of a validated neutralizer (90 g/L polysorbate 80, 9 g/L lecithin, and 3 g/L histidine and TSB) active against chlorhexidine [15], and gently massaged for 1 min; quantitative surface cultures were prepared on Tryptone soya agar plates (TSA plates; Caso agar°, Merck) using a sterile pipette tip and a sterile spreaders from all sampling solutions and their decimal dilutions.

The agar plates were incubated for up to 48 h at 36 °C ± 1 °C. After incubation, the colony forming unit (cfu) per mL was counted and recorded for each dilution step. The number of cfu per mL sampling fluid was calculated by multiplying the plate count by the dilution factor. In addition to recording cfu/mL counts, viable counts were transformed to decimal logarithms, where appropriate. For computational reasons, values of "0" ($\log_{10} 0 = -\infty$) was set at "1" ($\log_{10} 1 = 0$).

Statistical analysis

Logarithmic reduction factors ($\log_{10}$ RFs) were calculated as the intra-individual difference of $\log_{10}$ pre-treatment values minus $\log_{10}$ post-treatment values after 3 h for each glove type separately. $\log_{10}$ RFs were expressed as means ± standard deviation (±SD), with 95% confidence intervals (CIs) and range. Mean $\log_{10}$ RFs were tested for statistical significant difference between the tested groups (A/B; B/C; C/A) by using a paired two-tailed T-test. Negative values were corrected to positive values, if applicable. All tests for significance were run as two-sided tests with alpha was set at the 5% level.

Results

No significant differences were found between the means of the pre-treatment bacterial counts in any of the experimental test runs (data not shown). The means ranged between 4.39 and 4.55 $\log_{10}$ and therefore fulfilled the EN 12791 which requires pre-treatment values higher than 3.5 $\log_{10}$. After surgical hand antisepsis using 60% v/v n-propanol and a 3 h wear time of glove A (antimicrobial surgical glove) the $\log_{10}$ reduction was 2.67, and in the standard surgical gloves $\log_{10}$ 1.96 (glove B) and $\log_{10}$ 1.68 (glove C), respectively. Overall, after 3 h of wear, the antimicrobial surgical glove (glove A) demonstrated a higher $\log_{10}$ reduction, while the non-antimicrobial surgical gloves (glove B, glove C) showed a lower $\log_{10}$-reduction (Table 1).

The difference in the mean $\log_{10}$-reduction factors between antimicrobial surgical gloves and non-antibacterial gloves B or C was statistically significant ($\log_{10}$ reduction factor 0.71 and 0.99, respectively; $p = 0.001$ and $p < 0.001$, respectively). There was no statistical significant difference in the $\log_{10}$ reduction factors between the two non-

antimicrobial surgical gloves after a 3 h wear time ($\log_{10}$ reduction factor 0.28; $p = 0.056$, Table 2).

These results demonstrate that antibacterial surgical gloves were able to maintain a sustainable bacterial reduction on hands in a magnitude of almost 3 $\log_{10}$ ($\log_{10}$ 2.67 cfu) over 3 h wear time.

Discussion

SSI rates are influenced by multiple clinical variables. Nonetheless, bacteria may origin from a patient endogenously or may enter the sterile surgical site exogenously from the environment including the microbial flora of the surgical team, particularly in case of glove breach [8, 9, 14, 18]. The risk of glove defects is related to the type of surgery performed, ranging from 7% in urological surgery and 65% in cardio-thoracic surgery [19–23].

Previously, we were able to demonstrate that even after surgical hand antisepsis surgeons may harbour (again) between $\log_{10}$ 2.51 cfu to $\log_{10}$ 2.72 cfu of bacteria on their fingertips after 3 h wear time of non-antibacterial surgical gloves [14]. The aim of this study was to investigate a possibly present or absent suppressing effect of an antibacterial surgical glove in comparison to non-antibacterial surgical gloves on the skin flora after surgical hand treatment with the reference alcohol 60% (v/v) n-propanol of the European Norm EN 12791 [15], the European in vivo laboratory assay for testing bactericidal efficacy of surgical hand treatments, under standardized and reproducible laboratory conditions. Thus, in the present study, we were further able to demonstrate that wear of an antibacterial surgical glove coated with chlorhexidine-digluconate is able to suppress resident hand flora significantly over a period of 3 h and to maintain a sustainable bacterial reduction on hands in a magnitude of almost 3 $\log_{10}$ ($\log_{10}$ reduction factor 2.67 cfu).

Our study has a number of limitations. First, we were not able to state in exact numbers what happened immediately after surgical hand antisepsis and donning gloves. Second, we were also not able to state how many minutes of wearing an antimicrobial glove would have been needed to observe the first significant difference in cfu counts as compared to a non-antimicrobial glove. These questions can only be answered by conducting a

Table 1 Mean $\log_{10}$ reduction factors after 3 h wear time of three different surgical gloves

Group	N	Mean $\log_{10}$ RF	± SD	95%-Confidence Interval (CI) Lower	95%-Confidence Interval (CI) Upper	Min.	Max.
A	42	2.67	1.24	2.28	3.06	−1.19	5.37
B	42	1.96	1.31	1.55	2.37	−0.14	5.06
C	42	1.68	1.09	1.33	2.02	−0.23	3.85
Total	126	2.10	1.28	1.88	2.33	−1.19	5.37

RF reduction factor, *SD* Standard Deviation, *N* sample size, Group A: antimicrobial surgical glove; Group B and group C: non-antimicrobial standard surgical gloves

Table 2 Pair-wise ANOVA comparing differences in $\log_{10}$ RFs between glove types

	Paired differences				T	df	Significance
	Mean $\log_{10}$ RF	± SD	95%-Confidence Intervals of differences				
			Lower	Upper			
A – B	0.71	1.38	0.28	1.14	3.33	41	0.001
B – C	0.28	1.14	−0.07	0.64	1.62	41	0.056
C – A	0.99	1.20	0.62	1.37	5.37	41	0.000

df Degree of freedom, T Effect size for statistical test, SD Standard Deviation

bacterial elimination kinetic study with different measure points as compared to the strict time points required by the European reference method EN 12791. Although our study design would have been able to serve as basis for such an investigation on bacterial kinetics under antibacterial and non-antimicrobial gloves, it would require different sampling time points.

Interestingly, also in the standard glove groups we observed low bacterial counts on fingertips. In theory, the number of cfu on the hand donned with a non-antimicrobial glove should increase over time, while the number of cfu on antibacterially donned hands should remain low or increase only in minute counts. Therefore, the longer an antibacterial glove is worn, the larger the difference in cfu should be. However, by ascertaining that all tested groups were measured at the identical time, a possible influence based on such mechanisms may be ruled out.

Finally, when a new technology, drug, method or other procedure is introduced, it will be expected that a benefit is demonstrated with its use. Clearly, in case of antimicrobial devices, the primary intention to use this is prevention or treatment of infection. Therefore, it is logical that demonstration of prevention or treatment success is scientifically produced. However, concurrently with increasing awareness for infection control and implementation of bundle measures to decrease the burden of infection, demonstration of the clinical efficacy of antimicrobial devices is becoming also increasingly difficult because of the decreasing number of infection in individual surgical procedures. The required size of such randomized clinical trials automatically prohibits and attempt for such studies. If the efficacy of antimicrobial devices needs to be demonstrated clinically, one option would be to conduct such studies during episodes of highly increased incidences of SSI, such as during outbreak situations. Aside of the fact that outbreaks are rarely predictable and timely planning is impossible, the result of a randomized controlled trial performed in such a situation would not allow drawing conclusions for a device's efficacy in a normal patient population, and any effects would be subject to justified critique. Therefore, the only other two alternatives seem to be the establishment of huge international registries with

accepted definitions for SSI, or well-designed experimental clinical or in-vivo studies to evaluate and compare these concepts, preferably under the same test conditions and test methodology.

Conclusion

In conclusion, it was demonstrated that wear of an antibacterial surgical glove coated with chlorhexidine-digluconate is able to suppress resident hand flora significantly over a period of 3-h.

Funding
This study was funded by the Institute for Hygiene and Applied Immunology, Medical University of Vienna.

Authors' contributions
MS led study execution and was a major contributor to design, analysis and writing of the publication. MB performed all the analysis and helped writing the manuscript. OA led to the design, analysis and writing of the manuscript. KO and EP contributed to the writing of the manuscript. All authors read and approved the final manuscript.

Consent for publication
Not applicable.

Competing interests
The authors declare that they have no competing interests.

Author details
[1]Institute for Hygiene and Applied Immunology, Medical University of Vienna, Kinderspitalgasse 15, 1090 Vienna, Austria. [2]Department for Hospital Epidemiology and Infection Control, Medical University of Vienna, Vienna, Austria. [3]Institute for Skin Integrity and Infection Prevention, University of Huddersfield, Huddersfield, UK.

References
1. Smyth ET, McIlvenny G, Enstone JE, Emmerson AM, Humphreys H, Fitzpatrick F, et al. Four country healthcare associated infection prevalence survey 2006: overview of the results. J Hosp Infect. 2008;69:230–48.
2. Prospero E, Cavicchi A, Bacelli S, Barbadoro P, Tantucci L, D'Errico MM. Surveillance for surgical site infection after hospital discharge: a surgical procedure-specific perspective. Infect Control Hosp Epidemiol. 2006;27:1313–7.
3. Astagneau P, Rioux C, Golliot F, Brückner G, INCISO Network Study Group. Morbidity and mortality associated with surgical site infections: results from the 1997–1999 INCISO surveillance. J Hosp Infect. 2001;48:267–74.
4. Bayat A, McGrouther DA, Ferguson MW. Skin scarring. Br Med J. 2003;326:88–92.
5. McGarry SA, Engemann JJ, Schmader K, et al. Surgical-site infection due to staphylococcus aureus among elderly patients: mortality, duration of

hospitalization and cost. Infect Control Hosp Epidemiol. 2004;25:461–7.

6. Allegranzi B, Bischoff P, de Jonge S, Kubilay NZ, Zayed B, Gomes SM, et al. New WHO recommendations on preoperative measures for surgical site infection prevention: an evidence-based global perspective. Lancet Infect Dis. 2016;16:e276–e87.

7. Berríos-Torres SI, Umscheid CA, Bratzler DW, Leas B, Stone EC, Kelz RR, et al. Centers for Disease Control and Prevention guideline for the prevention of surgical site infection, 2017. JAMA Surg. 2017;152:784–91.

8. Misteli H, Weber WP, Reck S, Rosenthal R, Zwahlen M, Fueglistaler P, et al. Surgical glove perforation and the risk of surgical site infection. Arch Surg. 2009;144:553–8.

9. Hübner NO, Goerdt AM, Stanislawski N, Assadian O, Heidecke CD, Kramer A, Partecke LI. Bacterial migration through punctured surgical gloves under real surgical conditions. BMC Infect Dis. 2010;10:192.

10. Pittet D, Allegranzi B, Boyce J. World Health Organization world alliance for patient safety first global patient safety challenge Core Group of experts. The World Health Organization guidelines on hand hygiene in health care and their consensus recommendations. Infect Control Hosp Epidemiol. 2009;30:611–22.

11. Peterson AF, Rosenberg A, Alatary SD. Comperative evaluation of surgical scrub preparations. Surg Gynecol Obstet. 1978;146:63–5.

12. Rotter ML, Kampf G, Suchomel M, Kundi M. Population kinetics of the skin flora on gloved hands following surgical hand disinfection within 3 propanol-based hand rubs: a prospective, randomize, double-blinded trial. Infect Control Hosp Epidemiol. 2007;28:346–50.

13. Partecke LI, Goerdt AM, Langner I, Jaeger B, Assadian O, Heidecke CD, et al. Incidence of microperforation for surgical gloves depends on duration of wear. Infect Control Hosp Epidemiol. 2009;30:409–14.

14. Assadian O, Kramer A, Ouriel K, Suchomel M, McLaws ML, Rottman M, et al. Suppression of surgeons' bacterial hand flora during surgical procedures using a new antimicrobial surgical glove. Surg Infect. 2014;15:43–9.

15. European Norm (EN) 12791. Chemical disinfectants and antiseptics. Surgical hand disinfection – test method and requirement (phase 2/step 2). Brussels: Comité Européen de Normalisation; 2009.

16. EN ISO/IEC 17025. General requirements for the competence of testing and calibration laboratories. Brussels: Comité Européen de Normalisation; 2005.

17. Suchomel M, Weinlich M, Kundi M. Influence of glycerol and an alternative humectant on the immediate and 3-hours bactericidal efficacies of two isopropanol-based antiseptics in laboratory experiments in vivo according to EN 12791. Antimicrob Resist Infect Control. 2017;6:72.

18. Mangram AJ, Horan TC, Pearson ML, Silver LC, Jarvis WR. Guideline for prevention of surgical site infection, 1999. Hospital infection control practices advisory committee. Infect Control Hosp Epidemiol. 1999;20:250–78.

19. Laine T, Kaipia A, Santavirta J, Aarnio P. Glove perforations in open and laparoscopic abdominal surgery: the feasibility of double gloving. Scand J Surg. 2004;93:73–6.

20. Brough SJ, Hunt TM, Barrie WW. Surgical glove perforations. Br J Surg. 1988;75:317.

21. Kojima Y, Ohashi M. Unnoticed glove perforation during thoracoscopic and open thoracic surgery. Ann Thorac Surg. 2005;80:1078–80.

22. Pitten FA, Herdemann G, Kramer A. The integrity of latex gloves in clinical dental practice. Infection. 2000;28:388–92.

23. Manjunath AP, Shepherd JH, Barton DP, Bridges JE, Ind TE. Glove perforations during open surgery for gynaecological malignancies. BJOG. 2008;115:1015–9.

19

Clostridium difficile infection perceptions and practices: a multicenter qualitative study in South Africa

Laurel Legenza[1,2]*, Susanne Barnett[1], Warren Rose[1], Nasia Safdar[3], Theresa Emmerling[1], Keng Hee Peh[1] and Renier Coetzee[2]

Abstract

Background: *Clostridium difficile* infection (CDI) is understudied in limited resource settings. In addition, provider awareness of CDI as a prevalent threat is unknown. An assessment of current facilitators and barriers to CDI identification, management, and prevention is needed in limited resource settings to design and evaluate quality improvement strategies to effectively minimize the risk of CDI.

Methods: Our study aimed to identify CDI perceptions and practices among healthcare providers in South African secondary hospitals to identify facilitators and barriers to providing quality CDI care. Qualitative interviews (11 physicians, 11 nurses, 4 pharmacists,) and two focus groups (7 nurses, 3 pharmacists) were conducted at three district level hospitals in the Cape Town Metropole. Semi-structured interviews elicited provider perceived facilitators, barriers, and opportunities to improve clinical workflow from patient presentation through CDI (1) Identification, (2) Diagnosis, (3) Treatment, and (4) Prevention. In addition, a summary provider CDI knowledge score was calculated for each interviewee for seven components of CDI and management.

Results: Major barriers identified were knowledge gaps in characteristics of *C. difficile* identification, diagnosis, treatment, and prevention. The median overall CDI knowledge score (scale 0–7) from individual interviews was 3 [interquartile range 0.25, 4.75]. Delays in *C. difficile* testing workflow were identified. Participants perceived supplies for CDI management and prevention were usually available; however, hand hygiene and use of contact precautions was inconsistent.

Conclusions: Our analysis provides a detailed description of the facilitators and barriers to CDI workflow and can be utilized to design quality improvement interventions among limited resource settings.

Keywords: Healthcare associated infection, Infection control, Qualitative study, Antimicrobial stewardship, Global health

Background

Clostridium difficile infection (CDI) is an increasingly important healthcare-associated infection associated with long hospitalisations and high patient morbidity and mortality [1]. CDI often results from normal gut bacterial disruption due to broad-spectrum antimicrobial use, allowing for overgrowth of toxigenic *C. difficile*. CDI outbreaks have been reported extensively in the United States (US) and Europe over the last two decades. CDI in these hospitals is prevalent supporting extensive CDI prevention and control measures. However, CDI is understudied in low and limited resource settings, including nearly all African countries. Where limited data exists, a study at a tertiary hospital in Cape Town, South Africa found 22% of stool samples from patients with suspected CDI diarrhoea were *C. difficile* positive [2]. In addition, patients in South Africa are disproportionately affected by HIV and tuberculosis (TB) and therefore also experience known CDI risk factors of prior hospital and antibiotic exposure—exposures that

* Correspondence: Legenza@wisc.edu
[1]University of Wisconsin-Madison School of Pharmacy, 777 Highland Ave, Madison, WI 53705, USA
[2]University of the Western Cape School of Pharmacy, Robert Sobukwe, Cape Town 7535, South Africa
Full list of author information is available at the end of the article

can uniquely contribute to an increased risk of CDI and poor outcomes [3, 4].

Treatment of CDI requires a comprehensive approach that includes infection prevention and control (IPC) measures to limit transmission and prevent outbreaks. Although no CDI IPC guidelines exist specific to African countries, the Infectious Diseases Society of America (IDSA) and European Society of Clinical Microbiology and Infectious Diseases guidelines consistently recommend IPC components of antimicrobial stewardship programs (ASP) which include effective environment cleaning, patient isolation, use of personal protective equipment such as gowns and gloves, surveillance, and education [5]. These evidence-based recommendations are key to effective CDI management. The feasibility of using these recommendations in populations with limited healthcare resources has not been established. In addition, healthcare provider knowledge of CDI and the guidance to effectively mitigate and manage patient populations at higher risk for CDI is unknown.

Provider knowledge of CDI and treatment measures are essential to both successfully manage CDI and prevent disease transmission. An assessment of current facilitators and barriers to CDI identification, management, and prevention is needed to design and evaluate improvement strategies to effectively minimize the risk of CDI. To our knowledge, no comprehensive study of barriers and facilitators to CDI workflow (identification, diagnosis, treatment, and prevention) in Sub-Saharan Africa exists. Our study aims to fill this gap by eliciting CDI perceptions and management practices among healthcare providers in South African secondary hospitals to uncover facilitators and barriers to providing quality CDI care.

Methods
Data collection
We utilized a qualitative approach to elicit health care providers' perceptions of barriers and facilitators to CDI management because it provides detailed process oriented results. We conducted semi-structured interviews and focus groups among clinical providers at three secondary hospitals in South Africa. A Systems Engineering Initiative for Patient Safety (SEIPS) model served as a framework for the interview guide. The SEIPS framework connects work systems to patient and organizational outcomes, while including interactions in the work system between available tools, people, tasks, the internal environment, and the organization [6]. The semi-structured interview assessed each subject's CDI knowledge and traced workflow from patient presentation with CDI symptoms through CDI 1.) Identification, 2.) Diagnosis, 3.) Treatment, and 4.)

Prevention. Interview questions were structured to reveal facilitators and barriers to these CDI workflow steps and opportunities to improve CDI treatment. The interview guide included optional probes to use when appropriate to gather additional information. When participants revealed a lack of CDI knowledge from the preliminary questions, the interview was then modified to contain general questions about diarrhoea management. As a qualitative study, the interviewer could use information gathered from prior interviews to direct future interview discussions and build on emerging concepts. For example, asking for further detail and implications on processes mentioned with open-ended questions.

Participants
Providers working in three public secondary (district) level hospitals in the Western Cape, Cape Town Metropole, South Africa were invited to participate in this study. The three participating hospitals, averaging 265 inpatient beds overall, were previously selected to be included in a CDI quality improvement intervention. Our study aimed to interview, at minimum, 15 providers among five provider types including frontline nurses, nurse managers, pharmacists, junior physicians (registrars and medical officers), and senior physicians (consultants and department administrators). Semi-structured interviews and focus groups occurred August–November 2016.

Study investigators included healthcare providers from the US and South Africa with local hospital affiliations. The interviewers, a study investigator and a visiting US pharmacy resident, recruited front-line healthcare providers with convenience and snowball sampling, and recruited senior providers with purposive sampling. There were no participant exclusion criteria. Interviews were conducted as focus group discussions if preferred by participants. Participants were provided an informed consent document approved by the ethics committee prior to the interview and could decline participation at any time. Interviews were conducted by the interviewer in consultation rooms and offices. All interviews were conducted in English by one of the two interviewers with questions from a semi-structured interview guide and probing techniques by the interviewer. Interviews continued until thematic saturation was observed regarding barriers and facilitators for CDI treatment and management. The University of the Western Cape Research Ethics Committee granted approval for this qualitative study.

Data analysis
Interview audio recordings were transcribed verbatim and checked for accuracy. Data analysis included coding

to factors determined a priori (including key workflow steps: 1) Identification, 2) Diagnosis, 3) Treatment, and 4) Prevention) as well as inductive coding to emerging themes [7]. Two individuals from a team of three coders (LL, TE, and KP) conducted each coding phase. Paired coding with two coders per phase was performed to minimize bias. Coding schema was created to reconcile local medical terminology. Discrepancies in coding were resolved by consensus. Kappa scores were calculated to assess coding agreement at a mid-point and at the conclusion of coding. While we had initially planned to map results with the SEIPS framework, CDI management knowledge was significantly lower than expected and insufficient to frame the results in terms of tools, people, tasks, the internal environment, and the organization. Alternatively, we mapped coded themes to the workflow structure identified from the interviews.

After identifying large discrepancies in health care provider knowledge regarding CDI during the interview process, a scoring system was developed to categorize participants' CDI knowledge from their interview responses (Table 1). The intent of the assessment was to quantify the unexpected differences. With the knowledge assessment, one knowledge point was possible from each of the following seven CDI-related components: signs and symptoms (e.g. diarrhoea), characteristics of bacteria (e.g. microbiology, virulence mechanism, disruption of normal flora, opportunistic), hand hygiene (e.g. soap and water needed to clean hands, not just alcohol), treatment (e.g. metronidazole, oral vancomycin, fecal transplant, contraindication with loperamide), contact precautions/isolation (contagious), risk factors (e.g. healthcare

exposure, antibiotic use, immunocompromised by medication or illness [cancer, HIV status, CD4 count < 200] proton pump inhibitor use), and diagnosis (e.g. stool sample and testing methods, polymerase chain reaction[PCR]/toxin detection). The following responses did not receive a point allocation: 1) only stating 'bacterial infection' for characteristics of bacteria, 2) stating a non-specific sign and symptoms of infection or illness without stating diarrhoea, 3) stating rehydration (electrolytes) without specific antibiotic treatment name. Total knowledge score from each individual interview was further classified into four categories: 'no knowledge' (0–1 point), 'limited knowledge' (2–3 points), 'moderate knowledge' (4–5 points), and 'advanced knowledge' (6–7 points). Each CDI knowledge category was also scored across all interviewees. Researchers conducted subgroup analysis of knowledge level based on occupation and performed analysis of individual CDI assessment knowledge categories by participant and occupation. The two focus group interviews were excluded from the knowledge assessment analysis due to potential knowledge score overestimation. However, dialogue from the group interviews was included in the qualitative analysis. All analyses were conducted using NVIVO software (Version 11, QSR International).

Results

A total of 26 semi-structured interviews were conducted with healthcare providers (11 nurses, 4 pharmacists, 11 physicians) of various rankings (Table 2). In addition, two focus groups were conducted; one with seven nurses and the second with three pharmacists, resulting in 36 study participants (Table 2). Kappa scores indicated high intercoder agreement (midpoint kappa = 0.71, final kappa 0.63). The median overall CDI knowledge score from the 26 individual interviews was 3 [interquartile range 0.25, 4.75]. Subgroup median knowledge scores and an analysis of responders' knowledge of each category are presented in Table 3. Inductive themes were coded for processes required for CDI workflow and organizational culture (beliefs and attitudes) regarding change (i.e. the ease of positive change at the organization or 'change culture') in order to inform future interventions. Healthcare provider responsibility and accountability for components of CDI management emerged as an organizational culture theme from the interviews. Thematic saturation of barriers and facilitators to CDI management was reached across the health care provider types (i.e. no additional themes emerged after iterative analysis of 26 interview and two focus group transcripts) [8]. CDI workflow steps are presented along with corresponding knowledge scores, barriers, and facilitators, (Section I: Workflow) and followed by organizational culture themes (Section II: Organizational Culture).

Table 1 *Clostridium difficile* knowledge assessment

Criteria for *Clostridium difficile* knowledge	Points
Signs and symptoms (diarrhoea)	1
States characteristics of bacteria (any mention of: microbiology, virulence mechanism, disruption of normal flora, opportunistic)	1
Soap and water needed to clean hands, not just alcohol	1
Treatment options (any mention of: metronidazole, oral vancomycin, fecal transplant, contraindication with loperamide)	1
Contact isolation needed (or contagious)	1
Risk factors (immunocompromised, antibiotic use, proton pump inhibitors)	1
Diagnosis (stool sample, testing methods [PCR/toxins])	1
Total points	=

No knowledge = 0–1[a]
Limited knowledge = 2–3
Moderate knowledge = 4–5
Advanced knowledge = 6–7

[a]Point allocation of 1 is considered no knowledge because there are multiple diseases associated with any one of the criteria, unless person states characteristics of bacteria

Table 2 Occupations and stated titles of healthcare providers interviewed

Healthcare Provider Occupation	Participants	Interviews
Nurse		
Operational managers or Assistant manager	4	4
Registered nurse or unspecified nurse	4	4
Infection Prevention and Control Nurse	2	2
Nurse Training Clinical Program Coordinator	1	1
Ward Nurses Focus Group Interview	7	1
Subtotal:	18	12
Pharmacist		
Pharmacist	4	4
Pharmacist Focus Group Interview	3	1
Subtotal:	7	5
Physician		
Head of Department	2	2
Consultant	1	1
Unspecified physician	1	1
Registrar	1	1
Medical officer	5	5
Intern	1	1
Subtotal:	11	11
Total (N)	36	28

Section I: Workflow

Figure 1 presents workflow depicted from interview results, along with facilitators and barriers to CDI management summarized in the context of the CDI workflow, including the previously identified steps of CDI identification, diagnosis, treatment, and prevention. When CDI is suspected, a stool sample is sent to an offsite laboratory for *C. difficile* identification by PCR. Following CDI diagnosis, treatment and infection prevention and control measures are initiated. Processes were consistent between healthcare providers with knowledge of the workflow step.

Identification and healthcare provider knowledge

CDI identification requires knowledge of the bacteria, risk factors and clinical suspicion when patients present with CDI signs and symptoms. A major barrier to identification is low CDI knowledge. Ten interviews (6 nurses, 4 pharmacists) scored as 'no CDI knowledge' (Table 3). One participant candidly revealed the lack of CDI knowledge.

"It's actually the first time that I hear about it, to be honest" - Pharmacist

CDI signs and symptoms were most commonly known by healthcare providers ($n = 16$, 61.5%). Thirteen (50%) participants could not describe CDI risk factors that could prompt clinical inquiry for CDI; this knowledge gap creates a potential barrier for prompt identification. Two physicians reported extensive experience with CDI in the United Kingdom. A recurrent theme from the interviews among providers was that identification for

Table 3 *Clostridium difficile* infection (CDI) knowledge scores overall, by healthcare provider, and each CDI knowledge category

CDI knowledge sorted by healthcare provider

		Occupation			Overall
		Nurse (n = 11)	Physician (n = 11)	Pharmacist (n = 4)	All participants (n = 26)
Median Score (0–7), [1st, 3rd interquartile]		1 [0, 2.5]	5 [4, 6]	0.5 [0, 1]	3 [0.25, 4.75]
Knowledge Classification, n (%)					
No		6 (54.5)	0 (0.0)	4 (100.0)	10 (38.5)
Limited		4 (36.4)	0 (0.0)	0 (0.0)	4 (15.4)
Moderate		0 (0.0)	6 (54.5)	0 (0.0)	6 (23.1)
Advanced		1 (100.0)	5 (45.5)	0 (0.0)	6 (23.1)
Knowledge assessed in each CDI knowledge category					
Components of CDI knowledge assessment, n (%)					
1. Identification	1.1 Characteristics of bacteria	2 (18.2)	4 (36.4)	0 (0.0)	6 (23.1)
	1.2 Risk factors	3 (27.3)	10 (90.9)	0 (0.0)	13 (50.0)
	1.3 Signs and symptoms	3 (27.3)	11 (100.0)	2 (50.0)	16 (61.5)
2. Diagnosis	2.1 Diagnosis	1 (9.1)	10 (90.9)	0 (0.0)	11 (42.3)
3. Treatment	3.1 Treatment options	1 (9.1)	7 (63.6)	0 (0.0)	8 (30.8)
4. Prevention	4.1 Hand washing needed	4 (36.4)	7 (63.6)	0 (0.0)	11 (42.3)
	4.2 Need for contact isolation	4 (36.4)	8 (72.7)	0 (0.0)	12 (46.2)

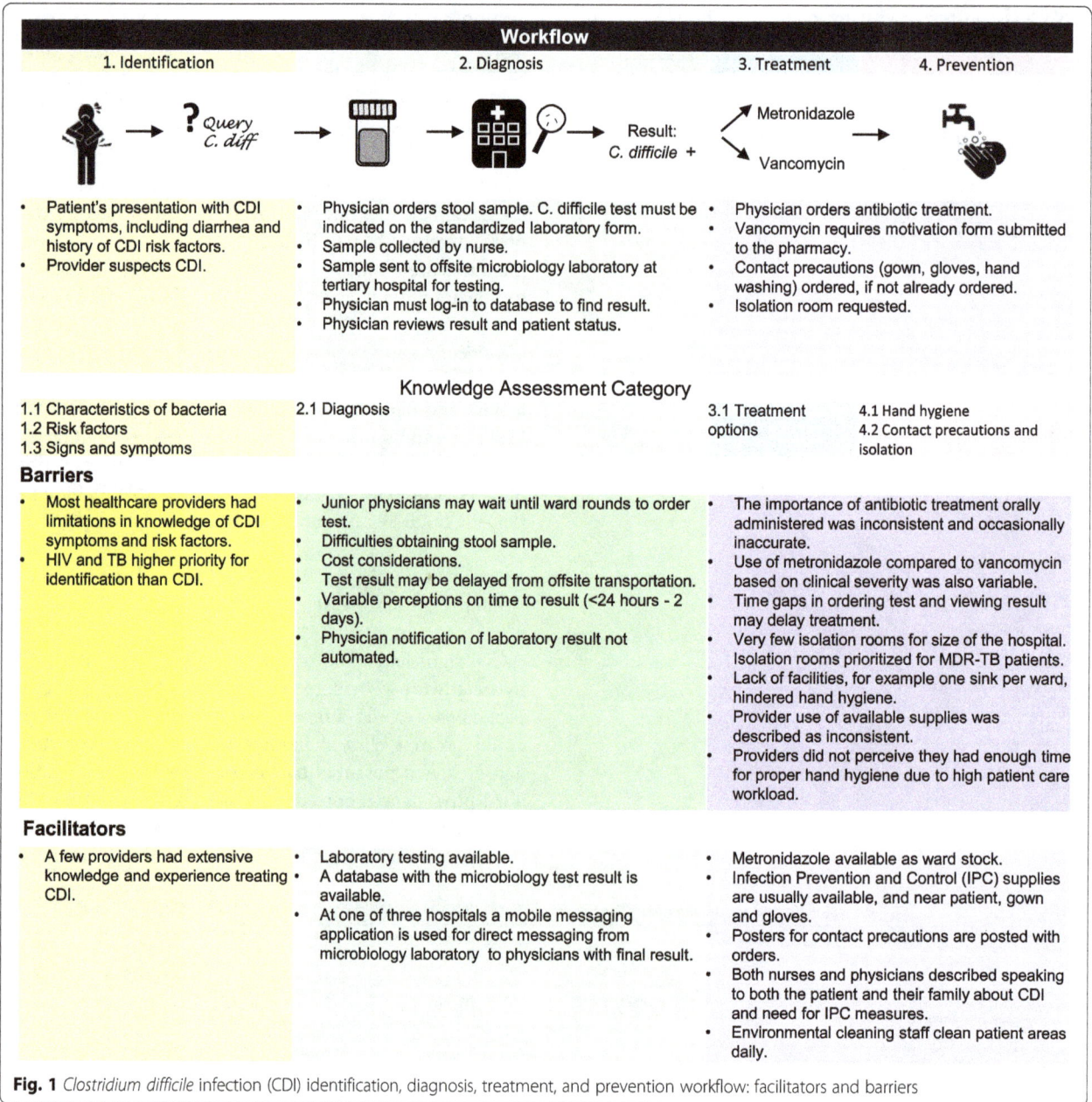

Fig. 1 *Clostridium difficile* infection (CDI) identification, diagnosis, treatment, and prevention workflow: facilitators and barriers

HIV and TB was prioritized over CDI. Physicians who have worked in the United Kingdom (U.K.) elaborated that the sense of urgency in South Africa for CDI was different than their previous experience due to competing attention of other prevalent disease.

"When I was in the UK [United Kingdom] years ago... [when] the manager mentioned C. diff the staff would jump up and down and get incredibly panicky... we just don't have that sense of urgency here... if you mention to someone in any hospital, they will go 'Okay, what is that?' [in cavalier tone]... however, if you tell them there is a patient with a potential XDR-

TB [Extensively drug-resistant TB], then they may jump up and down. So the whole thing with C. diff it's a reality... ...a lot of people just think it's a disease with the elderly, but we have a lot of immunocompromised patients..." - Physician

At one hospital, CDI awareness in senior staff only increased after an outbreak in the hospital. Awareness was lower for rotating junior staff who did not experience the outbreak.

"In terms of my junior staff, I think [CDI] ranks quite low. I think it's got to do with the way we've become

aware last year. We've had more cases making us aware that it's highly infectious." - Physician

While some providers conjectured CDI to be a national problem, others did not, and no providers were aware of CDI magnitude in South Africa. Facilitating CDI identification were the senior providers with higher CDI knowledge. At one of the hospitals, an ASP was referenced as attributing to low incidence.

Diagnosis

After identification, to inform diagnosis, a stool sample from the patient is tested at a laboratory for *C. difficile*. While all hospitals in our study had laboratory testing available to conduct a *C. difficile* PCR test, testing occurred offsite as there was not capacity for the PCR test at the onsite laboratory. In order to test for *C. difficile*, physicians must indicate the test on a standardized laboratory form. Perception of time to result varied widely and was attributed to delays in initiating treatment. Additional barriers identified included staff difficulties obtaining stool samples due to staff shortages and non-standardized collection of laboratory samples. Laboratory test costs were occasionally cited as reasons to not test for *C. difficile*. Eleven interview participants described CDI diagnosis (42.3%, Table 3).

"Most of the time they are not tested, because they come from the emergency, and because our emergency is so busy, then the patient is pushed up to the ward. So then only when the patient is in the ward, and then we are actually reporting the [diarrhoea] to them [post call]. And then report that the patient is having diarrhoea; then that's the only time that they collect a stool specimen, and then after some, a couple of days, they get the results: the patient is positive. See... It could be about a week." - Nurse Focus Group

Other attributes identified in delaying the time to diagnosis include waiting for a physician to suggest the *C. difficile* test or until ward rounds to order it. To find results, physicians must proactively login to the database—usually from their personal mobile phones, as computer stations are not easily available. One of three hospitals uses a mobile messaging application for direct messaging from the microbiology laboratory to physicians with the goal of reducing the result notification time.

"I think the one resource that we've shown very well is the communication system. I think we chose the cheapest one we could find which is WhatsApp and that does make a difference in terms of managing your patients and getting a quicker diagnosis. The thing about WhatsApp is if a patient had a positive result,

it would take the doctor another 2 days to figure it out that an infection exists. We actually have an alert system that works." - Physician

After observing the test result, the physician informs the nursing staff if the patient has a CDI. The IPC nurses are also informed of results and may, in turn, inform the medical team. However, there is not a timely and consistent pathway for this notification, especially during post-call hours. The IPC nurse sends physicians a report including positive *C. difficile* test results on a monthly basis.

Treatment

Antibiotic treatment options for antibiotic-associated diarrhoea included in South African treatment guidelines at the time of the interviews were oral metronidazole initially and oral vancomycin for diarrhoea not responsive to metronidazole; vancomycin must be oral to reach the infection. Of note, the interviews were conducted prior to the revised IDSA CDI guidelines in 2018 [3]. Eight (30.8%) respondents mentioned CDI treatment options, including treatment with metronidazole and vancomycin, though the importance of antibiotic treatment administered orally was reported inconsistently and occasionally inaccurately.

A few providers also discussed the clinical use of metronidazole compared to vancomycin, including patients' illness severity.

"So patients who don't respond to metronidazole would definitely be candidates for vancomycin or a metronidazole allergy." - Physician

Communication barriers were attributed to delays in treatment and included factors such as results being finalized while the physician was post call and drug order errors needing clarification.

Healthcare providers' high familiarity with metronidazole and its availability on the hospital floor as ward stock facilitated its use for CDI treatment. To order vancomycin and other antibiotics on the Essential Medicine List for Hospital Level Adults, providers needed to complete a pharmacy-approved motivation form that facilitates appropriate antibiotic use. Participants reported a time gap between ordering, sending the medication chart to the pharmacy, having the medication delivered to the ward, and administrating it to the patients. Some orders might be written up and not sent to the pharmacy. For stat orders, nurses may retrieve orders from the pharmacy. The pharmacies were closed during evenings and weekends. An emergency stock of inventory is kept in the emergency center. If the needed drug is unavailable, an on-call pharmacist is called-in to prepare it.

Occasionally medication was not administered and incorrectly documented as unavailable while drug was available in the emergency stock. Other reported barriers to patients receiving medications as ordered included: illegible handwriting, medication orders not including which ward an order came from, and physicians writing brand names when nurses only know the generic name. Additionally, sometimes a medication was given and not recorded; other times the patients missed doses because they were not present.

"The problem with this is ...that sometimes the results come back, the doctor is post call. Yes, and then he will only get the feedback the next day when he is actually coming to check on his patients. So that is the delay to start"- Nurse Focus Group

Prevention: Contact precautions, hand hygiene, isolation, environmental cleaning

Contact precautions CDI prevention procedures include contact precautions (e.g. gown, gloves) to reduce the risk of *C. difficile* spreading to other patients. Twelve (46.2%) participants reported the need for strict contact precautions when CDI was suspected or diagnosed. Supplies and procedures for IPC (included posters displaying orders for contact precautions) were usually available but not always utilised. Supplies (including gowns, gloves, masks, and hand sanitizer) were available in close proximity to a patient once contact precautions were ordered. Staff education and timely notification of need for infection control were the most common barriers to IPC measures. Pressure from patient bed shortages can lead to patients being placed near each other. Contact precautions with the first suspicion of CDI was described at one of the hospitals.

"...any patient with diarrhoea is placed with contact precaution; until we know if they have been exposed to any antibiotics, we put them as high risk." - Physician

At the three hospitals, the ward nurse in charge will enforce contact precautions with the nurses and the attending/consulting physicians will enforce junior physicians' contact precautions. The IPC team also enforces IPC practices. Both physicians and nurses inform patients about contact precautions; patients are told to inform their family members. While senior physicians reported informing patients of the need for IPC in the CDI setting, nurses considered themselves more approachable than the physicians and took a primary role in communicating with patients. One junior physician admitted his/her peers' shortfalling.

"I think that from all of it, that is where the biggest failing comes in—that we often don't tell patients enough of the stuff. So, I would like to think that once it's done there is a proper [communication] about the patient having things that can be transmitted, with words that they can understand and the importance of them not going around and touching lots of things and letting them know the reasons for gloving up and putting on gowns and stuff for their own peace of mind...It's apathy from the medical staff we forget to do these things..." - Physician

Hand hygiene Facilitators and barriers to hand hygiene were related to the treatment of patients with CDI and additional infections. Hand hygiene practices for patients with CDI should include hand washing with soap and water to remove *C. difficile* spores that are not killed by alcohol hand sanitizers. Supplies, including paper towels, soap, and hand sanitizer, were frequently available but not always utilised. Some stated that insufficient supplies were a barrier; others said that supplies were always available. Eleven (42.3%) participants acknowledged the importance of washing hands with soap and water when treating patients with CDI (Table 3).

"...have to use soap and water, we take [the] de-germ [alcohol based hand sanitizer] away from bedside so they are forced to use soap and water." - Physician

Some perceptions regarding this important hand hygiene practice were inaccurate.

"I would not say a normal hand soap is better for C. diff, I would say something alcohol based." - Physician

Staffing shortages and high workload were described as reasons for inconsistent hand hygiene practices.

"Can I tell you, all over the basins is that sign [WHO's "5 Moments of Hand Hygiene"]... but we don't practice it...We don't follow five moments of Hand Hygiene. We follow it when we go home... You can't afford to take that 5 min." – Nurse Focus Group

Participants described hand hygiene events (e.g. ultraviolent light, blue soap) in their hospitals that encouraged effective hand hygiene. Many stated that overcrowding and lack of facilities (e.g. one sink per ward) hindered hand hygiene as well as: the high ratio of patients to nurses, education limitations, and sometimes-empty alcohol and/or soap dispensers.

Isolation Infrastructure limitations were a major barrier to IPC, often preventing CDI patients from allocation to an isolation room. Isolation room availability ranged from two to four rooms. Isolation rooms were specifically prioritized for multidrug resistant tuberculosis (MDR-TB) patients, who may occupy the room for a month. CDI is viewed as a lower priority for isolation rooms.

"The fact that we have got a lot of immunocompromised patients in terms of our HIV rates and TB rates, a lot of our patients are at risk due to the use of antibiotics. In the UK we used to see a lot of elderly patients, but here you have got a different spectrum of patients, so C. diff is a huge risk... I think everyone focuses on MDR and very few people actually focus on C. diff ... C. diff is not something that is high on the radar." - Physician

Challenges for IPC included patient education regarding IPC, especially patients leaving isolation, walking around the hospital, and using shared bathrooms.

"The big problem that we have in our wards is a lack of isolation facilities. For an entire hospital, we've got only four isolation rooms [that] do not include isolation bathrooms. So a C. diff patient would have to use the same toilet as other patients." - Physician

Both nurses and physicians described speaking to patients and their family members about isolation. An elevated desire from patients to understand their condition was expressed when patients were moved to an isolation room.

"Sometimes you'll find the patient doesn't know what is going on, but when you move them into an isolation room then they want to know why." - Nurse

Environmental cleaning The ward managers inform cleaning staff verbally about room cleaning needs. Under supervision, the cleaners complete a written checklist for the bathrooms and patient rooms. Cleaning is sometimes rushed due to high bed demand, and the staff nurses will help.

"It's just that we are busy so the beds are always in demand so sometimes there is no opportunity for cleaning because everything is rush, rush, rush, rush. When the patient is waiting on discharge, others are waiting for that bed so we don't have the opportunity to do the spring cleaning of the unit. We aren't always able to do it in a calm environment." – Nurse

Section II: Organizational Culture

Themes related to organizational culture (beliefs and attitudes) and how leadership and administration respond to new ideas, specifically 'change culture', were analyzed in order to inform future interventions. Through this coding an additional organizational culture theme emerged related to healthcare provider responsibility and accountability.

Change culture: how leadership and administration respond to new ideas

The majority of respondents described leadership as being supportive of new ideas. Some respondents did not feel leadership was supportive of bottom-up ideas; others believed that ideas with evidence of positive impact would be supported. A few respondents noted a barrier to change related more to nursing staff and junior physician turnover than to administrative support. Progressive change is difficult when the same education concepts are repeated with rotating healthcare providers; institutional memory regarding CDI and CDI management was lost.

"Implementing change and practical change are very different, so we are able to change our practice so we can make lots of suggestions... but the difficulty comes in that our staff [is a] rotating staff." - Physician

A nurse new to a leadership position anticipated facing challenges in changing long-standing practices.

"The people above me, the specialist physicians or consultants, are quite open to change. If you can show clearly that an idea is going to work, the department is open to change and improving things. As you get higher up the leadership chain, it becomes more difficult to introduce change. I do find that on the face of it, the managers seem to be okay and accepting and are happy to listen." - Physician

Responsibility and accountability

While the interviewees described achievements of and challenges for patients and healthcare providers following IPC precautions, low adherence emerged as a compelling theme—sometimes in the context of IPC in general and for the treatment of TB, particularly when participants had limited CDI knowledge. Perception of the threats from infectious diseases and IPC prioritization also appear to be barriers to adherence when supplies are available. Accountability structures are not in place to properly encourage providers to remain knowledgeable about guidelines nor enforce IPC precautions.

"It seems we have many awareness days... we had spike last year, 2 years ago... we have had quite a few staff members contracted tuberculosis... people only get aware if their buddy gets it... It makes it real." - Physician

"Just to get the doctors to wear gloves—that for me is another thing where I can just say... like, 'Why are you not wearing gloves?' or, just tell them 'Your patient has TB. Can you put on your mask please?' ...together with the hand washing, and at the end of the day, it is part of the IPC principles to have full personal protection equipment available in the unit, but there's hand sanitizers, soap, and water, available in the unit, so no one has an excuse." - Physician

Informal structures for peer accountability were discussed as a helpful strategy from two interviews. First, accountability for hand hygiene occurred on the ASP ward round at one hospital. Second, an Operational Manager in the Operating Room (Theater) described nursing and cleaning staff who speak up about needs and follow cleaning expectations.

"The cleaning staff and the nursing staff is quite well informed as to what is supposed to happen, because sometimes they can tell you. 'Sister, this was not done yet; You can't really put your patient here'... Those are the people that I work with... that I come across, that will tell me. Doesn't matter if you are the cleaner, you can tell me, 'Sister, it's not ready yet.' You understand. It's that relationship that we have [of a] multidisciplinary team, to do what is expected of us."
– Nurse

Discussion
Principal findings
This is the first qualitative study of CDI in Sub-Saharan Africa, and the results provide novel insight into CDI treatment and workflow in a limited resource setting. The context of CDI in Africa is especially important to consider given the high HIV and tuberculosis prevalence and high risk of *C. difficile* associated mortality in this population. This study reveals significant barriers and facilitators to CDI treatment in public district (secondary) level South African hospitals. Major barriers included knowledge gaps in CDI management, especially regarding awareness of the infection, transmission, treatment, and IPC practices among health care providers. Physician CDI knowledge was higher than nurse and pharmacist knowledge. The results reveal opportunities for healthcare provider education related to CDI. Our study affirms that healthcare providers have an awareness of evidence-based IPC precautions but

barriers to following them include perceptions of priority and time availability.

Implications: perceptions and knowledge
Based on quantitative results from the overall CDI knowledge assessment, participants had limited CDI knowledge. Gaps in CDI knowledge may delay clinical suspicion and all workflow steps in CDI identification, diagnosis, treatment and prevention. While physicians scored higher, some physicians were less confident regarding when to order the *C. difficile* test resulting in delayed diagnosis. Physicians with high CDI knowledge noted an urgency surrounding CDI not observed in junior physicians and other healthcare providers.. This, together with a high risk of mortality in patients with positive *C. difficile* test results, underscores an urgent need for education and intervention tailored to relevant aspects of healthcare providers' job responsibilities.

Overall, participants scored well in areas of identifying CDI risk factors, signs, and symptoms. However, improvement is needed in terms of educating healthcare professionals in South Africa about other aspects of CDI. In the occupation subgroup analysis, nurses and pharmacists appear to be less knowledgeable about CDI characteristics, with response rates of 50% or less in all the knowledge assessment categories. The identified areas for potential development relevant to nurses and pharmacists are: CDI patients' need for contact isolation, the importance of hand washing instead of using alcohol gel in preventing the spread of CDI, and CDI treatment options. Nurses can also be educated to suspect CDI when monitoring bowel movements.

This study reveals a more complicated process for obtaining and administering vancomycin compared to metronidazole that may be hindering healthcare providers' use of vancomycin. In an epidemiology, treatment, and outcomes study in the same setting, vancomycin was rarely ordered (2%) as initial CDI treatment [4]. One strategy is to incorporate treatment options for CDI into pharmacist education and teach pharmacists what to look for on physician-submitted motivation forms. Pharmacist education about treatment options is especially important considering the role pharmacists have in the approval process for vancomycin use. The healthcare team should be educated on the clinical use of vancomycin for CDI with an emphasis on timely preparation and delivery.

How results relate to other studies
Our study affirms current literature's described need for improved CDI identification in settings with extensive CDI experience. Despite a history of substantial CDI outbreaks in Europe, a study identified persistent underdiagnoses of CDI when all diarrhoea samples were tested at 482 hospitals across 20 European countries; 23% of *C.*

difficile positive results were not identified at the local hospital. Authors attributed the underdiagnoses to a lack of clinical suspicion and suboptimal laboratory diagnostic methods [9]. Meanwhile, in the US, a regulatory climate that reduces hospital reimbursement for patients who develop hospital-acquired infections is driving efforts to refine testing protocols to avoid *C. difficile* over testing and inappropriate diagnosis [10]. These studies emphasize the importance of appropriate testing for diagnosis.

A global review of CDI guidelines found antimicrobial stewardship (ASPs) to be universally recognized as an essential evidence-based component of CDI IPC [5]. Continued development of interdisciplinary ASPs in limited resource settings is necessary to facilitate effective CDI management and IPC measures.

One barrier to hand hygiene identified in this study was the perception that there is insufficient time available for thorough hand cleaning. Indeed, in a study conducted in the US about healthcare providers' compliance with IPC practices for patients with CDI, full compliance was very low and time-consuming with a mean time for full compliance greater than 5 min for patients in single isolation rooms [11]. Patient care workload continues to be a barrier to full compliance with CDI contact precautions in high resource settings [12]. Therefore, improving full compliance of IPC practices in limited resource settings will require both a workload adjustment to allow more time per patient and education on the importance of CDI-related IPC practices.

Significant challenges for the implementation of IPC programs and practices exist in low and limited resource settings, including infrastructural constraints with a limited number of isolation rooms and variable staff compliance with hand hygiene practices. A similar qualitative study in India found perceived workload and nursing staff turnover to be barriers to infection control [13]. This relates to our study's previously referenced finding that perceived workload hindered infection control practices, especially regarding hand hygiene. Our respondents reported high turnover of both nursing staff and junior physicians as barriers to implementing change. The secondary hospitals included in our study did not have an IPC team as developed as the one in the tertiary hospital in India. The study in India also found participants reporting the availability of IPC supplies but experiencing challenges with compliance, while an international study of healthcare settings representing 30 countries identified inadequate supplies as a barrier to infection control of multidrug resistant organisms in some high and middle income countries [13, 14].

Limitations

As a qualitative study, the results are not generalizable to a larger population but may be transferable to similar settings. Visiting researchers' presence conducting the interviews may have affected responses; stated practices are not necessarily the reality of practice. While all interviews were conducted in English, English was a second language for some participants. This may have limited the respondents' understanding of some questions and ability to articulate responses. Furthermore, we may have underestimated facilitators to CDI management in an attempt to identify improvement opportunities. Our analysis was not a systematic audit of workflow and practices, and some inaccuracies may exist. To mitigate bias, multiple researchers of the study team reviewed the results. Finally, as we developed the knowledge assessment after the interviews were completed, the assessment is not yet validated and results are limited. Our knowledge assessment measured breadth of CDI knowledge and not depth. For example, some providers gave detailed explanations for some of the knowledge components, such as advantages of different testing protocols, yet these explanations were still only assigned one point for that component.

Conclusions

Our analysis provides a detailed description of the facilitators and barriers to CDI workflow, including the need for increased healthcare provider knowledge of CDI management. Interventions should increase CDI knowledge and utilization of the available systems and supplies by addressing the identified barriers and championing the identified facilitators. Increasing CDI knowledge alone is unlikely to be effective without addressing the need to create a sense of urgency around CDI and appropriate IPC practices. The results provide context for technical intervention and implementation strategies in low-resource public healthcare settings. This study serves as a baseline and supplements quantitative CDI patient data from ongoing CDI research including provider education and a clinical intervention to improve CDI quality of care in South Africa. The results of this workflow and provider knowledge analysis identify areas of need and are useful to design interventions to improve the quality of care for CDI patients in this population and similar limited resource settings.

Abbreviations
ASP: Antimicrobial stewardship programs; CDI: *Clostridium difficile* infection; IPC: Infection prevention and control; MDR(-TB): Multidrug resistant(–tuberculosis); PCR: Polymerase chain reaction; SEIPS: Systems Engineering Initiative for Patient Safety; TB: Tuberculosis; UK: United Kingdom; US: United States; XDR-TB: Extensively drug-resistant TB

Acknowledgements
We thank South African Department of Health for their collaboration. We also thank the Western Cape hospitals participating in this study. We appreciate the ongoing collaboration between the University of the Western Cape and the University of Wisconsin-Madison.

Funding
There was no funding for this study. LL was supported by an internal endowment at the University of Wisconsin-Madison.

Authors' contributions
LL designed the study, designed data collection, monitored data collection for the whole study, conducted interviews, transcribed audio, analysed the data, drafted and revised the paper. SB provided guidance on the study and revised the paper. WR provided guidance on the study and revised the paper. NS provided guidance on the study and revised the paper. TE transcribed audio, analysed data, and revised the paper. KHP transcribe audio, analysed data, and revised the paper. RC facilitated the collaborative project between the University of the Western Cape and the University of Wisconsin, provided guidance on the study and revised the paper. All authors read and approved the final manuscript.

Consent for publication
Not applicable.

Competing interests
The authors declare that they have no competing interests.

Author details
[1]University of Wisconsin-Madison School of Pharmacy, 777 Highland Ave, Madison, WI 53705, USA. [2]University of the Western Cape School of Pharmacy, Robert Sobukwe, Cape Town 7535, South Africa. [3]University of Wisconsin School of Medicine and Public Health, 750 Highland Ave, Madison, WI 53726, USA.

References
1. Steiner C, Barrett M, Sun Y. HCUP Projections: Clostridium Difficile Hospitalizations 2004-2015. Projections Report #2015-02 2015 [Available from: https://www.hcup-us.ahrq.gov/reports/projections/2015-02.pdf.
2. Rajabally N, Kullin B, Ebrahim K, Brock T, Weintraub A, Whitelaw A, et al. A comparison of Clostridium difficile diagnostic methods for identification of local strains in a South African centre. J Med Microbiol. 2016;65(4):320-7.
3. McDonald LC, Gerding DN, Johnson S, Bakken JS, Carroll KC, Coffin SE, et al. Clinical Practice Guidelines for Clostridium difficile Infection in Adults and Children: 2017 Update by the Infectious Diseases Society of America (IDSA) and Society for Healthcare Epidemiology of America (SHEA). Clin Infect Dis. 2018.
4. Legenza L, Barnett S, Rose W, Bianchini M, Safdar N, Coetzee R. Epidemiology and outcomes of Clostridium difficile infection among hospitalised patients: Results of a multicentre retrospective study in South Africa. BMJ Global Health. 2018;3(4).
5. Balsells E, Filipescu T, Kyaw MH, Wiuff C, Campbell H, Nair H. Infection prevention and control of Clostridium difficile: a global review of guidelines, strategies, and recommendations. J Glob Health. 2016;6(2):020410.
6. Carayon P, Schoofs Hundt A, Karsh BT, Gurses AP, Alvarado CJ, Smith M, et al. Work system design for patient safety: the SEIPS model. Qual Saf Health Care. 2006;(15 Suppl 1):i50-8.
7. Bradley EH, Curry LA, Devers KJ. Qualitative data analysis for health services research: developing taxonomy, themes, and theory. Health Serv Res. 2007; 42(4):1758-72.
8. Glaser BG. The discovery of grounded theory : strategies for qualitative research: New Brunswick, N.J. : Aldine Transaction, [1999] ©1999; 1999.
9. Davies KA, Longshaw CM, Davis GL, Bouza E, Barbut F, Barna Z, et al. Underdiagnosis of Clostridium difficile across Europe: the European, multicentre, prospective, biannual, point-prevalence study of Clostridium difficile infection in hospitalised patients with diarrhoea (EUCLID). Lancet Infect Dis. 2014;14(12):1208-19.
10. Fang FC, Polage CR, Wilcox MH. Point-Counterpoint: What Is the Optimal Approach for Detection of Clostridium difficile Infection? J Clin Microbiol. 2017;55(3):670-80.
11. Yanke E, Zellmer C, Van Hoof S, Moriarty H, Carayon P, Safdar N. Understanding the current state of infection prevention to prevent Clostridium difficile infection: a human factors and systems engineering approach. Am J Infect Control. 2015;43(3):241-7.
12. Yanke E, Moriarty H, Carayon P, Safdar N. A qualitative, interprofessional analysis of barriers to and facilitators of implementation of the Department of Veterans Affairs' Clostridium difficile prevention bundle using a human factors engineering approach. Am J Infect Control. 2018;46(3):276-84.
13. Barker AK, Brown K, Siraj D, Ahsan M, Sengupta S, Safdar N. Barriers and facilitators to infection control at a hospital in northern India: a qualitative study. Antimicrob Resist Infect Control. 2017;6:35.
14. Safdar N, Sengupta S, Musuuza JS, Juthani-Mehta M, Drees M, Abbo LM, et al. Status of the Prevention of Multidrug-Resistant Organisms in International Settings: A Survey of the Society for Healthcare Epidemiology of America Research Network. Infect Control Hosp Epidemiol. 2017;38(1):53-60.

20

Do wearable alcohol-based handrub dispensers increase hand hygiene compliance?

Jonas Keller[1†], Aline Wolfensberger[1*†] ⓘ, Lauren Clack[1], Stefan P. Kuster[1], Mesida Dunic[1], Doris Eis[2], Yvonne Flammer[1,3], Dagmar I. Keller[2] and Hugo Sax[1]

Abstract

Background: Hand Hygiene (HH) compliance was shown to be poor in several studies. Improving the availability of alcohol-based hand rub (ABHR) is a cornerstone for increasing HH compliance.

Methods: In this study, we introduced wearable dispensers for ABHR in an Emergency Department (ED) well equipped with mounted ABHR dispensers and accompanied this single-modal intervention by a quasi-experimental mixed-method study. The study was performed in the ED of the University Hospital Zurich, Switzerland, a 950-bed tertiary teaching hospital. During a five-week baseline period and a seven-week intervention period, we observed HH compliance according to the WHO 'Five Moments' concept, measured ABHR consumption, and investigated perceived ABHR availability, self-reported HH compliance and knowledge of HH indications by questionnaire. Multivariable logistic regression was used to identify independent determinants for HH compliance. In addition, semi-structured interviews were conducted and thematically analyzed to assess barriers and facilitators for the use of the newly introduced dispensers.

Results: Across 811 observed HH opportunities, the HH compliance for all moments was 56% (95% confidence interval (CI), 51–62%) during baseline and 64% (CI, 59–68%) during intervention period, respectively. In the multivariable analysis adjusted for sex, profession, and WHO HH moment, there was no difference in HH compliance between baseline and intervention (adjusted Odds ratio: 1.22 (0.89–1.66), $p = 0.22$), No significant changes were observed in consumption and perceived availability of ABHR. During intervention, 7.5% ABHR was consumed using wearable dispensers. HCP perceived wearable dispensers as unnecessary since mounted dispensers were readily accessible. Poor ergonomic design of the wearable dispenser emerged as a main barrier, especially its lid and fastening mechanism. Interviewees identified two ideal situations for wearable dispensers, HCP who accompany patients from ED to other wards, and HCP approaching a patient from a non-patient areas in the ED such as the central working station or the meeting room.

Conclusion: The introduction of wearable dispensers did not increase observed hand hygiene compliance or ABHR consumption in an ED already well equipped with mounted dispensers. For broader acceptance and use, wearable dispensers might benefit from an optimized ergonomic design.

Keywords: Hand hygiene, Compliance, Wearable dispensers, Pocket dispensers, Clip on dispensers, Emergency room, Availability, Point of care

* Correspondence: aline.wolfensberger@usz.ch
†Jonas Keller and Aline Wolfensberger contributed equally to this work.
[1]Division of Infectious Diseases and Hospital Epidemiology, University Hospital Zurich, University of Zurich, Rämistrasse 100, CH-8091 Zurich, Switzerland
Full list of author information is available at the end of the article

Background

Despite significant advances in infection control, healthcare-associated infections represent a major challenge to modern medicine [1]. Appropriate hand hygiene (HH) is considered crucial to reduce the transmission of nosocomial pathogens and helps to prevent hospital-acquired infections [2, 3]. However, HH compliance has been shown to be poor in a multitude of studies [4, 5]. Data about HH compliance in Emergency Departments (ED) is limited, and results vary greatly [6]. ED physicians had a higher risk for non-adherence to HH compared to physicians working in other departments [7]. The mean rate of HH indications is higher in the ED than in medical or surgical wards [8], and high workload has been identified as a risk factor for low HH compliance [5].

To improve HH compliance, WHO names two strategies with known effectiveness: introducing widely accessible alcohol based hand rub (ABHR), and multifaceted interventions [4]. Again, in multifaceted approaches, improving the availability of ABHR is often an element of success [7]. Providing ABHR at the 'point of care' – requiring ABHR to be easily accessible and as close as possible (e.g. within arm's reach), where patient care or treatment is taking place – is a cornerstone of the WHO strategy to improve HH compliance [4]. Accessibility can be achieved by introducing wearable dispensers with ABHR [9, 10]. But, in a single intervention study in 2008, Haas et al. showed that availability of wearable ABHR dispensers alone was not associated with a significant improvement in HH compliance in an ED [11].

For many years, ED personnel in our hospital expressed the wish to benefit from wearable dispensers. All wards of the University Hospital Zurich (UHZ), including the ED, are well equipped with mounted ABHR dispensers in close vicinity of patients, and up to this study, wearable dispensers were only available for staff in a few selected wards, e.g. in neonatology. In spring 2016, the infection prevention and control (IPC) team decided to meet the ED's wish for wearable dispensers. The introduction was accompanied by a mixed-method study to investigate HH compliance, ABHR consumption, and the attitude of healthcare providers (HCP) towards wearable dispensers.

Methods

Study setting and population

The study was conducted between April and June 2016 at the ED of the UHZ, Switzerland. The UHZ is a 950-bed tertiary hospital covering all medical specialties except pediatrics and orthopedics. The ED holds 17 beds, and a mean of 44'000 patients are admitted to the ED yearly. The ED staff consists of 100 nurses, 13 staff emergency physicians, 25 medical interns, and various other professions (e.g. maintenance and nursing assistants). Non-ED consulting physicians and surgeons regularly visiting the ED. The study population for HH observation and interviews consisted of ED staff only, ABHR consumption was measured overall, thus including also HCP visiting the ER. The ED has an open floor plan with a central nursing and working station, and single patient bays separated by privacy curtains. Mounted dispensers are available in or immediately outside every patient room/bay. In total, there are 34 wall-mounted or table-top dispensers available in close proximity, i.e. below 2 m, of each patient bed. Additional dispensers exist in the staff lounge, storage rooms, and restrooms.

Study design and endpoints

This mixed-method quasi-experimental before-after study evaluated the effect of introducing wearable ABHR dispensers, i.e. the intervention, by multiple measures. The main outcome was the observed HH compliance, defined as the proportion of individual HH indications met by a HH action [12]. Secondary outcomes were the measured consumption of ABHR and self-reported HH compliance. In addition, we investigated the perception and attitude of ED HCP regarding wearable dispensers by self-applied questionnaires and semi-structured interviews.

Intervention

The study consisted of a five-week baseline period and a seven-week intervention period that started with the introduction of wearable dispensers. The wearable dispenser (B Braun®, 100 ml, dimensions 7x8x2.2 cm) included clips to attach the dispensers to the hospital apparel. Promotion of the wearable dispensers occurred in several staff-meetings, by user information via email, and by distribution of dispensers to HCP in person. The number and position of the mounted dispensers remained unchanged.

Effect evaluation

HH compliance, the main outcome parameter, was assessed according to the WHO 'My 5 moments for hand hygiene' observation method through direct observation by two trained and validated members of the IPC team (MD and JK) [13, 14]. They recorded HH opportunities, HH actions, and HCP profession and sex in an anonymized form. During the last three weeks of the intervention period, the usage of either wearable dispensers or mounted dispensers was additionally noted during observations. Observations were done during weekdays at different time points between 8 am and 6 pm. Consumption of ABHR from mounted dispensers and wearable dispensers was assessed by weekly weighing the dispensers and counting the stock to calculate consumption.

Perceived ABHR availability, self-reported HH compliance, and knowledge of the WHO 'My five moments for HH' was assessed through a self-administered 3-item questionnaire using a 5-item Likert scale (Table 1). Additionally, participants indicated their profession and sex. Questionnaires were distributed to physicians' physical mailboxes and were made available in the nurses' common room after the baseline period and at the end of the intervention period.

Sample size calculation and statistical analysis

The needed number of HH opportunities in baseline and intervention was calculated on the assumption that HH at baseline would be 50%, based on earlier observations using the same observation method. A clinically meaningful increase in HH compliance was judged to be at least 15 percentage points, i.e. from 50 to 65%. Requiring equal sample sizes for baseline and intervention, and assuming an average cluster size of three, a two-sided alpha of 0.05, and a power of 80% resulted in twice 339 opportunities.

Descriptive statistics were used to summarize data on HH compliance, ABHR consumption, and results of the questionnaire. Chi-square test was used to test differences in categorical variables. For comparison of continuous variables we used students t-test or anova, as appropriate. Multivariable logistic regression was used to adjust the effect of the intervention on HH compliance for potential confounders. We included the variables intervention period, sex, profession, hand hygiene moment and their respective subcategories in the multivariable model. We applied a chi-square test for trend to evaluate the change in consumption of ABHR from wearable dispensers as a proportion of overall ABHR consumption over time ('ptest', trend analysis for proportions). A p-value of $<.05$ was considered statistically significant. All statistical analysis were performed with STATA version 15 (Stata Corp., College Station, TX, USA).

Semi-structured interviews and qualitative analysis

Semi-structured interviews were conducted with a convenience sample of nurses and physicians working in the ED at the end of the intervention period. The interview guide is displayed in Table 2. All interviews were audio-taped after obtaining oral informed consent and transcribed verbatim. Data analysis of anonymized interviews was conducted inductively, following a grounded theory approach [15]. Two researchers (JK and AW) independently read transcripts and identified emerging themes. Emerging themes were then discussed and final categories were established through consensus. Quotes about barriers and facilitators were semi-quantified by a scoring system: three points for quotes mentioned by a majority of participants, two points for quotes mentioned by a minority but two or more, one point for quotes mentioned by a single participant.

Results

Hand hygiene compliance

A total of 811 HH opportunities were observed, 328 (40.4%) in the baseline period and 483 (59.6%) in the intervention period. The average HH compliance rose from 56% during baseline to 64% during intervention with a univariable odds ratio of 1.36 (1.02–1.81; p = .035). When adjusted for HH moment, sex and profession in the multivariable logistic regression model, odds ratio was 1.22 (0.89–1.66; p = .218) (Table 3). Weekly compliance across all indications are displayed in Fig. 1. In intervention, 7.3% (95% confidence interval (CI), 3.6–13.0) of observed HH actions were performed using wearable dispensers.

Table 1 Questionnaire for self-evaluation of participants

No.	Question	Likert-Scale
1.	Have you memorized the "WHO five moments for hand hygiene" so that you utilize them automatically in daily routine?	1 = no
		2 = some of them
		3 = many of them
		4 = most of them
		5 = yes, completely
2.	How often do you correctly conduct hand hygiene according to the "WHO five moments for hand hygiene"?	1 = never
		2 = sometimes
		3 = often
		4 = most of the time
		5 = always
3.	Is ABHR sufficiently available to conduct hand hygiene according to the "WHO five moments for hand hygiene"?	1 = never
		2 = sometimes
		3 = often
		4 = most of the time
		5 = always

Abbreviations: *ABHR* alcohol based hand rub, *No.* Number, *WHO* World Health Organisation

Table 2 Interview guide for the semi-structured interviews

No.	Question
1.	What do you think of the recently introduced wearable dispensers?
2.	How frequently have you used the wearable dispensers?
3.	What are the advantages/disadvantages of the wearable dispensers?
4.	Are there any situations where you prefer using either the wearable dispensers or the mounted dispensers?
5.	Do you have ideas to improve the wearable dispensers?

Table 3 Univariable and multivariable analysis of predictors for hand hygiene compliance

	Baseline period		Intervention period		Univariable analysis	Multivariable analysis
	HH opportunities	HH actions (%)	HH opportunities	HH actions (%)	Odds ratio (CI95%)	Odds ratio (CI95%)
Intervention period (vs. baseline period)	328	185 (56)	483	308 (64)	1.36 (1.02–1.81)	1.22 (0.89–1.66)
WHO HH moment						
Before touching patient	87	31 (36)	106	39 (37)	1	1
Before aseptic procedure	21	12 (57)	47	37 (79)	4.53 (2.47–8.30)	3.10 (1.66–5.79)
After body fluid exposure risk	38	27 (71)	59	47 (80)	5.65 (3.25–9.82)	4.49 (2.54–7.95)
After touching patient	162	109 (67)	254	180 (71)	4.00 (2.79–5.73)	4.05 (2.80–5.86)
After touching patient surroundings	20	6 (30)	17	5 (29)	0.74 (0.35–1.60)	0.61 (0.28–1.35)
Sex						
Female	206	125 (61)	360	245 (68)	1	1
Male	122	60 (49)	123	63 (51)	0.53 (0.39–0.72)	0.72 (0.50–1.02)
Profession						
Physician	114	57 (50)	156	74 (47)	1	1
Nurse	210	128 (61)	313	224 (72)	2.18 (1.62–2.95)	1.92 (1.34–2.76)
Other	4	0 (0)	14	10 (71)	1.33 (0.51–3.46)	0.93 (0.34–2.51)

Abbreviations: *CI* confidence interval, *n.a.* not applicable, *HH* hand hygiene

Consumption of alcohol-based hand rub

Figure 1 shows the weekly consumption of ABHR, which was 25.6 ml per patient admission during baseline, and 25.2 ml per patient admission during intervention. During the intervention period, 7.5% of the total ABHR consumption resulted from use of wearable dispensers, confirming the abovementioned 7.3% of observed use. Consumption of ABHR from wearable dispensers did increase over the seven-week intervention period (p < .001).

Perceived ABHR availability, self-reported hand hygiene compliance, and knowledge of HH moments

A total of 87 questionnaires were returned, 51 during baseline (20 (39%) by physicians, 27 (53%) by nurses, and 4 (8%) by others), and 36 during intervention (12 (33%) by physicians, 22 (61%) by nurses, and 2 (6%) by others).

The perceived availability of ABHR did not increase from baseline to intervention (4.47 vs 4.64, p = .31). Self-reported HH compliance did not differ between baseline and intervention (4.12 vs 4.03, p = .56), neither between sex (female vs male, 4.14 vs 3.97, p = .28), nor profession (physician vs nurse vs other, 4.09 vs 4.08 vs 4.0, p = .96). Mean self-reported knowledge of HH indications did not differ between baseline and intervention (4.27 vs. 4.28, p = .98). Overall, women's perception of their own knowledge was better than men's (4.40 vs 4.03, p = .024), whereas profession had no impact on the self-reported knowledge (physician vs nurse vs others, 4.31 vs 4.29 vs 4.0, p = .61).

Semi-structured interviews

Overall, 24 participants took part in the interviews, 14 (58%) nurses, nine physicians (38%), and one (4%) nursing assistant; six (25%) participants were male. The interviews had a mean duration of 10 min. Thirteen of the interviewees (54%) had a negative overall impression of the wearable dispensers, eight (33%) were neutral, and three (13%) were positive.

We identified four categories of barriers and facilitators for the use of the wearable dispensers: *usability* characteristics of the current wearable dispenser, *availability* of ABHR, *cues to action/cognition* (i.e. subconscious or conscious activation towards use), and perceptions about the *safety* of wearable dispensers. Selected typical interview quotes are listed in Table 4. A majority of facilitators was categorized to "availability". HCPs liked the principal idea of carrying the hand rub on them and also mentioned certain situations in which the wearable dispenser was of use, e.g. heading towards a patient from an area without mounted dispensers, and accompanying patient to wards where location of mounted dispensers was not familiar. In addition, interviewees perceived the wearable dispenser as a reminder to perform hand hygiene. Barriers were more often mentioned than facilitators, and arguments from all thematic groups emerged. Concerning usability, interviewees did not like the way the wearable dispensers were attached to the uniform because it made the dispenser dangle back and forth, and the fastening mechanism often

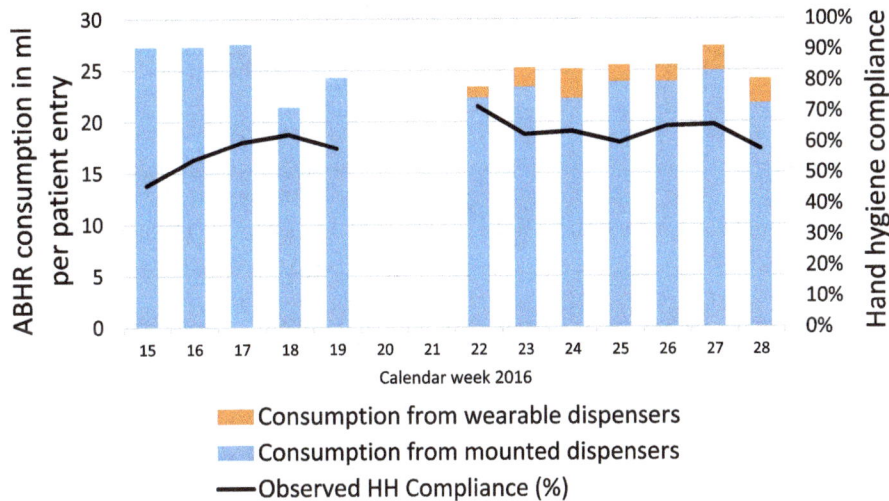

Fig. 1 Hand hygiene compliance and consumption of alcohol based hand rub. Legend: The bar graph depicts consumption of ABHR in milliliters by mounted dispensers (blue bars) and wearable dispensers (orange bars). The line graph depicts HH compliance in percent. The five-week baseline period (weeks 15 to 19) and the seven-week intervention period (weeks 22 to 28) are separated by a two-week (weeks 20 and 21) period dedicated to preparing the intervention. Abbreviations: ABHR = Alcohol-based hand rub; HH = hand hygiene; ml = milliliters

failed, dropping the dispenser. HCP perceived the wearable dispensers as an additional item to carry around, while they already carried a multitude of other items such as stethoscopes and notes in their pockets, especially when wearing scrubs without coat. Wearable dispensers were mainly perceived to be unnecessary, given that a mounted dispenser was in easy reach during the vast majority of HH indications. HCPs were used to the mounted dispensers and habitually used them instead of the wearable dispensers. The outer surface of the wearable dispensers was perceived as risk factor for contaminating patients and hospital surroundings.

Interviewees made numerous suggestions about how to improve the wearable dispenser, including reducing its size to make it better fit in coat pockets, modifying the bottle outlet, e.g. by replacing it by a membrane, to avoid the need to open its cap, and improving the attaching mechanism.

Discussion

The purpose of this study was to examine whether a single intervention approach of introducing wearable ABHR dispensers in addition to existing mounted dispensers would increase observed HH compliance and ABHR consumption in our ED. Additionally, we aimed to explain the findings by qualitative and quantitative data on HCP perceptions and attitude. We found that the intervention did not improve HH compliance and consumption of ABHR. Less than a tenth of ABHR was consumed using wearable dispensers. Two main 'barriers' for the acceptance of the wearable dispensers explained this unexpectedly low uptake, namely the habitual use and perceived

sufficient access to mounted dispensers and the flawed ergonomic design of the wearable dispensers.

Increasing availability of ABHR is an often-mentioned facilitator for HH compliance and the "WHO Guidelines on Hand Hygiene in Health Care" declare ABHR availability as a prerequisite for good HH compliance [16–18]. Introducing wearable dispensers is one possibility to increase availability. Many researchers introduce wearable dispensers as part of multifaceted interventions. Yeung et al. found that the introduction of wearable dispensers with education led to increased HH compliance in long-term care facilities [10] and Koff et al. found improvement in HH compliance of anesthesia providers through the use of wearable dispensers with an audible alarm [19]. Only rarely introduction of wearable dispensers was studied as single intervention. Parks et al. were able to show that HH compliance of a regional anesthesia team increases when wearable dispensers are worn on person [20]. In contrast, the introduction of wearable dispensers in the ED of our hospital did not significantly increase HH compliance. Our results confirm the findings of Haas et al. in 2008, who did not find an improvement in ABHR consumption after introducing wearable dispensers in an ED [11].

Our ED is well equipped with mounted dispensers, making ABHR available within maximum 2 m distance from every patient bed. Interviewees mentioned the abundant availability of dispensers as one of the most important reasons for not using wearable dispensers and did not perceive an increase in availability of ABHR during intervention. Nevertheless, prior to this study, HCPs in the ED had repetitively been expressing the wish to get access to wearable dispensers. The low uptake in this investigation came therefore

Table 4 Typical quotes about barriers and facilitators for use of wearable dispensers

	Facilitators	Barriers
Usability	Fastening mechanism ●○○ - "I generally like the possibility to attach the wearable dispensers to one's trousers." - Dimensions ●○○ - "The size and weight of the wearable dispenser is perfect. If it was bigger, it couldn't be put it in my pockets anymore."	Fastening mechanism ●●● - "During a CT scan of a patient I accompanied, the wearable dispenser came off four times." - "The wearable dispenser dangles constantly, and its weight pulls on my trousers which is really uncomfortable." Opening and closing mechanism ●●○ - "It is difficult to close the bottle with one hand only." - Dosing of ABHR ●○○ - "It is more difficult to dose the appropriate amount of ABHR compared to wall-mounted dispensers" - Dimensions ●○○ - "The wearable dispenser is so small that you have to exchange it too often." Burden ●●● - "The wearable dispenser is just something more to carry around, and I have to carry many other things with me already."
Availability	General ●●● - "I generally like the idea that I carry the ABHR with me and have it available all the time." Specific situations ●●○ - "Sometimes the next wall-mounted dispenser is 10 m away, then the wearable dispenser is of use." - "I can use the wearable dispenser and do HH while heading to a patient." - "The wearable dispenser is of use, when I shift a patient to a ward and do not know the locations of ABHR dispensers."	General ●●● - "No, I do not see any advantage of the wearable dispenser. We do have enough ABHR available in the ER."
Cues to action / Cognition	Habitualness ●○○ - "Yes, I did use the wearable dispenser. I was used to wearable dispensers from the hospital I worked before." Reminder ●●○ - "The wearable dispenser is a good reminder for HH."	Habitualness ●●○ - "I'm so used to all the wall-mounted dispensers… [that I did not use the wearable dispenser]."
Safety	n.a.	Dispensers perceived as risk factor for contamination ●●○ - "The problem is that the bottle has to be opened with contaminated hands and afterwards closed with clean hands." - "The dirty bottle in contact with my clean clothes all the time."

Abbreviations: *ABHR* alcohol based hand rub, *CT* Computer tomography, *ER* emergency room, *HH* hand hygiene, ●●● Mentioned by a majority of participants. ●●○ Mentioned by ≥2 participants. ●○○ Mentioned by one single participant

as a surprise. Interviewees did not comment on the ED's anecdotal wish for wearable dispensers, but we hypothesize that it was voiced mainly by HCPs who were used to wearable dispensers from other hospitals or was triggered by rare events where ABHR was not accessible, corresponding to a classical reporting bias. Yet, interviewees identified two situations where ABHR was not easily accessible: first, when approaching a patient from a non-patient area in the ED such as the central working station or the meeting room and second, when accompanying patients to locations with unfamiliar localization of mounted dispensers.

Poor usability of the wearable dispensers was seen as a main barrier for application and several HCP interviewees expressed safety concerns as the outer surface of the dispensers was perceived to contaminate clean hands and patients surroundings. The design of a medical device affects compliance and behavior. Human factors engineering principles like 'affordance' (i.e. making use intuitive) and 'minimizing physical effort' (i.e. making adherence convenient) were found to improve adherence when applied in the development of medical devices [21, 22]. Good usability of medical products was shown to improve patient safety, e.g.

by reducing errors using blood glucose meters and increase compliance using hand sanitizers [23, 24]. Properties of a medical product can act as 'forcing functions'. These 'forcing functions' limit user errors by prohibiting or facilitating specific actions, and stand at the top of scale of the 'hierarchy of intervention effectiveness' - structural and technological interventions are more reliable in shaping people's behavior than human based interventions such as training and education [25]. Therefore, the wearable dispensers might benefit from an optimized design to encourage use and dismantle safety concerns.

Our study has limitations. First, the intervention period might have been too short to change a year-long habit. Second, although we were not aware of any other infection prevention and control promotional activity in the ER during the study periods we cannot fully exclude a time dependent bias. Third, as we only provided wearable dispensers to the ED staff and not to healthcare providers 'visiting' the ER (e.g. consultation service), the percentage of consumption from wearable dispensers might have been underestimated. Still, the amount of ABHR consumed by 'visiting' HCP is probably negligible. Forth, the Hawthorne effect and HH observation only during daytime, excluding night-shifts and weekends, might have skewed the HH observation results. Our results were, however, triangulated by ABHR consumption and the qualitative and quantitative investigation of perception and attitude of ED collaborators, which are strengths of the mixed-method study approach we used [26].

Conclusion

In conclusion, we found that the a single intervention of introduction of wearable ADHR dispensers in a busy ED, that had already been well equipped with mounted ABHR dispensers, did not significantly improve hand hygiene compliance or ABHR consumption. The main barriers for their use according to HCPs were the competing benefit of well-placed and abundant mounted dispensers and the flawed ergonomic design.

Abbreviations
ABHR: Alcohol-based hand rub; CI: Confidence interval; ED: Emergency Department; HCP: Healthcare provider; HH: Hand Hygiene; IPC: Infection prevention and control; UHZ: University Hospital Zurich; WHO: World health organization

Acknowledgements
We would like to acknowledge the contribution of the health care providers of the Emergency Department of the University Hospital Zurich, Switzerland, who took part in the study.

Funding
This study was partially funded by the Swiss National Science Foundation, grant 32003B_149474.
AW is supported by the academic career program "Filling the gap" of the Medical Faculty of the University of Zurich.
300 Clips for attaching the wearable dispensers were sponsored by B Braun, Switzerland.

Authors' contributions
JK, YF, HS, LC and AW designed the study. JK, YF, MD acquired the data, and JK, AW, and SPK performed the statistical analysis. JK, AW, and LC performed qualitative analysis of the interviews. AW, JK, LC, and HS analyzed and interpreted the data. JK and AW drafted the manuscript, and HS, LC, SPK, YF, DE, DIK and MD provided critical review of the manuscript for important intellectual content. All authors agree with the content and conclusions of this manuscript.

Consent for publication
Not applicable.

Competing interests
The authors declare that they have no competing interests.

Author details
[1]Division of Infectious Diseases and Hospital Epidemiology, University Hospital Zurich, University of Zurich, Rämistrasse 100, CH-8091 Zurich, Switzerland. [2]Emergency Department, University Hospital Zurich, University of Zurich, Zurich, Switzerland. [3]Baraka Health Centre, German Doctors Nairobi, Nairobi, Kenya.

References
1. Zimlichman E, et al. Health care-associated infections: a meta-analysis of costs and financial impact on the US health care system. JAMA Intern Med. 2013;173(22):2039–46.
2. Pittet D, et al. Evidence-based model for hand transmission during patient care and the role of improved practices. Lancet Infect Dis. 2006; 6(10):641–52.
3. Allegranzi B, Pittet D. Role of hand hygiene in healthcare-associated infection prevention. J Hosp Infect. 2009;73(4):305–15.
4. WHO. Guide to implementation: a guide to the implementation of the WHO Multimodal Hand Hygiene Improvement Strategy. 2009 [cited 2018 Jan 14]; Available from: http://www.who.int/gpsc/5may/Guide_to_ Implementation.pdf.
5. Erasmus V, et al. Systematic review of studies on compliance with hand hygiene guidelines in hospital care. Infect Control Hosp Epidemiol. 2010; 31(3):283–94.
6. Scheithauer S, et al. Improving hand hygiene compliance in the emergency department: getting to the point. BMC Infect Dis. 2013;13:367.
7. Pittet D, et al. Hand hygiene among physicians: performance, beliefs, and perceptions. Ann Intern Med. 2004;141(1):1–8.
8. Goodliffe L, et al. Rate of healthcare worker-patient interaction and hand hygiene opportunities in an acute care setting. Infect Control Hosp Epidemiol. 2014;35(3):225–30.
9. Pittet D, et al. Effectiveness of a hospital-wide programme to improve compliance with hand hygiene. Infection Control Programme Lancet. 2000; 356(9238):1307–12.
10. Yeung WK, Tam WS, Wong TW. Clustered randomized controlled trial of a hand hygiene intervention involving pocket-sized containers of alcohol-based hand rub for the control of infections in long-term care facilities. Infect Control Hosp Epidemiol. 2011;32(1):67–76.
11. Haas JP, Larson EL. Impact of wearable alcohol gel dispensers on hand hygiene in an emergency department. Acad Emerg Med. 2008;15(4):393–6.
12. Sax H, et al. The World Health Organization hand hygiene observation method. Am J Infect Control. 2009;37(10):827–34.
13. WHO. In WHO Guidelines on Hand Hygiene in Health Care. Geneva: First Global Patient Safety Challenge Clean Care Is Safer Care; 2009.
14. Sax H, et al. My five moments for hand hygiene': a user-centred design approach to understand, train, monitor and report hand hygiene. J Hosp Infect. 2007;67(1):9–21.
15. Strauss AL, Corbin JM. Grounded theory in practice. Thousand Oaks: Sage Publications; 1997.
16. Hugonnet S, Perneger TV, Pittet D. Alcohol-based handrub improves compliance with hand hygiene in intensive care units. Arch Intern Med. 2002;162(9):1037–43.
17. Picheansathian W. A systematic review on the effectiveness of alcohol-based solutions for hand hygiene. Int J Nurs Pract. 2004;10(1):3–9.

18. WHO Guidelines on Hand Hygiene in Health Care - First Global Patient Safety Challenge Clean Care is Safer Care. WHO 2009. http://apps.who.int/iris/bitstream/10665/44102/1/9789241597906_eng.pdf. Last Accessed 24 Feb 2018.

19. Koff MD, et al. Reduction in intraoperative bacterial contamination of peripheral intravenous tubing through the use of a novel device. Anesthesiology. 2009;110(5):978–85.

20. Parks CL, Schroeder KM, Galgon RE. Personal hand gel for improved hand hygiene compliance on the regional anesthesia team. J Anesth. 2015;29(6): 899–903.

21. Drews FA, Bakdash JZ, Gleed JR. Improving central line maintenance to reduce central line-associated bloodstream infections. Am J Infect Control. 2017;45(11):1224–30.

22. Drews FA. Adherence engineering. a new approach to increasing adherence to protocols Ergon Des. 2013;21:19–25.

23. Cure L, Van Enk R. Effect of hand sanitizer location on hand hygiene compliance. Am J Infect Control. 2015;43(9):917–21.

24. Rogers WA, Mykityshyn AL, Cambell RH, Fisk AD. Analysis of a "simple" medical device. Ergon Des. 2001;9(1):6–14.

25. Cafazzo, J.A. and O. St-Cyr, From discovery to design: the evolution of human factors in healthcare. Healthc Q, 2012. 15 Spec No: p. 24–29.

26. Jick TD. Mixing qualitative and quantitative methods - triangulation in action. Adm Sci Q. 1979;24(4):602–11.

21

Antibiotic use on paediatric inpatients in a teaching hospital in the Gambia

Pa Saidou Chaw[1,2*], Kristin Maria Schlinkmann[1,3], Heike Raupach-Rosin[3], André Karch[1,3,4], Mathias W. Pletz[5], Johannes Huebner[6], Ousman Nyan[7] and Rafael Mikolajczyk[2,3,4,8]

Abstract

Background: Antibiotics are useful but increasing resistance is a major problem. Our objectives were to assess antibiotic use and microbiology testing in hospitalized children in the Gambia.

Methods: We conducted a retrospective analysis of paediatric inpatient data at The Edward Francis Small Teaching Hospital in Banjul, The Gambia. We extracted relevant data from the admission folders of all patients (aged > 28 days to 15 years) admitted in 2015 (January–December), who received at least one antibiotic for 24 h. We also reviewed the microbiology laboratory record book to obtain separate data for the bacterial isolates and resistance test results of all the paediatric inpatients during the study period.

Results: Over half of the admitted patients received at least one antibiotic during admission (496/917) with a total consumption of 670.7 Days of Antibiotic Therapy/1000 Patient-Days. The clinical diagnoses included an infectious disease for 398/496, 80.2% of the patients on antibiotics, pneumonia being the most common (184/496, 37.1%). There were 51 clinically relevant bacterial isolates, *Klebsiella species* being the most common (12/51, 23.5%), mainly from urine (11/12, 91.7%). Antibiotic resistance was mainly to ampicillin (38/51, 74.5%), mainly reported as *Coliform species* 11/51, 21.6%.

Conclusions: More than half of the admitted patients received antibiotics. The reported antibiotic resistance was highest to the most commonly used antibiotics such as ampicillin. Efforts to maximize definitive antibiotic indication such as microbiological testing prior to start of antibiotics should be encouraged where possible for a more rational antibiotic use.

Keywords: Paediatrics, Antibiotic use, Microbiology, Antibiotic resistance, Antibiotic stewardship

Background

Antibiotic resistance is a major problem especially in resource-limited countries where the burden of infectious diseases is high, with often higher resistance rates than in industrialized countries [1]. Children have higher risk of developing infectious diseases than adults [2, 3], and accurate aetiological diagnosis is often difficult due to the non-specific manifestation of infections in this age group [4, 5]. Microbiological investigations are therefore especially useful to confirm definitive indication of antibiotics and for their rational use on children [6], but this is a challenge in developing countries where limited laboratory testing is available [2]. In developing countries, shortages of drug supplies also often restrict prescribers to the available drugs [7].

Inappropriate antibiotic use is well described in developed countries but not as well studied in developing countries [8]. Local data on antibiotic consumption and resistance profile is useful in helping formulate policies and recommendations on antibiotic use both at local and regional levels [7]. Inappropriate prescription of

* Correspondence: pasaidouchaw@helmholtz-hzi.de
[1]PhD Programme, Epidemiology"Braunschweig-Hannover, Department of Epidemiology, Helmholtz Centre for Infection Research, 38124 Braunschweig, Germany
[2]Institute for Medical Epidemiology, Biometry, and Informatics (IMEBI), Medical Faculty of the Martin-Luther University Halle-Wittenberg, 06112 Halle (Saale), Germany
Full list of author information is available at the end of the article

antibiotics has been reported elsewhere in Africa such as in Ethiopia where a study reported up to 86.6% of antibiotics prescribed for the treatment of cough and diarrhoea among less than 60 months old children attending to hospitals were inappropriate [9]. Within the sub region, a study in Senegal reported prescription indication errors mainly with antibiotic and antimalarial drugs, and dosage errors mainly with antibiotics and antifungal drugs [10]. In the Gambia, over prescription of antibiotics among children less than 60 months old have been reported in the outpatient setting of health centres [11], but to our knowledge, data on appropriateness of antibiotic prescribing is lacking. In addition, antibiotic resistance patterns have been reported for *Streptococcus species* [12, 13], *Salmonella* [14], *Helicobacter pylori* [15], and for specific disease conditions such as severe malnutrition [16], within smaller health facilities and population. Microbiological test patterns for neonates treated with antibiotics have also been reported [17]. But national and international data on antimicrobial resistance patterns in the paediatric setting is still limited, thus affecting the development of evidence based policies and guidelines [7]. As far as we know there has been no published study examining antibiotic prescribing and microbiological testing patterns in the general paediatric inpatients in the Gambia.

Different bacteria use different mechanisms to develop antibiotic resistance as defined by Munita et al. [18], who classified antibiotic resistance into four major biochemical mechanisms as follows: a) modifications of the antimicrobial molecule (by chemical alterations of antibiotics and destruction of antibiotic molecule), b) prevention of antibiotics to reach target (by decreasing antibiotic penetration and increasing efflux), c) change or bypass of target sites (through target protection and modifying the target site), and d) resistance due to global cell adaptive processes. While the process of prevention of antibiotics to reach target by decreasing antibiotic penetration is mainly for gram-negative bacteria due to the presence of an outer membrane, classical antibiotics affected by resistance due to global cell adaptive processes are usually used for treating gram-positives (vancomycin and daptomycin). In developed countries, the dynamic spread of antibiotic resistance has led to the establishment of antibiotic stewardship (ABS) programs fostering prudent use of antibiotics [19–21]. Such programs are currently rare and more difficult to implement in developing countries due to limited resources [22]. In order to estimate the expected impact of an ABS-program, prior analysis of antibiotic prescribing behaviour is required. Therefore, the objectives of our study were to assess the antibiotic consumption, the antibiotic indication and dosage, and use of microbiological testing on paediatric inpatients

at a teaching hospital in The Gambia. This would enable us to test our hypothesis that in addition to other possible factors, limited microbiology use contributes to limited definitive antibiotic indication and high antibiotic consumption in The Gambia. Our results would provide up-to-date information on current practice on antibiotic prescribing and antibiotic resistance patterns in the paediatric setting, and other countries are likely to face similar problems. Thus the findings support the need and would contribute evidence, for the establishment of national, regional, and global guidelines and policies to promote rational antibiotic use.

Methods
Setting
The study was a retrospective analysis of paediatric inpatient data from The Edward Francis Small Teaching Hospital in Banjul (EFSTH), The Gambia's largest hospital referral centre. The hospital serves as the country's main tertiary care centre receiving patients from the whole country. The team of medical doctors responsible for the management of patients include specialists, medical officers, and house officers.

Data collection
We extracted the required data from the admission folders of patients aged > 28 days to 15 years admitted in 2015 (January–December), who received at least one antibiotic for at least 24 h, using Microsoft Access 2010. We excluded records of patients discharged against medical advice and admission folders with missing dates or loss of documents containing antibiotic or diagnoses details. Data extracted included: age, weight, height, sex, clinical diagnosis, antibiotic treatment (name, treatment duration, route and frequency of administration), and microbiology workup. All the included patients had at least one diagnosis at the time of admission; the diagnoses were mostly clinically based. All the diagnoses included were as documented on the patients' records. We also obtained information on the total admissions during this period. In addition, we reviewed the microbiology laboratory record book to obtain separate data for the bacterial isolates and resistance test results of all the paediatric inpatients during the study period.

Assessment of antibiotic consumption
Antibiotic consumption was assessed based on qualitative indicators which assess appropriateness of antibiotic use, and quantitative indicators which assess the volume or cost of antibiotics used [23]. For the qualitative assessment of antibiotic consumption, we used a World Health Organization (WHO) guideline to assess compliance to indication and dosing. Because under 5 year old children with community acquired pneumonia (CAP) have been

reported to have the highest percentage of encounter with an antibiotic prescribed in an outpatient study in The Gambia [11], we used the clinical diagnoses of CAP to assess the antibiotics indicated, and the prescribed dosages for ampicillin and penicillin-G for treating the cases among children less than 5 years old, by comparing them to the dosage recommendations by the WHO for the treatment of severe pneumonia in this age group [24]. We restricted this analysis to clinical diagnoses of pneumonia but excluded the cases of pneumonia with other underlying diseases such as sickle cell disease or HIV, superimposed pneumonia, or cases of pneumonia with possible non-infectious causes such as aspiration pneumonia, as indicated on the clinical diagnoses records. We excluded anti-Tuberculosis drugs from the analysis of the antibiotics. We also used two of the common infectious disease diagnoses in children (sepsis and urinary tract infections (UTI)) [25, 26] to assess the use of microbiological culture results to guide definitive antibiotic indication.

For the quantitative assessment of antibiotic consumption for inpatients, we used the recommended Days of Antibiotic-Therapy (DoT)/1000 Patient-Days (PD) to assess the volume of antibiotics used in the paediatric inpatient setting [19], since the defined daily dose (DDD) is mainly indicated for adults [27] and poorly estimates antibiotic consumption in paediatrics [28]. We found DoT to be a good option to estimate antibiotic use density since it considers each antibiotic and the number of days it was used, therefore every antibiotic contributes independently to the DoT [28]. This provides a better estimate of the overall antibiotic volume and comparable with other settings [19, 23]. In addition, we also calculated the proportion of antibiotics used by any patient during the study period.

Bacterial cultures and antibiotic resistance testing
To assess the bacteria isolates and resistance test results for the study period, we used the data we obtained from the laboratory records since we assumed that this data may be more complete than those in the admission folders. However, due to lack of the hospital numbers for some of the records, matching of these patients with the admission data was not feasible.

Data analysis
We analyzed the data with Stata version 12 (StataCorp., College Station, TX, USA) using a complete case approach. We summarized the results into proportions, ratios, and medians. Where applicable, we compared children under 5 and those over 5 years of age. To make comparisons and test for associations for antibiotic use, we used Chi square test (for all admitted children) and

Fisher's exact test (for CAP, sepsis, and UTI diagnoses). We set statistical significance at ≤0.05.

Results
Diagnoses and antibiotic use
For the year 2015 (January–December), 917 patients were admitted, 496 (54.1%) received at least one antibiotic and fulfilled the other inclusion criteria for the analysis, 181/496, 36.5% of these also received antibiotics on discharge. The total antibiotic consumption was 670.7 DoT/1000 PD. Most of the patients treated with antibiotics had at least one infectious disease diagnosis (80.2%) (Table 1), the most common were pneumonia (184/496, 37.1%) and sepsis (70/496, 14.1%). The most common antibiotics used were ampicillin (179/917, 19.5%), gentamicin (133/917, 14.5%), and ceftriaxone (117/917, 12.8%). Table 2 shows antibiotics prescribed for admitted patients during the study period, classified according to the Anatomical Therapeutic Chemical (ATC) classification system by the WHO Collaborating Centre for Drug Statistics Methodology [27]. Fig.1 compares the DoT of each antibiotic to the proportion of patients treated with each antibiotic.

Antibiotic indication and dosage
Most of the children with CAP were treated with ceftriaxone-monotherapy (16/69, 23.2%), penicillin-G (12/69, 17.4%), or ampicillin and gentamicin (11/69, 15.9%) as recommended by the WHO: using ampicillin (or penicillin) with gentamicin as first-line or ceftriaxone as second-line for treatment of severe CAP among children aged 2 to 59 months. Other antibiotic combinations used included penicillin-G and chloramphenicol (6/69, 8.7%), ceftriaxone and cloxacillin (4/69, 5.8%), and ampicillin and cloxacillin (2/69, 2.8%). Ampicillin was dosed at 50 mg/kg for eight patients, one patient received a lower dose; penicillin-G was dosed at 50,000 units/kg for 19 patients, two patients received a higher dosage. There was no use of macrolides, tetracyclines or fluoroquinolones.

Forty-eight (68.6%) of the patients with sepsis (70) had cultures requested, of which four (8.3%) had bacteria isolated and respectively treated with ceftriaxone and ciprofloxacin (*Acinetobacter baumanii*, from cerebrospinal fluid, with no reported resistance); ampicillin and gentamicin combination, which were changed to ciprofloxacin (*Coliform species*, from oral-swab, with resistance reported to ampicillin and gentamicin); ampicillin and gentamicin combination, which were changed to ceftriaxone, and later to ciprofloxacin (*Salmonella species*, from stool, with resistance reported to ampicillin); ceftriaxone and cloxacillin (*Staphylococcus aureus*, from blood, with no reported resistance). Nine (81.8%) of the patients with UTI (11) had cultures requested, of which

Table 1 General characteristics of admitted patients aged > 28 days to 15 years from January–December 2015

Variable	Categories	Frequency
Total admissions		$n = 917$, %
Age	Under 5	630, 68.7%
	Over 5	287, 31.3%
Patients treated with antibiotic		$n = 496$, %
Sex	Male	302, 61.1%
	Female	192, 38.9%
Type of clinical diagnosis*	Infectious disease diagnosis	398, 80.2%
	Non-infectious disease diagnosis	300, 60.5%
	Both Infectious disease and non-infectious disease diagnosis	202, 40.7%
Age	Under 5	366, 73.8%
	Over 5	130, 26.2%
Length of hospital stay	<=7 days	264, 53.2%
	8–14 days	150, 30.2%
	> 14 days	82, 16.5%
Duration of antibiotic treatment	<=7 days	361, 72.8%
	7–14 days	100, 20.2%
	> 14 days	35, 7.1%

*not mutually exclusive, based on admission diagnosis

two (22.2%) had bacteria isolated from urine and were treated with ampicillin and gentamicin combination, later changed to ceftriaxone, with additions of nitrofurantoin and ciprofloxacin during the course of treatment (*Escherichia coli and Klebsiella species*, with resistance reported to ampicillin for both organisms); ampicillin and gentamicin combination (*Coliform species*, with resistance reported to ampicillin). Thus all the resistant bacteria reported (five) were to ampicillin (5/5, 100%) and gentamicin (1/5, 20%). The difference in the choice of antibiotics between these patients with or without positive cultures was not significant.

Bacterial cultures and antibiotic resistance testing

At least one culture request was indicated in the admissions records for 266/496, 53.6% of the patients who were on antibiotics. There were 51 clinically relevant bacterial isolates from the laboratory records. The most common were *Klebsiella species* (14/51, 27.5%, from urine 13/14, 92.9% and aspirate 1/14, 7.1%), *Coliform species* (11/51, 21.6%, from urine 7/11, 63.6%, swabs 2/ 11, 18.2%, and for each specimen (sputum and aspirate) 1/11, 9.1%), and *S. aureus* (9/51, 17.6%, from swabs 7/9, 77.8%, and for each specimen (blood and aspirate) 1/9, 11.1%) (Fig. 2).

Antibiotic resistance was mainly to ampicillin (38/51, 74.5%, mainly reported as *Coliform species* 11/51, 21.6%, *S. aureus* 6/51, 11.8%, and *E. coli* 5/51, 9.8%. The proportion of the reported resistance of *Klebsiella species* to ampicillin was excluded due to its intrinsic resistance to

ampicillin), co-trimoxazole (27/51, 52.9%, mainly reported as *Coliform species* and *Klebsiella species* 10/51, 19.6% for each organism, *E. coli* 3/51, 5.9%, and *Salmonella species* 2/51, 3.9%), and gentamicin (22/51, 43.1%, mainly reported as *Klebsiella species* 12/51, 23.5%, for each organism (*Coliform species* and *E. coli*) 3/51, 5.9%, and *S. aureus* 2/51, 3.9%) (Fig. 3). Fig. 3b illustrates the reported antibiotic resistant bacteria to all the tested antibiotics. Antibiotic resistance to third generation cephalosporin was 6/51, 11.7%, all were Enterobacteriaceae thus suggestive of extended spectrum beta lactamase producing (ESBL), isolated from urine (3/6, 50%) and for each specimen (blood, aspirate, and swabs) 1/6, 16.7%.

Discussion

Our retrospective study conducted amongst paediatric inpatients in the highest referral hospital in the Gambia shows more than half of the admitted patients received at least one antibiotic and slightly more than half of these patients had microbiological cultures indicated. Antibiotic resistance was high for the most commonly used antibiotics (ampicillin and gentamicin).

We observed an overall higher antibiotic consumption (670.7 DoT/1000 PD) when compared to that observed from a pre-interventional phase of an ABS study conducted in a paediatric unit in a developed country (483.6 DoT/1000 PD) [19]. The volume of antibiotic used in our study was higher for all comparable antibiotics except for metronidazole, ciprofloxacilln and vancomycin. The proportion of patients treated with antibiotics was

Table 2 Antibiotics used on inpatients aged > 28 days to 15 years during the period January – December 2015

Antibiotic	DoT	DoT/1000PD (Total PD = 4045)	Proportion of patients treated with the antibiotic (n = 917, %)	Age		P Value*
				under 5 years n = 630, %	5 years and more n = 287, %	
J01G aminoglycosides						
Gentamicin	664	164.2	133, 14.5%	121, 19.2%	12, 4.2%	< 0.001
Neomycin	33	8.2	5, 0.5%	5, 0.8%	0	0.154
J01D cephalosporins						
Cefriaxone	490	121.1	117, 12.8%	86, 13.7%	31, 10.8%	0.982
Cefalexin	16	4.0	3, 0.3%	3, 0.5%	0	0.231
Cefpodoxime	1	0.2	1, 0.1%	1, 0.2%	0	0.551
J01C Beta-lactam antibacterials, Penicillins						
Ampicillin	416	103.0	179, 19.5%	140, 22.2%	39, 13.6%	0.003
Penicillin-G	416	103.0	92, 10.0%	64, 10.2%	28, 9.8%	0.077
Cloxacillin	200	49.4	44, 4.8%	39, 6.2%	5, 1.7%	0.054
Amoxicillin	150	37.1	31, 3.4%	21, 3.3%	10, 3.5%	0.847
Amoxicillin-clavulanic	16	4.0	1, 0.1%	0	1, 0.3%	0.017
Flucloxacillin	6	1.4	1, 0.1%	1, 0.2%	0	0.551
J01B Amphenicols						
Chloramphenicol	129	31.9	50, 5.5%	33, 5.2%	17, 5.9%	0.078
J01XD Imidazole derivatives						
Metronidazole	73	18.0	9, 1.0%	5, 0.8%	4, 1.4%	0.209
J01 M Quinolones						
Ciprofloxacin	35	8.7	10, 1.1%	3, 0.5%	7, 2.4%	< 0.001
J01A Tetracyclines						
Tetracycline	26	6.4	1, 0.1%	0	1, 0.3%	0.093
J01XA glycopeptides						
Vancomycin	24	5.9	1, 0.1%	1, 0.2%	0	0.551
J01FA macrolides						
Erythromycin	7	1.7	3, 0.3%	2, 0.3%	1, 0.3%	0.398
J01E Sulfonamides and Trimethoprim						
Co-trimoxazole	6	1.4	1, 0.1%	1, 0.2%	0	0.551
J01XE Nitrofuran derivatives						
Nitorfurantoin	5	1.2	1, 0.1%	0	1, 0.3%	0.093
Total	2713	670.7	–	–	–	–

*Chi-squared
DoT: Days of Antibiotic-Therapy
PD: Patient-Days

as similarly observed at the health-center outpatient level among children under 5 years old (63.4%), and higher among admitted neonates (94%) in the Gambia [11, 17]. In other developing countries, a similar proportion of children received antibiotics during admission, ranging from 63.6% in Indonesia to 71.1% in Nigeria [3, 21]. The wide difference in the use of antibiotics between developing and developed countries could be related to multiple factors such as the higher rate of infectious diseases in developing countries [3, 29], the limited access to diagnostic parameters to confirm definitive need for antibiotic use,

the limited access to support from specialists such as infectious disease specialists, and lack of local antibiotic policies in developing countries [1, 30]. From our study, the availability of microbiology results was useful in guiding the selection of the right antibiotic class as demonstrated in the treatment of sepsis and UTI, although the limited available results may have affected the statistical significance.

Empirical antibiotic indication and dosage for the treatment of severe CAP were as recommended by WHO for most of the patients [24]. A smaller proportion of patients

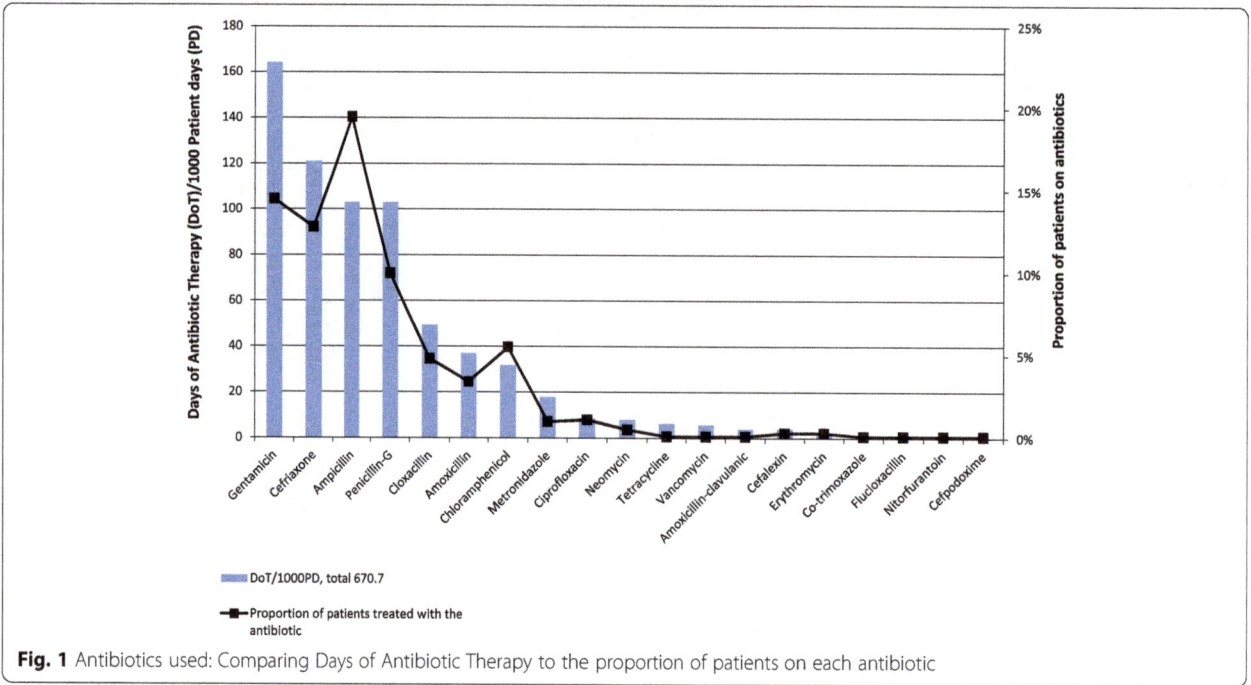

Fig. 1 Antibiotics used: Comparing Days of Antibiotic Therapy to the proportion of patients on each antibiotic

were treated with penicillin-G and chloramphenicol combination although this has been reported in the WHO recommendation as inferior to ampicillin and gentamicin combination for treating severe CAP. This may be partly explained by availability of penicillin and chloramphenicol. The other antibiotics used for few of the patients are however not in the WHO recommendations, possibly based on specific clinical judgement such as failure of first and second-line therapies started from a referral hospital, high clinical suspicion for a specific organism based on the clinical presentation, or drug availability. The disruption of drug supply in developing countries affecting drug availability and appropriate antibiotic use has been reported [7, 31]. Ceftriaxone, which belongs to the WHO WATCH group of antibiotics often used as second-line treatment [32] was one of the most common antibiotics used, with a higher density of use than ampicillin which is a first line drug. Although at our study site the prescription of this drug is controlled, as it has to be countersigned by a specialist, the limited availability of other second-line drugs may have contributed to its frequent use.

About half of the patients treated with antibiotics had at least one microbiology test requested. A high proportion

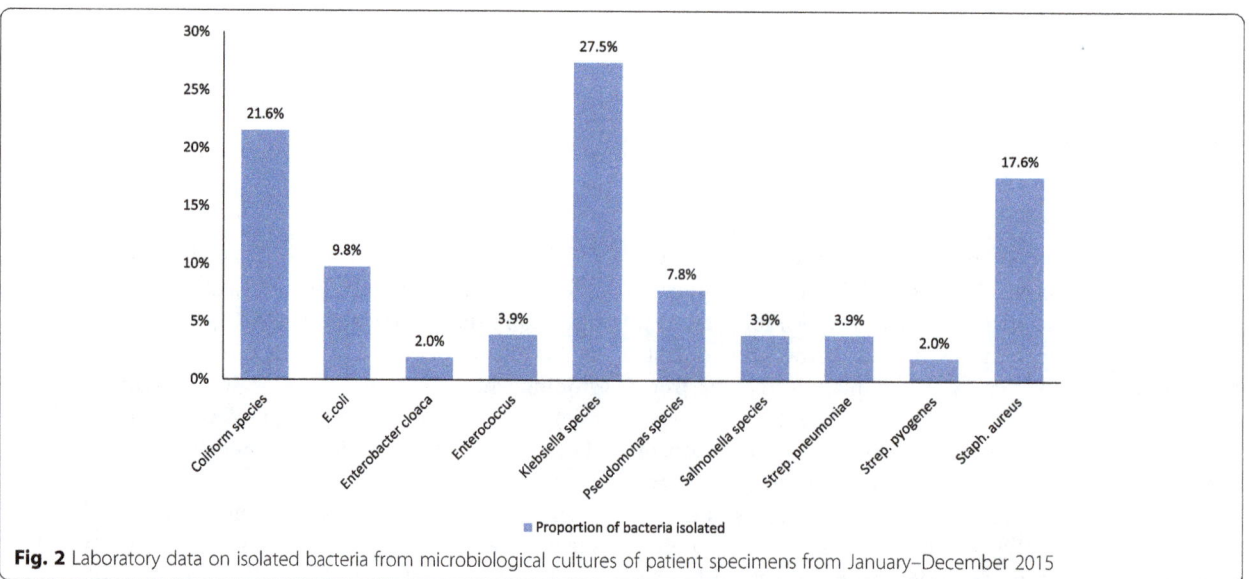

Fig. 2 Laboratory data on isolated bacteria from microbiological cultures of patient specimens from January–December 2015

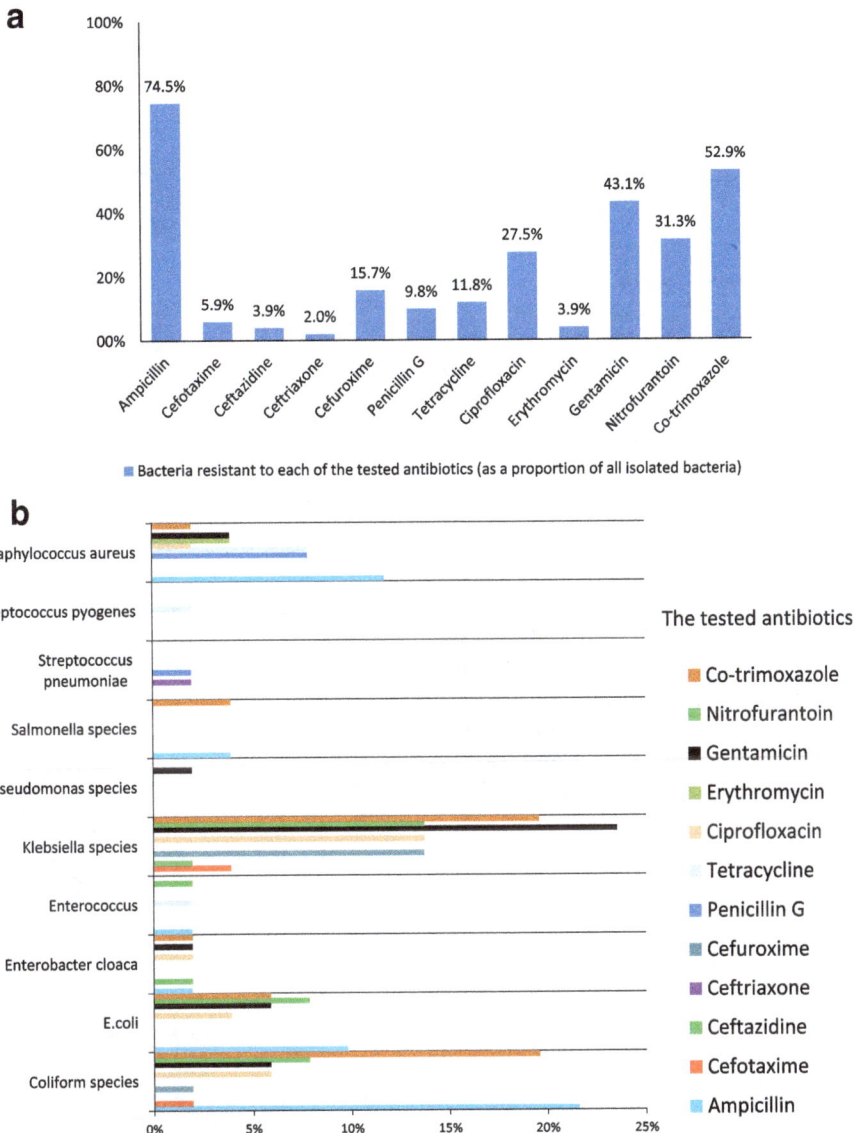

Fig. 3 a Laboratory data on antibiotic resistance testing from January–December 2015. **b** The distribution of the reported antibiotic resistant bacteria to all the tested antibiotics

of empirical antibiotic use based on clinical judgement was also reported in The Gambia among neonatal admissions [17], and elsewhere in Africa [29]. This limited microbiological laboratory use in developing countries may also reflect a lack of trust into the value of microbiological results, possibly due to the limited laboratory services, delays in the provision of results, amongst others [33, 34]. Clinical suspicion of co-infections or severe infections such septicemia may have also warranted the immediate administration of relevant antibiotics, pending later microbiological investigation.

Although the species for many of the organisms were not identified, the bacteria belong to the groups of the most dangerous resistant pathogens including both gram positive and negative organisms as reported by Fair et al. [35]. They also reported stability in the resistance rates of gram positive organisms, on the contrary, gram negative organisms' resistance rates tend to be on the rise. This finding is similar to our results, as most of the reported resistant pathogens were gram negatives and multi-drug resistant as defined by Magiorakos et al. [36]. The more difficulty in treating gram negatives could be explained by their resistant mechanisms especially their added mechanism of inhibiting antibiotic penetration due to the existence of an outer membrane, and the higher presence of efflux pumps over-expression compared to gram positives, in the presence of the other possible mechanisms [18, 35]. The recorded resistance towards the commonly used antibiotics (ampicillin and gentamicin), and considering that some of the isolates are suggestive of ESBL Enterobacteriaceae which is one of the 12 important bacteria families highlighted by the WHO needing more attention [37], conducting microbiological workup prior to the onset of empirical treatment could encourage a more rational antibiotic use and limit resistance. A review on antibiotic resistance in Africa also reported a high bacterial resistance to the first line antibiotic therapy and Enterobacteriaceae to third generation cephalosporin [38]. Although use of co-trimoxazole in our study was low, the resistance reported was among the highest. This could be explained by the high use of this antibiotic in the outpatient health centers where availability of the other antibiotics maybe limited [11].

Limitations

The possibility of missing data from the admission records especially the microbiology data makes it difficult to make absolute judgements on the use of antibiotics based on laboratory findings. The data we obtained from the laboratory could not resolve this problem because some of the records lack hospital numbers thus matching this data with the admission data was not feasible. Many of the organisms were reported as genus without identification to the species level, making it difficult to compare with other settings and specify the resistant organism more appropriately.

Conclusion

Our study shows that more than half of the admitted patients received antibiotics although most of the available results showed no microbiological evidence for their indication, suggesting that most of the antibiotics were empirically prescribed. Although several other factors in such settings could contribute to use of antibiotics for patients without microbiological evidence, the availability of microbiology results was a useful guide for choosing the class of antibiotic. Thus, in addition to the use of standards to guide empirical antibiotic therapy such as that of the WHO, microbiological use to guide antibiotic prescribing should be encouraged. This is probably achievable through better access to laboratory services and the establishment of ABS and its promotion for acceptance. Our study has shown high bacterial resistance to commonly used antibiotics, including ESBL bacteria, warranting the need for further research on the local antibiotic resistance patterns of bacteria as well as setting up an antibiotic resistance surveillance system.

Acknowledgements

We would like to thank the staff of the Edward Francis Small Teaching Hospital (EFSTH) especially those working at the paediatric department for their support during the study. We thank Mrs. Rohey Awe and Mr. Modou Lamin Camara, Data Entry Clerks, EFSTH, for their contributions during the data collection. We thank Dr. Dado Jabbie, Medical Officer, Bundung Maternal & Child Health Hospital, for the technical support she provided during the course of the study.

Funding

The first author is a student (from The Gambia) of the PhD Programme "Epidemiology "Braunschweig-Hannover, Germany, and this study is part of his PhD research project funded by the Government of The Gambia.

Authors' contributions

PSC designed the study, collected and analyzed the data, and drafted the paper. KMS contributed on the study design and data collection. HRR contributed on the study design. AK contributed on the study design and statistical analysis. MWP, JH, and ON reviewed the study design and contributed on the interpretation of the data. RM provided technical expertise, contributed on the study design of the paper, and supervised the overall work. All authors contributed to the manuscript. All authors have accepted the final version of the manuscript.

Consent for publication

Not applicable.

Competing interests

The authors declare that they have no competing interests.

Author details

[1] PhD Programme, Epidemiology"Braunschweig-Hannover, Department of Epidemiology, Helmholtz Centre for Infection Research, 38124 Braunschweig, Germany. [2] Institute for Medical Epidemiology, Biometry, and Informatics (IMEBI), Medical Faculty of the Martin-Luther University Halle-Wittenberg, 06112 Halle (Saale), Germany. [3] Department of Epidemiology, Helmholtz Centre for Infection Research, 38124 Braunschweig, Germany. [4] German Center for Infection Research (DZIF), Hannover-Braunschweig site, 30625 Hannover, Germany. [5] Center for Infectious Diseases and Infection Control, Jena University Hospital, Am Klinikum 1, 07747 Jena, Germany. [6] Division of Paediatric Infectious Diseases, Dr. Von Hauner Children's Hospital, Ludwig Maximilian University Munich, 80337 Munich, Germany. [7] Department of Medicine, School of Medicine and Allied Health Sciences, University of the Gambia, Edward Francis Small Teaching Hospital, Banjul, The Gambia. [8] Hannover Medical School, 30625 Hannover, Germany.

References

1. Bartoloni A, Gotuzzo E. Bacterial-resistant infections in resource-limited countries. In: *Antimicrobial Resistance in Developing Countries*. Edn: Springer New York; 2010. p. 199–231.
2. Lee AC, Chandran A, Herbert HK, Kozuki N, Markell P, Shah R, Campbell H, Rudan I, Baqui AH. Treatment of infections in young infants in low- and middle-income countries: a systematic review and meta-analysis of frontline health worker diagnosis and antibiotic access. PLoS Med. 2014;11(10): e1001741.
3. Fadare J, Olatunya O, Oluwayemi O, Ogundare O. Drug prescribing pattern for under-fives in a paediatric clinic in south-western Nigeria. Ethiopian J Health Sci. 2015;25(1):73–8.
4. Thaver D, Zaidi AK. Burden of neonatal infections in developing countries: a review of evidence from community-based studies. Pediatr Infect Dis J. 2009;28(1 Suppl):S3–9.
5. Darmstadt GL, Saha SK, Choi Y, El Arifeen S, Ahmed NU, Bari S, Rahman SM, Mannan I, Crook D, Fatima K, et al. Population-based incidence and etiology of community-acquired neonatal bacteremia in Mirzapur, Bangladesh: an observational study. J Infect Dis. 2009;200(6):906–15.
6. Levy-Hara G, Amábile-Cuevas CF, Gould I, Hutchinson J, Abbo L, Saxynger L, Vlieghe E, Lopes Cardoso FL, Methar S, Kanj S, et al. 'Ten commandments'

for the appropriate use of antibiotics by the practicing physician in an outpatient setting. Front Microbiol. 2011;2(NOV)

7. Le Doare K, Barker CI, Irwin A, Sharland M. Improving antibiotic prescribing for children in the resource-poor setting. Br J Clin Pharmacol. 2015;79(3): 446–55.

8. Fisher BT, Meaney PA, Shah SS, Irwin SA, Grady CA, Kurup S, Malefho KC, Jibril H, Steenhoff AP. Antibiotic use in pediatric patients admitted to a referral hospital in Botswana. Am J Trop Med Hyg. 2009;81(1):129–31.

9. Tekleab AM, Asfaw YM, Weldetsadik AY, Amaru GM. Antibiotic prescribing practice in the management of cough or diarrhea among children attending hospitals in Addis Ababa: a cross-sectional study. Pediatric Health Med Ther. 2017;8:93–8.

10. Camara B, Faye PM, Fall AL, Diagne GN, Sbaa HC, Ba M, Sow HD. Prescription errors in a pediatric hospital department in Dakar Senegal. Medecine tropicale : revue du Corps de sante colonial. 2011;71(1):33–6.

11. Risk R, Naismith H, Burnett A, Moore SE, Cham M, Unger S. Rational prescribing in paediatrics in a resource-limited setting. Arch Dis Child. 2013;98(7):503–9.

12. Ashu EE, Jarju S, Dione M, Mackenzie G, Ikumapayi UN, Manjang A, Azuine R, Antonio M. Population structure, epidemiology and antibiotic resistance patterns of Streptococcus pneumoniae serotype 5: prior to PCV-13 vaccine introduction in eastern Gambia. BMC Infect Dis. 2016;16:33.

13. Foster-Nyarko E, Kwambana B, Ceesay F, Jawneh K, Darboe S, Mulwa SN, Ceesay B, Secka OO, Adetifa I, Antonio M. Incidence of macrolide-lincosamide-streptogramin B resistance amongst beta-haemolytic streptococci in the Gambia. BMC Res Notes. 2017;10(1):106.

14. Kwambana-Adams B, Darboe S, Nabwera H, Foster-Nyarko E, Ikumapayi UN, Secka O, Betts M, Bradbury R, Wegmuller R, Lawal B, et al. Salmonella infections in the Gambia, 2005-2015. Clin Infect Dis. 2015;61(Suppl 4):S354–62.

15. Secka O, Berg DE, Antonio M, Corrah T, Tapgun M, Walton R, Thomas V, Galano JJ, Sancho J, Adegbola RA, et al. Antimicrobial susceptibility and resistance patterns among helicobacter pylori strains from the Gambia, West Africa. Antimicrob Agents Chemother. 2013;57(3):1231–7.

16. Okomo UA, Garba D, Fombah AE, Secka O, Ikumapayi UN, Udo JJ, Ota MO. Bacterial isolates and antibiotic sensitivity among Gambian children with severe acute malnutrition. Int J Pediatr. 2011;2011:825123.

17. Okomo UA, Dibbasey T, Kassama K, Lawn JE, Zaman SMA, Kampmann B, Howie SRC, Bojang K. Neonatal admissions, quality of care and outcome: 4 years of inpatient audit data from the Gambia's teaching hospital. Paediatr Int Child Health. 2015;35(3):252–64.

18. Munita JM, Arias CA. Mechanisms of antibiotic resistance. Microbiol Spectr. 2016;4(2)

19. Kreitmeyr K, von Both U, Pecar A, Borde JP, Mikolajczyk R, Huebner J. Pediatric antibiotic stewardship: successful interventions to reduce broad-spectrum antibiotic use on general pediatric wards. Infection. 2017;45(4): 493–504.

20. Dik JW, Hendrix R, Lo-Ten-Foe JR, Wilting KR, Panday PN, van Gemert-Pijnen LE, Leliveld AM, van der Palen J, Friedrich AW, Sinha B. Automatic day-2 intervention by a multidisciplinary antimicrobial stewardship-team leads to multiple positive effects. Front Microbiol. 2015;6:546.

21. Murni IK, Duke T, Kinney S, Daley AJ, Soenarto Y. Reducing hospital-acquired infections and improving the rational use of antibiotics in a developing country: an effectiveness study. Arch Dis Child. 2015;100(5):454–9.

22. Shankar RP, Partha P, Shenoy NK, Easow JM, Brahmadathan KN. Prescribing patterns of antibiotics and sensitivity patterns of common microorganisms in the internal medicine ward of a teaching hospital in western Nepal: a prospective study. Ann Clin Microbiol Antimicrob. 2003;2:7.

23. D-ADriradara: QUALITY INDICATORS & QUANTITY METRICS OF ANTIBIOTIC USE, http://drive-ab.eu/wp-content/uploads/2014/09/WP1A_Final-QMs-QIs_final.pdf.

24. WHO: Revised WHO classification and treatment of childhood pneumonia at health facilities • EVIDENCE SUMMARIES • Available at: http://apps.who.int/iris/bitstream/10665/137319/1/9789241507813_eng.pdf. 2014:34.

25. Carcillo JA. Reducing the global burden of sepsis in infants and children: a clinical practice research agenda. Pediatr Crit Care Med. 2005;6(3 Suppl): S157–64.

26. Masika WG, O'Meara WP, Holland TL, Armstrong J. Contribution of urinary tract infection to the burden of febrile illnesses in young children in rural Kenya. PLoS One. 2017;12(3):s.

27. Methodology WCCfDS: ATC/DDD Index, https://www.whocc.no/atc_ddd_index/?code=J01. 2017.

28. (DASON) DASON: DUKE ANTIMICROBIAL STEWARDSHIP OUTREACH NETWORK (DASON), https://dason.medicine.duke.edu/sites/dason.medicine.duke.edu/files/march_2016_dason-newsletter_au_metrics_rwm.pdf. 2016, 4(3):5.

29. Kebede HK, Gesesew HA, Woldehaimanot TE, Goro KK. Antimicrobial use in paediatric patients in a teaching hospital in Ethiopia. PLoS One. 2017;12(3): e0173290.

30. Kariuki S, Dougan G. Antibacterial resistance in sub-Saharan Africa: an underestimated emergency. Ann N Y Acad Sci. 2014;1323:43–55.

31. Ndihokubwayo JB, Yahaya AA, Desta AT, Ki-Zerbo G, Odei AE, Keita B, Pana PA, Nkhoma W. Antimicrobial resistance in the African region: issues, challenges and actions proposed. African Health Monitor. 2013;16

32. WHO: WHO Model List of Essential Medicines. Available at: http://www.who.int/medicines/publications/essentialmedicines/20th_EML2017.pdf?ua=1. 2017, 20th List:62.

33. Chaw PS, Maria Schlinkmann K, Raupach-Rosin H, Karch A, Pletz MW, Huebner J, Mikolajczyk R. Knowledge, attitude and practice of Gambian health practitioners towards antibiotic prescribing and microbiological testing: a cross-sectional survey. Trans R Soc Trop Med Hyg. 2017;111(3): 117–24.

34. Adorka M, Dikokole M, Mitonga KH, Allen K. Healthcare providers' attitudes and perceptions in infection diagnosis and antibiotic prescribing in public health institutions in Lesotho: a cross sectional survey. Afr Health Sci. 2013; 13(2):344–50.

35. Fair RJ, Tor Y. Antibiotics and bacterial resistance in the 21st century. Perspect Medicin Chem. 2014;6:25–64.

36. Magiorakos AP, Srinivasan A, Carey RB, Carmeli Y, Falagas ME, Giske CG, Harbarth S, Hindler JF, Kahlmeter G, Olsson-Liljequist B, et al. Multidrug-resistant, extensively drug-resistant and pandrug-resistant bacteria: an international expert proposal for interim standard definitions for acquired resistance. Clin Microbiol Infect. 2012;18(3):268–81.

37. WHO. Global priority list of antibiotic-resistant bacteria to guide research, discovery, and development of new antibiotics. In: Available at: http://www.who.int/medicines/publications/WHO-PPL-Short_Summary_25Feb-ET_NM_WHO.pdf, vol. 7; 2017.

38. Tadesse BT, Ashley EA, Ongarello S, Havumaki J, Wijegoonewardena M, Gonzalez IJ, Dittrich S. Antimicrobial resistance in Africa: a systematic review. BMC Infect Dis. 2017;17(1):616.

22

Hydrogen peroxide and sodium hypochlorite disinfectants are more effective against *Staphylococcus aureus* and *Pseudomonas aeruginosa* biofilms than quaternary ammonium compounds

Caitlinn B. Lineback[1], Carine A. Nkemngong[1], Sophie Tongyu Wu[1], Xiaobao Li[2], Peter J. Teska[2] and Haley F. Oliver[1]* ⓘD

Abstract

Background: Antimicrobial disinfectants are used as primary treatment options against pathogens on surfaces in healthcare facilities to help prevent healthcare associated infections (HAIs). On many surfaces, pathogenic microorganisms exist as biofilms and form an extracellular matrix that protects them from the antimicrobial effects of disinfectants. Disinfectants are used as all-purpose antimicrobials though very few specifically make biofilm efficacy claims. The objective of this study was to evaluate the efficacy of eight registered disinfectants (six registered by the Environmental Protection Agency and two products registered in by the European Chemical Agency) with general bactericidal claims, but currently no biofilm efficacy claims, against *Staphylococcus aureus* ATTC-6538 and *Pseudomonas aeruginosa* ATCC-15442 biofilms. We hypothesized that hydrogen peroxide and sodium hypochlorite disinfectant products would be more effective than quaternary ammonium chlorides.

Methods: This study tested the bactericidal efficacy of eight registered disinfectant products against *S. aureus* ATCC-6538 and *P. aeruginosa* ATCC-15442 grown on glass coupons using a Center for Disease Control (CDC) biofilm reactor and EPA MLB SOP MB-19. Bactericidal efficacy was determined after treating coupons with disinfectants following standard EPA MLB SOP MB-20.

Results: Overall, sodium hypochlorite and hydrogen peroxide disinfectants had significantly higher bactericidal efficacies than quaternary ammonium chloride disinfectants. We also found that all tested disinfectants except for quaternary ammonium chloride disinfectants met and exceeded the EPA standard for bactericidal efficacy against biofilms.

Conclusion: In general, bactericidal efficacy against biofilms differed by active ingredient. The efficacies of sodium hypochlorite and hydrogen peroxide disinfectants did not vary between strains, but there were significant differences between strains treated with quaternary ammonium chloride disinfectants.

Keywords: Disinfectant, Biofilms, Efficacy

* Correspondence: hfoliver@purdue.edu
[1]Department of Food Science, Purdue University, 745 Agriculture Mall Drive, West Lafayette, IN 47907, USA
Full list of author information is available at the end of the article

Background

Healthcare associated infections (HAIs) are reported to occur in one out of 25 patients daily on average in the US [1] with over 2 million patients contracting HAIs annually [2]. In the USA, the overall incidence of HAIs is estimated to have increased by 36% in the last two decades [3]. Bacterial biofilms account for 65 and 80% of microbial and chronic infections, respectively [4]. A 2012 study suggested that biofilms may serve as a source of infections by periodically releasing planktonic bacterial cells into the environment [5]. The use of disinfectants is critical to preventing transmission of infectious pathogens from contaminated surfaces and medical equipment to patients [6, 7]. Despite emphasis on surface disinfection, pathogenic microorganisms are routinely isolated from the hospital environment [5, 7].

Within healthcare facilities, *Staphylococcus aureus* and *Pseudomonas aeruginosa* are amongst the most problematic pathogens [8] with *S. aureus* being the second most common pathogen that caused HAIs [9]. These pathogens grow on hard non-porous surfaces such as metal pipes and floor drains [10] and develop an extracellular polymeric matrix that protects the cells from adverse conditions [4, 11]. It has also been shown that the biofilm matrix enhances tolerance to disinfectants by encasing the underlying cells [12, 13] and by limiting diffusion of disinfectants into the biofilm matrix [14]. In fact, the bactericidal efficacy of disinfectants on biofilms is much lower compared to the efficacy of the same disinfectants against planktonic cells [8, 15–17]. The tolerance of biofilms to disinfectants is dependent on

disinfectant active, temperature, and the type of surface [13]. Surface roughness, surface humidity, and the availability of nutrients influence the establishment of biofilms on surfaces [18]. Moist surfaces have been shown to be more favorable for biofilm growth even though biofilms have also been reported to grow on dry surfaces [4, 14].

Disinfectants are primary intervention options against pathogenic organisms on surfaces in healthcare facilities [7, 14] and are used as broad-spectrum antimicrobials [19]. Common antimicrobials used for disinfecting surfaces in healthcare facilities include quaternary ammonium compounds, hydrogen peroxide, and chlorine-based products [6, 17]. There are few published studies that investigate the efficacy of disinfectants on bacterial biofilms at label use concentrations. The objective of this study was to evaluate the efficacy of eight registered disinfectants with general bactericidal claims, but no current biofilm efficacy claims, against *S. aureus* ATTC-6538 and *P. aeruginosa* ATCC-15442 biofilms. We hypothesized that accelerated hydrogen peroxide disinfectant products would be more effective than quaternary ammonium compounds and that sodium hypochlorite disinfectants would be the most effective at eliminating biofilms.

Methods

Disinfectants and bacteria strains used in this study

This study tested the bactericidal efficacy of eight registered disinfectant products (Table 1) against *S. aureus* ATCC-6538 and *P.s aeruginosa* ATCC-15442. These

Table 1 Active ingredients and contact times for disinfectant products tested in this study

Disinfectant Product "Name" (used in the manuscript or figures)[a]	Disinfectant Active Ingredient(s)[c]	Dilution	Active Level at Use[e]	Label Contact Time (mins)[f]
HP1	0.5% hydrogen peroxide	RTU[d]	0.5%	1
HP2	0.5% Hydrogen Peroxide	RTU	0.5%	1
HP3[b]	7.0% hydrogen peroxide	RTU	7.0%	1
HP4[b]	7.2% hydrogen peroxide	1:20	0.36%	5
HP5	4.25% hydrogen peroxide	1:16	0.27%	5
Q1	6.67% octyl decyl ammonium chloride; 2.67% docctyl dimethyl ammonium chloride; 4.00% didecyl dimethyl ammonium chloride; 8.90% alkyl (C_{14}, 50%; C_{12}, 40%; C_{16}, 10%) dimethyl benzyl ammonium chloride	1:256	0.087%	3
Q2	8.704% didecyl dimethyl ammonium chloride; 8.190% n-alkyl (C_{14}, 50%; C_{12}, 40%; C_{16}, 10%) dimethyl benzyl ammonium chloride	1:256	0.066%	10
SH1	1.312% sodium hypochlorite	RTU	1.312%	4

[a] Naming scheme abbreviates the active ingredients of the products used in this study and differentiates products with the same class of active ingredients by numbers
[b] ECHA registered products
[c] Active ingredient concentration
[d] Ready to Use
[e] Active ingredient concentration after dilution
[f] Defined EPA label contact time in minutes

strains are EPA-defined strains required for biofilm disinfectant efficacy registration claims [20]. Disinfectants were tested at label contact times and concentrations. Phosphate buffered saline (PBS) was used as a control.

Biofilm development on borosilicate glass coupons

Biofilms were grown using EPA Standard Operation Procedure (SOP) MB-19 for biofilms using a Center for Disease Control (CDC) biofilm reactor (Biosurfaces Technologies, Inc., Bozeman, MT). Borosilicate glass coupons (1.27 ± 0.013 cm; Biosurface Tech, Inc.) were used as carriers in the CDC biofilm reactor. The borosilicate glass coupons were placed in rods each containing three coupons. The biofilm reactor was positioned on a hotplate stirrer (Talbays, Thorofare, NJ) and filled with 500 mL of first phase growth media (Table 2). The media was inoculated with 1 mL of bacterial culture greater than or equal to 10^7 CFU/mL (Table 2). This formed the batch phase. Each of the test microbes began to adhere to the coupons for 24 h under the conditions defined in Table 2. The cells were subsequently grown in a continuous stirred tank reactor (CSTR) growth phase; 20 L of growth media (detailed in Table 2; TSB; Becton, Dickinson and Company, Sparks, MD) was pumped (Cole-parmer, Barrington, IL) through the reactor at a rate of 30 ± 2 min residence time for both S. aureus and P. aeruginosa.

Disinfectant efficacy testing

The efficacy of disinfectants against single strain biofilms was determined using EPA MLB SOP MB-20 [20]. Each rod contained three coupons and was rinsed by dipping in dilution water (1.25 mL KH_2PO_4 + 5.0 mL $MgCl_2 \cdot 6H_2O$). The target density for each coupon was 7.5–9.0 CFU/coupon for S. aureus and 8.0–9.5 CFU/coupon for P. aeruginosa per EPA MLB SOP MB-20. Coupons were placed in a 50 mL sterile conical tube (Corning Science, Mexico) for treatment and enumeration; coupons were individually evaluated. Five biological replicates were conducted for quaternary ammonium compounds due to known high variability [21]. Three biological replicates were conducted for sodium hypochlorite and hydrogen peroxide testing based on previous work conducted by our group [22]. Each biological replicate for all test products was composed of five technical replicates. Three control coupons were used for each test. Disinfectant product (four mL)

was added to each sterile conical tube containing a coupon. Coupons were dipped in dilution water prior to transferred into the tube to remove planktonic cells. Disinfectants were left in contact with the coupons for the label contact times at room temperature (Table 1). Four mL of PBS was added to control coupons. Disinfectant products were neutralized at the label-defined contact time with 36 mL neutralizing buffer solution (1 L H_2O + 5.2 g Difco neutralizing buffer; Becton, Dickinson and Company Sparks, MD). The treated coupons underwent a rotational series of vortexing (30 s) and sonication using an ultra-sonic water bath (Cole-Parmer Instrument Company, Chicago, IL) at 45 Khz for 30 s three times to release the biofilms from the coupons and suspend the bacteria in solution [20].

The control samples were quantified by serial dilution and spread plating on Tryptic Soy Agar (TSA; BD Biosciences, San Jose, CA) for S. aureus and Reasoner's 2a Agar (R2a; Becton, Dickinson and Company Sparks, MD) for P. aeruginosa following EPA MLB SOP MB-20 [20]. Coupons treated with quaternary ammonium chloride disinfectants were serially diluted and plated due to high cell recovery; coupons treated with hydrogen peroxide and sodium hypochlorite-based disinfectants were not serially diluted. Ten mL aliquots from each diluted sample were vacuum-filtered onto a membrane filter (0.2 μm pore; Pall Corporation, Port Washington, NY). Membrane filters were plated onto TSA and R2a agar for S. aureus and P. aeruginosa, respectively, and incubated at 37 °C for 48 ± 4 h prior to estimation.

Statistical analyses

All statistical analyses were performed using SAS 9.4 (SAS Institute, Cary, NC). CFU $\log_{10}$ reductions were calculated and normalized relative to the number of CFUs on control coupons. Disinfectant products were grouped based on the main active ingredients: sodium hypochlorite (1 product), hydrogen peroxide (5 products), and quaternary ammonium compounds (2 products). The data were fitted in a generalized linear mixed model with Proc Glimmix procedure to determine if there were significant differences in $\log_{10}$ reductions among disinfectants both by active category and product ($n = 56$; $\alpha = 0.05$). Least Squares Means with Tukey's adjustment were used to elucidate the trend of the identified significant differences.

Table 2 Growth conditions for S. aureus and P. aeruginosa biofilms

Bacteria Strain	Hotplate Stirrer Settings	Test Culture preparation	Batch phase growth medium 24 h	CSTR[a] growth medium 24 h
S. aureus ATCC-6538	60 ± 5 rpm at 36 ± 1 °C	Frozen stock with 10 ml TSB (30 g TSB/L) overnight at 36 ± 1 °C	3 g/L TSB	1 g/L TSB
P. aeruginosa ATCC-15442	125 ± 5 rpm at 21 ± 2 °C	Frozen stock with 10 mL TSB (300 mg TSB/L) overnight at 36 ± 1 °C	300 mg/L TSB	100 mg/L TSB

[a] Continuously stirred tank reactor (CSTR) phase

Results

Hydrogen peroxide- and sodium hypochlorite-based disinfectant products had similar bactericidal effects against both *S. aureus* and *P. aeruginosa* biofilms

Regardless of bacterial strain, hydrogen peroxide and sodium hypochlorite disinfectants achieved a greater overall bactericidal efficacy than quaternary ammonium disinfectants, both by active ingredient category ($P <$ 0.0001) (Fig. 1) and by individual product ($P < 0.0001$) (Fig. 2). Overall, *S. aureus* biofilms had a greater overall log reduction than *P. aeruginosa* biofilms after disinfection regardless of active ingredient category ($P < 0.0001$; Fig. 1) or the specific product applied ($P = 0.0002$; Fig. 2). A comparison of disinfectants by active ingredient category showed a significantly higher log reduction of *S. aureus* biofilms (4.37 log reduction) than *P. aeruginosa* biofilms (0.82 log reduction) by quaternary ammonium products ($P < 0.0001$; Fig. 1). Coupons disinfected with quaternary ammonium chloride products had on average 4.75 ± 1.69 *S. aureus* CFU/coupon (4.37 log reduction) and 8.02 ± 0.60 *P. aeruginosa* CFU/coupon (0.82 log reduction) post-treatment. There were no significant differences in bactericidal efficacy against *S. aureus* and *P. aeruginosa* biofilms after disinfection by hydrogen peroxide or sodium hypochlorite products. *S. aureus* and *P. aeruginosa* biofilms had an average log density of 0.33 ± 0.06 CFU/coupon (8.73 log reduction) and 0.30 CFU/coupon (8.51 log reduction) after disinfection with hydrogen peroxide disinfectants, respectively (Fig. 1) per EPA MLB SOP MB-20, 0.30 CFU/coupon is the reported detection limit when no cells are recovered thus there is no calculable standard deviation. *S. aureus* and *P. aeruginosa* coupons disinfected with the sodium hypochlorite product had mean log densities of 0.30 CFU/coupon (8.73 log reduction) and 0.33 ± 0.08 CFU/coupon (8.75 log reduction), respectively (Fig. 1).

When evaluating each disinfectant individually, both quaternary ammonium products exhibited significant differences in bactericidal efficacy against *S. aureus* and *P. aeruginosa* biofilms (Fig. 2). Specifically, *S. aureus* biofilms were significantly more reduced than the *P. aeruginosa* biofilms when treated with Q1 ($P < 0.0001$) and Q2 ($P = 0.0001$) (Fig. 2). No other significant differences were observed between *S. aureus* and *P. aeruginosa* biofilms disinfected by hydrogen peroxide or sodium hypochlorite products.

Hydrogen peroxide and sodium hypochlorite disinfectants had significantly higher bactericidal efficacy against *S. aureus* biofilms than quaternary ammonium products

There were significant differences in bactericidal efficacy among tested disinfectants against *S. aureus* both by active ingredient category ($P < 0.0001$; Fig. 1) and by individual product ($P < 0.0001$; Fig. 2). Products with hydrogen peroxide and sodium hypochlorite as active ingredients achieved significantly higher *S. aureus* log reduction than quaternary ammonium-based products ($P < 0.0001$; (Fig. 1). Specifically, sodium hypochlorite disinfectant SH1 and all hydrogen peroxide disinfectants (HP1, HP2, HP3, HP4, and HP5) individually by product were more effective against *S. aureus* biofilms than either of the two tested quaternary ammonium products ($P < 0.0001$; Fig. 2). There was no significant difference in bactericidal efficacy against *S. aureus* biofilms treated with Q1 compared to Q2 ($P > 0.05$; Fig. 2). There were no significant differences in disinfection performance among the aforementioned hydrogen peroxide and sodium hypochlorite products collectively ($P > 0.05$; Fig. 2).

Hydrogen peroxide and sodium hypochlorite disinfectants were more bactericidal against *P. aeruginosa* biofilms compared to quaternary ammonium compounds

Bactericidal efficacy was significantly different among disinfectants applied to *P. aeruginosa* biofilms both by active ingredient category ($P < 0.0001$; Fig. 1) and by

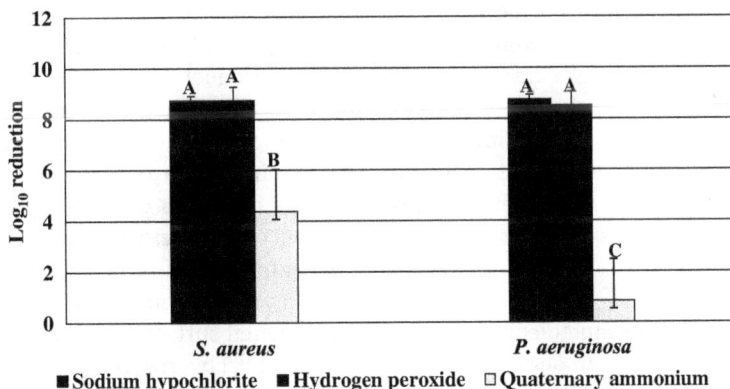

Fig. 1 Comparison of active ingredient class by strain

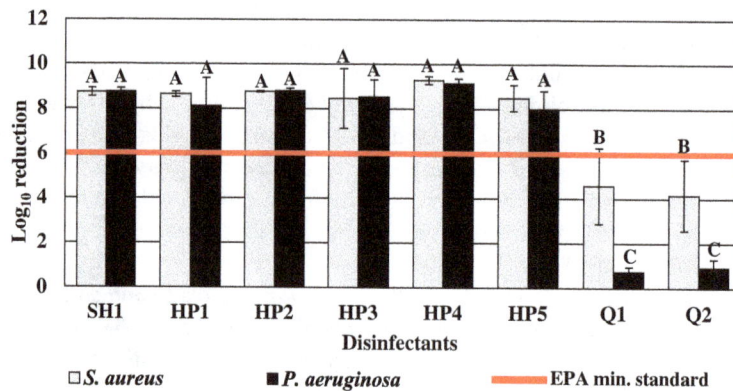

Fig. 2 Comparison of EPA registered disinfectants by strain

specific product ($P < 0.0001$; Fig. 2). Hydrogen peroxide and sodium hypochlorite-based disinfectants were more effective against *P. aeruginosa* biofilms than quaternary ammonium products ($P < 0.0001$; Fig. 1). Specifically, sodium hypochlorite disinfectant (SH1) and all hydrogen peroxide disinfectants (HP1, HP2, HP3, HP4, and HP5) by product individually achieved significantly higher bactericidal efficacy against *P. aeruginosa* than either of the quaternary ammonium chloride products Q1 and Q2 ($P < 0.0001$; Fig. 2). There were no significant differences among hydrogen peroxide products or between sodium hypochlorite disinfectant and hydrogen peroxide products ($P > 0.05$). There was no statistically significant difference in efficacy between the two quaternary ammonium products ($P > 0.05$).

Discussion

In this study, we tested eight registered disinfectants under label use conditions against *S. aureus* and *P. aeruginosa* biofilms using EPA methods MB-19 and MB-20. We found statistically significant quantitative differences among disinfectant active ingredients and products against *S. aureus* and *P. aeruginosa*. Specifically, we found (i) statistically significant differences in disinfectant efficacy among disinfectants, (ii) similar performance of hydrogen peroxide and sodium hypochlorite-based products against *S. aureus* and *P. aeruginosa* biofilms, and iii) significantly higher bactericidal efficacy of quaternary ammonium-based products against *S. aureus* than *P. aeruginosa*. Bacterial biofilms are common on a wide range of surfaces made of different materials and have been reported to be present in drains, metal pipes [10], sanitizing bottles, trolleys and clipboards [23] thus are potential sources of HAIs.

Disinfectant efficacy varies by active ingredient

We found significant differences among quaternary ammonium compound disinfectants compared to hydrogen peroxide and sodium hypochlorite disinfectants. The

quaternary ammonium compounds did not achieve the current EPA regulation minimum stating that the disinfectant must decrease the bacterial load by 10^6 CFU [24]. The findings in this study underscoring low quaternary ammonium compound efficacy against laboratory-grown biofilms. This raises concerns for healthcare facilities as quaternary ammonium disinfectants are reported to be among the most commonly used disinfectants in healthcare facilities [25, 26]. Quaternary ammonium compounds are cationic in nature [27, 28] and their interaction with a negatively charged biofilm matrix could inhibit their bactericidal efficacy [29]. Tseng et al. found that the efficacy of tobramycin, a positively charged antibiotic, was decreased as it was sequestered at the surface of the negatively charged biofilm matrix thus did not penetrate the matrix to contact underlying viable *P. aeruginosa* cells [29]. In addition, the bactericidal efficacy of quartenary ammonium compounds may fluctuate because they have been shown to be biogradeble under aerobic condictions [30].

Hydrogen peroxide and sodium hypochlorite disinfectants were effective against *P. aeruginosa* and *S. aureus* biofilms at the EPA required reduction levels. Hydrogen peroxide and sodium hypochlorite disinfectants have been reported to destroy both the biofilm matrix and the bacteria cells within, making them better anti-biofilm agents [31, 32]. Specifically, sodium hypochlorite disinfectant products irreversibly kill bacterial cells in biofilms by denaturing proteins in the biofilm matrix and inhibiting major enzymatic functions in bacterial cells. Although sodium hypochlorite disinfectants at concentrations as low as 0.0219% are effective against the formation of *S. aureus* biofilms [33], the use of sub-lethal concentrations of some sodium containing disinfectants could actually promote the formation of biofilms on environmental surfaces [34]. In a study conducted by West et al. [22], hydrogen peroxide products and sodium hypochlorite products were more effective against both *S. aureus* and *P. aeruginosa* planktonic cells compared to quaternary ammonium. On another note, surfaces disinfected with hydrogen peroxide based antimicrobials have demonstrated significantly lower chances of bacterial regrowth than those disinfected with quaternary ammonium compounds [35]. To this effect, the study by Boyce et al. [35] concluded that the risk of the incidence of HAIs was lower with hydrogen peroxide disinfectants than with the use of quaternary ammonium compounds. Our data suggest that hydrogen peroxide or sodium hypochlorite products should be used in healthcare facilities for routine use, particularly on surfaces prone to biofilm development. However, hydrogen peroxide disinfectants have also been reported to be corrosive on medical equipment such as flexible endoscopes [36] and can discolor metal finishes [37]. Despite these limitations, Alfa et al. [38] also demonstratated that a 0.5% hydrogen peroxide antimicrobial is highly efficient at disinfecting medical devices. Moreover, hydrogen peroxide disinfectants are neither irritating or malodorous [37].

The ability of biofilm matrices to prevent contact between disinfectant products and bacterial cells is complex [39]. Biofilms are characterized by high cell population densities that supply large amounts of polymeric substances, which consequently enables the formation of well-structured, functional matrices [39]. Moreover, biofilm cells are genetically primed to better tolerate disinfectant products compared to plaktonic cells [39, 40]. These features prevent the diffusion of disinfectants and limit bactericidal efficacy [41]. While our study emphasized the efficacy of disinfectants at label concentration and contact time, it did not investigate the efficacy of disinfectants at off label use or with varying environmental effects. Monoculture biofilms will be rare in healthcare environments and soil levels and surface type will vary. Further, this work was conducted on glass coupons per the EPA protocol, which does not necessarily represent how cells will grow on other surfaces (e.g. hard plastics, stainless steel). Recognizing these limitations, more work is needed to investigate other variables that can impact disinfectant efficacy (e.g. dry biofilms) as well as applications in healthcare settings.

Conclusion

We found that hydrogen peroxide and sodium hypochlorite products are effective against *S. aureus* and *P. aeruginosa* biofilms, which can be common in healthcare facilities. However, quaternary ammonium chloride compounds are not as effective against *S. aureus* and *P. aeruginosa* biofilms grow on hard non-porous surfaces and did not achieve a minimum 6 $\log_{10}$ CFU reduction. While further research is warranted to evaluate more complex biofilms in hospital environments, test the efficacy of disinfectants against dry biofilms, and to optimize the bactericidal effects of a combination of

different ready to use antimicrobials, infection preventionists should consider the use of hydrogen peroxide and sodium hypochlorite products on surfaces at risk of biofilm development to prevent HAIs.

Abbreviations
ATCC: American type Culture collection; CFU: Colony forming unit; EPA: Environmental Protection Agency; HAI: Healthcare-associated infection; HP1: 0.5% hydrogen peroxide; HP2: 0.5% hydrogen peroxide; HP3: 7.0% hydrogen peroxide; HP4: 7.2% hydrogen peroxide; HP5: 4.25% hydrogen peroxide; PBS: Phosphate buffered saline; Q1: 22.24% quaternary ammonium compounds; Q2: 16.89% quaternary ammonium; RTU: Ready-to-use; SH1: 1.312% sodium hypochlorite sodium hypochlorite; TSB: Tryptic soy broth

Acknowledgements
Dr. Oliver is supported by the USDA National Institute of Food and Agriculture Hatch project 2016-67017-24459.

Funding
This work was supported by Diversey Inc., Charlotte, NC, USA.

Authors' contributions
CL, CN, and STW performed the disinfectant efficacy testing, analysed and interpreted the data generated, and wrote the manuscript. XL provided industry experience, designed elements of the experimental protocol, and was a contributor in writing and editing the manuscript. PT provided testing materials, industry experience, and was a contributor in writing and editing the manuscript. HO served as the principle investigator for the study and was a contributor in writing and editing the manuscript. All authors read and approved the final manuscript.

Consent for publication
Not applicable.

Competing interests
CL, HO, CN, STW report grants from Diversey, Inc. during the conduct of the study. PT and XL reports grants from Diversey, Inc. during the conduct of the study; personal fees from Diversey, Inc., outside the submitted work.

Author details
[1]Department of Food Science, Purdue University, 745 Agriculture Mall Drive, West Lafayette, IN 47907, USA. [2]Diversey Inc., Charlotte, NC 28273, USA.

References
1. Center for Disease Control. Healthcare associated infection progress report. CDC. 2014. https://www.cdc.gov/hai/surveillance/progress-report/index.html. Published 2016. Accessed 5 July 2018.
2. Vallès J, Ferrer R. Bloodstream infection in the ICU. Infect Dis Clin N Am. 2009;23:557–69.
3. Stone PW. Economic burden of healthcare-associated infections: an American perspective. Expert Rev Pharmacoecon Outcomes Res. 2009;9(5):417–22.
4. Jamal M, Ahmad W, Andleeb S, Jalil F, Imran M, Nawaz MA, Hussain T, Ali M, Rafiq M, Kamil MA. Bacteria biofilms and associated infections. J Chin Med Assoc. 2017;81(1):7–11.
5. Vickery K, Deva A, Jacombs A, Allan J, Valente P, Gosbell IB. Presence of biofilm containing viable multiresistant organisms despite terminal cleaning on clinical surfaces in an intensive care unit. J Hosp Infect. 2012;80(1):52–5.
6. Rutala WA, Weber DJ. Disinfection, sterilization, and control of hospital waste. In Mandell, Douglas, and Bennett's principles and practice of

infectious diseases. Vol. 2. Elsevier Inc. 2014. p. 3294–3309.e1; https://doi.org/10.1016/B978-1-4557-4801-3.00301-5.

7. Quinn MM, Henneberger PK, National Institute for Occupational Safety and Health (NIOSH), National occupational research agenda (NORA) cleaning and disinfecting in healthcare working group, Braun B, Delclos GL, Fagan K, Huang V, Knaack JL, Kusek L, Lee SJ, Le Moual N, Maher KA, SH MC, Mitchell AH, Pechter E, Rosenman K, Sehulster L, Stephens AC, Wilburn S, Zock JP. Cleaning and disinfecting environmental surfaces in health care: toward an integrated framework for infection and occupational illness prevention. Am J Infect Control. 2015;43(5):424–34.

8. Smith K, Hunter IS. Efficacy of common hospital biocides with biofilms of multi-drug resistant clinical isolates. J Med Microbiol. 2008;57:966–73.

9. Dantes R, Mu Y, Belflower R, Aragon D, Dumyati G, Harrison LH, Lessa FC, Lynfield R, Nadle J, Petit S, Ray SM, Schaffner W, Townes J, Fridkin S. Emerging infections program–active bacterial Core surveillance MRSA surveillance investigators. National burden of invasive methicillin-resistant Staphylococcus aureus infections, United States, 2011. JAMA Intern Med. 2013;173:1970–8.

10. Liu J, Luo Z, Liu K, Zhang Y, Peng H, Hu B, Ren H, Zhou X, Qiu S, He X, Ye P, Bastani H, Lou L. Flushing on the detachment of biofilms attached to the walls of metal pipes in water distribution systems. J Zhejiang Univ-Sci A. 2017;18:313–28.

11. Kramer A, Schwebke I, Kampf G. How long do nosocomial pathogens persists on inanimate surfaces? A systemic review. BMC Infect Dis. 2006;6:130.

12. Percival S, Cutting K, Thomas J, Williams D. An introduction to the world of microbiology and biofilmology. In: Percival S, Cutting K, editors. Microbiology of wounds. Boca Raton: CRC Press; 2010.

13. Abdallah M, Khelissa O, Ibrahim A, Benoliel C, Heliot L, Dhulster P, Chihib NE. Impact of growth temperature and surface type on the resistance of Pseudomonas aeruginosa and Staphylococcus aureus biofilms to disinfectants. Int J Food Microbiol. 2015;214:38–47.

14. Bridier A, Briandet R, Thomas V, Dubois-Brissonnet F. Resistance of bacterial biofilms to disinfectants: a review. Biofouling. 2011;27:1017–32.

15. Buckingham-Meyer K, Goeres DM, Hamilton MA. Comparative evaluation of biofilm disinfectant efficacy tests. J Microbiol Methods. 2007;70:236–44.

16. Davison WM, Pitts B, Stewart PS. Spatial and temporal patterns of biocide action against Staphylococcus epidermidis biofilms. Antimicrob Agents Chemother. 2010;54:2920–7.

17. Fagerlund A, Møretrø T, Heir E, Briandet R, Langsrud S. Cleaning and disinfection of biofilms composed of Listeria monocytogenes and background microbiota from meat processing surfaces. Appl Environ Microbiol. 2017. https://doi.org/10.1128/AEM.01046-17.

18. Donlan RM. Biofilms: microbial life on surfaces. Emerg Infect Dis. 2002;8:881–90.

19. Meyer B, Cookson B. Does microbial resistance or adaptation to biocides create a hazard in infection prevention and control? J Hosp Infect. 2010;76:200–5.

20. Environmental Protection Agency. Methods and guidance for testing the efficacy of antimicrobial products against biofilms on hard, non-porous surfaces. EPA. 2017. https://www.epa.gov/pesticide-analytical-methods/methods-and-guidance-testing-efficacy-antimicrobial-products-against#efficacy-data. Accessed 2 Nov 2018.

21. Hong Y, Teska PJ, Oliver HF. Effects of contact time and concentration on bactericidal efficacy of 3 disinfectants on hard nonporous surfaces. Am J Infect Control. 2017. https://doi.org/10.1016/j.ajic.2017.04.015.

22. West AM, Teska PJ, Oliver HF. There is no additional bactericidal efficacy of EPA-registered disinfectant towelettes post-surface drying or beyond label contact time. Am J Infect Control. 2018;7:122. https://doi.org/10.1016/j.ajic.2018.07.005.

23. Ledwoch K, Dancer SJ, Otter JA, Kerr K, Roposte D, Rushton L, Weiser R, Mahenthiralingam E, Muir DD, Maillard JY. Beware biofilms! Dry biofilms containing bacterial pathogens on multiple healthcare surfaces; a multiple center study. J Hosp Infect. 2018;100:e47–56.

24. Environmental Protection Agency. Efficacy testing standards for product data call in responses. EPA; 2015. https://www.epa.gov/sites/production/files/2017-05/documents/reregistration_efficacy_standards.pdf. Accessed 1 Aug 2018.

25. McBain AJ, Ledder RG, Moore LE, Catrenich CE, Gilbert P. Effects of quaternary ammonium-based formulations on bacterial community dynamics and antimicrobial susceptibility. Appl Environ Microbiol. 2004;70(6):3449–56.

26. Gerba CP. Quaternary ammonium biocides: efficacy in application. 2015. Appl Environ Microbiol. 2015;81(2):464–9.

27. Nasioudis A, Joyce WF, Van Velde JW, Heeren RMA, Van den Brink OF. Formation of low charge state ions of synthetic polymers using quaternary ammonium compounds. Anal Chem. 2010;82:5735–42.

26. Gerba CP. Quaternary ammonium biocides: efficacy in application. 2015. Appl Environ Microbiol. 2015;81(2):464–9.

27. Nasioudis A, Joyce WF, Van Velde JW, Heeren RMA, Van den Brink OF. Formation of low charge state ions of synthetic polymers using quaternary ammonium compounds. Anal Chem. 2010;82:5735–42.

28. Velpandian T, Jayabalan N, Arora B, Ravi AK, Kotnala A. Understanding the charge issues in mono and di-quaternary ammonium compounds for their determination by LC/ESI-MS/MS. Anal Lett. 2012;45(16):2367–76.

29. Tseng BS, Zhang W, Harrison JJ, Quach TP, Song JL, Penterman J, Singh PK, Chopp DL, Packman AI, Parsek MR. The extracellular matrix protects Pseudomonas aeruginosa biofilms by limiting the penetration of tobramycin. Environ Microbiol. 2013;15:2865–78.

30. Tezel U, Spyros GP. Quatenary ammonium disinfectants: microbial adaptation, degradation and ecology. Environ Biotech. 2015;33:296–304 https://doi.org/10.1016/j.copbio.2015.03.018.

31. DeQueiroz GA, Day DF. Antimicrobial activity and effectiveness of a combination of sodium hypochlorite and hydrogen peroxide in killing and removing Pseudomonas aeruginosa biofilms from surfaces. J Appl Microbiol. 2007. https://doi.org/10.1111/j.1365-2672.2007.03299.x.

32. Tiwari S, Rajak S, Mondal DP, Biswas D. Sodium hypochlorite is more effective than 70% ethanol against biofilms of clinical isolates of Staphylococcus aureus. Am J Infect Control. 2018;46:e37–42.

33. Barnes TM, Greive KA. Use of bleach baths for the treatment of infected atopic eczema. Australas J Dermatol. 2013;54:251–8.

34. Cincarova L, Polansky O, Babak V, Kulich P, Kralik P. Changes in the expression of biofilm-associated surface proteins in Staphylococcus aureus food-environmental isolates subjected to sublethal concentrations of disinfectants. Biomed Res Int. 2016. https://doi.org/10.1155/2016/4034517.

35. Boyce MJ, Guercia KA, Sullivan L, Havill NL, Fekieta R, Kozakiewicz J, Goffman D. Prospective cluster controlled crossover trial to compare the impact of an improved hydrogen peroxide disinfectant and a quaternary ammonium-based disinfectant on surface contamination and health care outcomes. Am J Infect Control. 2017;45:1006–10.

36. Omidbakhsh N. A new peroxide-based flexible endoscope–compatible high-level disinfectant. Am J Infect Control. 2006;34:571.

37. Rutala WA, Weber DJ. Disinfection of endoscopes: review of new chemical sterilants used for high-level disinfection. Infect Control Hosp Epidemiol. 1999;20:69.

38. Alfa MJ, Jackson M. A new hydrogen peroxide–based medical-device detergent with germicidal properties: comparison with enzymatic cleaners. Am J Infect Control. 2001;29:168.

39. Mitchell KF, Zarnowski R, Sanchez H, Edward JA, Reinicke EL, Nett JE, Mitchell AP, Andes DR. Community participation in biofilm matrix assembly and function. Proc Natl Acad Sci U S A. 2015;112:4092–7.

40. Al-Jailawi M, Ameen R, Al-Jeboori MR. Effect of disinfectants on antibiotics susceptibility of Pseudomonas aeruginosa. J Appl Biotechnol. 2013. https://doi.org/10.5296/jab.v1i1.4038.

41. Gilbert P, Das JR, Jones MV, Allison DG. Assessment of resistance towards biocides following the attachment of microorganisms to, and growth on, surfaces. J Appl Microbiol. 2001;91:248–54.

23

Self-contamination during doffing of personal protective equipment by healthcare workers to prevent Ebola transmission

Lorna K. P. Suen[1]* , Yue Ping Guo[1], Danny W. K. Tong[2], Polly H. M. Leung[3], David Lung[4], Mandy S. P. Ng[5], Timothy K. H. Lai[1], Kiki Y. K. Lo[1], Cypher H. Au-Yeung[1] and Winnie Yu[6]

Abstract

Background: Healthcare workers (HCWs) use personal protective equipment (PPE) in Ebola virus disease (EVD) situations. However, preventing the contamination of HCWs and the environment during PPE removal crucially requires improved strategies. This study aimed to compare the efficacy of three PPE ensembles, namely, Hospital Authority (HA) Standard Ebola PPE set (PPE1), Dupont Tyvek Model, style 1422A (PPE2), and HA isolation gown for routine patient care and performing aerosol-generating procedures (PPE3) to prevent EVD transmission by measuring the degree of contamination of HCWs and the environment.

Methods: A total of 59 participants randomly performed PPE donning and doffing. The trial consisted of PPE donning, applying fluorescent solution on the PPE surface, PPE doffing of participants, and estimation of the degree of contamination as indicated by the number of fluorescent stains on the working clothes and environment. Protocol deviations during PPE donning and doffing were monitored.

Results: PPE2 and PPE3 presented higher contamination risks than PPE1. Environmental contaminations such as those originating from rubbish bin covers, chairs, faucets, and sinks were detected. Procedure deviations were observed during PPE donning and doffing, with PPE1 presenting the lowest overall deviation rate (%) among the three PPE ensembles ($p < 0.05$).

Conclusion: Contamination of the subjects' working clothes and surrounding environment occurred frequently during PPE doffing. Procedure deviations were observed during PPE donning and doffing. Although PPE1 presented a lower contamination risk than PPE2 and PPE3 during doffing and protocol deviations, the design of PPE1 can still be further improved. Future directions should focus on designing a high-coverage-area PPE with simple ergonomic features and on evaluating the doffing procedure to minimise the risk of recontamination. Regular training for users should be emphasised to minimise protocol deviations, and in turn, guarantee the best protection to HCWs.

Introduction

Ebola virus disease (EVD) is a severe infectious disease with a high fatality rate of approximately 50% [1]. The virus in the blood and body fluids of a patient can enter another person's body through skin lesions or mucous membranes of the eyes, nose or mouth. Therefore, health care workers (HCWs) should wear protective gear and adopt strict infection control measures when caring for suspected patients [2, 3].

The EVD outbreak has recently prompted interest in personal protective equipment (PPE) apparel and their use [4]. PPE comprise gowns, gloves, hood, face shield, boots, masks or respirators, which are used to protect HCWs from contact with infectious agents. However, although equipped with protective clothing, HCWs can be contaminated if the PPE apparel is improperly removed [3]. PPE

* Correspondence: lorna.suen@polyu.edu.hk
[1]School of Nursing, The Hong Kong Polytechnic University, Hung Hom, Hong Kong, Special Administrative Region of China, China
Full list of author information is available at the end of the article

must be removed slowly, deliberately and in the correct sequence to reduce the possibility of self-contamination or exposure to EVD [5].

Several healthcare organisations developed PPE protocols based on the best locally available components. However, HCWs may be hesitant to use a PPE with no empirical validation [4]. Thus, crucial precautions during PPE removal must be determined to effectively protect HCWs [6].

The Hospital Authority (HA) of Hong Kong is a statutory body that manages Hong Kong's public hospital services [7]. The HA recommends a PPE ensemble with a neck-to-ankle overall without skin exposure to meet the current recommendations of the Centers for Diseases Control and Prevention (CDC) on the PPE to be used by HCWs during management of patients with confirmed EVD [5]. A waterproof hood and a water-resistant gown were designed to cover the head, neck and body of HCWs. Previous studies [8, 9] reported that a water-resistant gown can provide a good physical barrier via preventing the absorption of liquid contaminants, and thus, conferring protection to HCWs who come in contact with body fluids and secretions of patients with EVD. Our previous study has shown that the barrier protection performance and usability of PPEs are affected by the covered area and ergonomic features [8]. However, systematic data on the risk of self-contamination of different PPE types for Ebola prevention remain lacking. In the present study, three types of PPEs, namely, Hospital Authority Standard Ebola PPE set (PPE1), Dupont Tyvek Model, style 1422A (PPE2) and HA isolation gown for routine patient care and performing aerosol-generating procedures (PPE3), were tested. We compared the PPE ensembles used to prevent EVD transmission in terms of protocol deviations during usage and the degree of contamination during doffing.

Materials and methods
This research was an experimental study of one group using multiple comparisons.

Study participants
A total of 59 HCWs were recruited for this study. The sample size was determined as previously described by Guo et al. [8], who have examined body-contamination rates and environmental-contamination levels during doffing of different PPE types in accordance with the protocol recommended by the HA. Pregnant females and participants suffering from upper respiratory tract infection and respiratory diseases requiring treatment were excluded.

Among the participants, 57.60% ($n = 34$) were female with an age range of 21–60 years old. The participants were either registered nurses ($n = 50$, 84.80%), advanced practicing nurses ($n = 4$, 6.80%), nursing officers ($n = 3$, 5.10%) or nurse educators ($n = 2$, 3.40%). The participants worked

in units with high infection risk, including the intensive care unit, emergency department, infection control units and respiratory wards, accounting for 47.50% ($n = 28$), whilst the rest worked in units with relatively low infection risk (i.e., other clinical units apart from the units mentioned above [$n = 31$, 52.50%]). All the participants have not yet worn PPE2 because this ensemble is generally not adopted in local hospitals for HCWs. Participants who are currently working in high-infection -risk units have more opportunities to wear PPE1 and PPE3 in daily practice.

PPE ensembles under testing
Three PPE ensembles were tested (Additional file 1: Figure S1, Additional file 2: Figure S2, Additional file 3: Figure S3, Additional file 4: Figure S4, Additional file 5: Figure S5, Additional file 6: Figure S6). (1) HA standard Ebola PPE set (PPE1) is a neck-to-ankle overall with an overlying water-resistant gown (Halyard, AAMI Level 4 Liquid Barrier Standard), double and long nitrate gloves, boots, hood, disposable face shield and N95 respirator. A bow was tied at the lateral of the waist to minimise the risk of front contamination. (2) DuPont™ Tyvek®, Model 1422A (PPE2) is commonly adopted in clinical settings to prevent Ebola transmission in countries, such as the US [10, 11] and South Korea [3]. Its protective clothing is also fluid resistant, but the design is a one-piece head-to-ankle overall with a zipper on the front. The whole outfit includes double gloves, boots, disposable face shield and an N95 respirator. A plastic apron was used to cover up the front zipper before use. (3) PPE3 is a HA isolation gown (Medicom®) for routine patient care and performing aerosol-generating procedures. PPE3 was selected as the reference PPE in the present study. A commercially available pure cotton surgical scrub suit (upper and lower working clothes) was worn inside the individual PPE ensembles during testing. Participants were free to select the appropriate size of gowns and gloves and the known best-fitted respirator model (3 M 1860, 1860s and 1870). Table 1 shows the comparison of the three PPE ensembles.

Procedures
Data collection was performed in an air-conditioned room with an average temperature of 23 °C ± 2 °C and a relative humidity of 60% ± 3%. Information about the purpose and procedures of the study was provided to the participants, and written consent was obtained prior to the study.

The participants' socio-demographic data, including gender, age, educational background, specialty, working units and clinical experience, were collected. Each subject received a 30 min briefing from a trained research personnel. The donning and doffing procedures for PPE1 and PPE3 were designed based on the recommendations by the HA, whilst the World Health Organisation (WHO)

Table 1 Comparison of the three PPE ensembles

Hospital Authority Standard Ebola PPE set (PPE1)	DuPont™ Tyvek®, Model 1422A (PPE2)	Hospital Authority isolation gown for routine patient care and performing aerosol-generating procedures (PPE 3) [As a reference]
Neck-to-ankle outfit	Head-to-ankle coverall	Neck-to-ankle outfit
N95 respirator	N95 respirator	N95 respirator
Hood (Kimberly Clark, model no. 25797)	Hood with elasticated facial opening	No hood
Disposable face shield	Disposable face shield	Disposable face shield
MICROCOOL Breathable High Performance Surgical Gown (Halyard, AAMI Level 4 Liquid Barrier Standard)[a]	Tyvek, a brand of flash spun high-density polyethylene fibers, a synthetic material. Apparel with elasticated wrists and ankles.	Water resistant isolation gown (Medicom®)
No zipper; the bow of the water-resistant gown is tied at the lateral side of the waist.	Zipper along the center front of the coverall, covered by a plastic apron.	No zipper; the bow of the water-resistant gown is tied at the lateral side of the waist.
Boots	Boots	Shoes
Double, long nitrate gloves	Double, long nitrate gloves	Single, latex gloves

[a]AAMI: The Association for the Advancement of Medical Instrumentation

protocol was followed for PPE2 doffing [12]. On the testing day, the participants watched a video about donning and doffing of the PPE ensembles to familiarise themselves with the procedures. The total duration for donning and doffing of PPEs in the videos was 8.74, 10.68 and 4.59 min for PPE1, PPE2 and PPE3, respectively. Posters related to donning and doffing procedures were pinned up in the venue. Participants with long hair were asked to tie up their mane. Watch and jewellery were removed to minimise the risk of exposure during the procedures. Afterwards, the participants donned and doffed the three PPEs in a random order as decided by a computer-generated randomised table.

The experiment was sequentially conducted in three areas. Area A was the 'clean zone', where the participants donned the working clothes and clean PPE ensemble in front of a mirror. Area B was the 'preparation zone', where the PPE of the participants was contaminated with a fluorescent solution (UV GERM Hygiene Spray, Glow Tec Ltd., London, England) that mimics contaminated bodily fluids or secretions spread via contact route. Fluorescent solution was sprayed onto the face shield, two upper limb/gloves and anterior surfaces of the gown at a distance of 60 cm from the participants, which represents the length of a stethoscope, simulating the usual working distance between a patient and an HCW [8], with an average of 1.99 g fluorescent solution/per stroke [9]. This value was determined using an electronic analytical balance with a precision of 0.1 g (NJW-3000, Xiangxin, Taipei, Taiwan) via obtaining the average of 20 trial cases. A standard of three strokes was sprayed on each body part with a total of 12 strokes made for each case. The weight of the splash in 1 stroke was 1.99 g in this study when the density of the solution was assumed as 1. Area C is the 'degown and test zone', wherein the participants were required to doff the PPE. A video camera with a high-density capability was set up for subsequent evaluation of protocol deviations

during donning and doffing. Protocol deviations are defined as accidental or noncompliance with the donning and doffing procedures of the PPEs under testing. The performance of the participants was monitored using a checklist. The participants were notified immediately of any deviation being committed. For evaluation, all protocol deviations were recorded. The participants were timed and videotaped whilst donning and doffing the PPE. The timer was stopped when the participants removed the final item of the protective clothing.

During the procedures, hand washing with liquid soap and water was performed according to the procedures of individual PPEs. Immediately after doffing, the participants were scanned for the presence of fluorescent solution. The participants' body (hair and head, face, anterior/posterior neck, left/right arms, hands or wrists, upper/lower working clothes and clogs) and the surrounding environment (rubbish bin cover, chair, faucet and sink) were examined using an ultraviolet lamp (CheckPoint, 220–240 V/50 Hz; Glow Tec Ltd., London, England) under dim light. Areas of contamination were counted and measured in square centimetres, and the fluorescent patches of different sizes were counted. Contaminated stains were defined as either small- ($\leq 1 cm^2$), medium- ($1 cm^2$ to $<3 cm^2$), large- ($\geq 3 cm^2$ to $5 cm^2$) or extra-large patch ($\geq 5 cm^2$) [8, 13, 14]. The number of contaminated patches and the time consumed by the participants during donning and doffing were recorded. The environment was thoroughly cleaned, and the areas were rechecked for any contamination with the ultraviolet lamp before the next trial. A 15 min break was given, and water was provided to the participants before testing the next PPE to prevent fatigue, which may affect performance.

Statistical analyses

All data were analysed with IBM SPSS Statistics 23. Descriptive statistics were used for all independent variables, including the subjects' age, gender, position, working specialty and clinical experience in years. The contamination sites among the PPEs were compared with χ^2 or Fisher's exact test as required. The degree of contamination during doffing and the time for PPE donning and doffing were compared using one-way ANOVA. Protocol deviations were expressed as the deviation rate (%). All differences reported were considered significant at the $p < 0.05$ level.

Results

Degree of contamination during doffing

Contamination by small patches on the working clothes of the wearers occurred less frequently during PPE1 removal than during PPE2 and PPE3 removal (median: 5.00 versus 7.00 versus 7.00, $p < 0.05$). The degree of contamination by large patches occurred less frequently during the removal of PPE1 and PPE2 than during the removal of PPE3 (median: 1.00 versus 1.00 versus 2.00, $p < 0.05$). No significant difference in medium-contaminated patches and number/area of extra-large contaminated patches was observed among the three PPEs. The older staff (aged 41–50 and 51–60 years old) featured significantly less-small contaminated patches than that of the younger staff (aged 21–30 and 31–40 years old) ($p < 0.05$). No gender differences were observed in the degree of contamination among the ensembles under testing. Moreover, HCWs working in units with relatively low infection risk showed significantly less small contaminated patches than those working in units with high infection risk (median: 5.00 versus 8.00, $p < 0.001$).

Contamination sites during doffing

Table 2 shows the distribution of contaminated sites on the body and the surrounding environment during doffing. The overall contamination of PPE1 during doffing is relatively less than those of PPE2 and PPE3, as indicated by either small- or extra-large contaminated patches. PPE2 is relatively more heavily contaminated than PPE1 during doffing in sites, such as hands and wrists, working clothes and the environment (chair). Meanwhile, PPE3 is more easily contaminated in the neck regions, clogs and arms than PPE1.

Donning and doffing protocol deviations

Procedure deviations during donning and doffing of the PPEs were observed, with PPE1 exhibiting the lowest overall deviation rate among the three PPE ensembles during doffing (2.95, 9.48 and 3.52% for PPE1, PPE2 and PPE3, respectively). The top three highest deviation percentages in each type of PPE are in bold (Table 3). Participants working in units with high infection risk presented significantly lower deviation rate than those working in units with low infection risk during donning

of PPE1 and PPE2, but no significant differences in the deviation rates can be observed among the groups during doffing of the three PPEs.

Timing for PPE donning and doffing

On the average, the participants used the longest time to don and doff PPE2, followed by PPE1 and PPE3. Donning PPE1, PPE2 and PPE3 required an average of 6.61 (range: 4.00–14.41 min), 7.29 (range: 4.48–14.52 min) and 3.28 min (range: 1.34–7.36 min), respectively, whereas doffing required 6.97 (range: 3.28–14.33 min), 10.37 (range: 5.43–23.53 min) and 4.42 min (range: 2.08–12.23). The HCWs working in units with relatively low infection risk showed significantly longer donning time when wearing PPE2 and PPE3 than those working in units with high infection risk. However, no significant differences were observed in the time used for doffing all PPEs under testing (Table 4).

Discussion

Self-contamination during doffing

Our study demonstrated considerable self-contamination during doffing. This result raised concerns on pathogen contamination of the skin or clothes of HCWs during PPE removal, which may result in self-inoculation and spread of the virus to patients and other HCWs through contaminated body fluids, including blood, urine, vomitus and stool. Gastrointestinal fluid losses of patients with EVD can be massive (5–10 L/day), droplet dispersion can be greater than 10 ft. and serum viral loads of dying patients with EVD can reach 10 billion copies/mL [15]. Given that no licensed vaccines nor proven effective antiviral therapies for EVD are currently available, PPE plays a crucial role in mitigating the risk of HCW exposure to contaminated body fluids in the care of patients with EVD [16].

The frequent occurrence of self-contamination during PPE doffing is also consistent with the findings of previous studies [6–8, 13–21]. The most likely contaminated areas include the neck, hands and fingers, arms and wrists and face [14, 17]. A study conducted in South Korea that estimated the degree of contamination during PPE doffing of HCWs reported that the most vulnerable processes comprise the removal of the respirator, shoe cover and hood [3].

The current study indicated that contamination of the working clothes occurred less frequently during PPE1 removal than during the removal of PPE2 and PPE3, which may be due to the ergonomic features of individual PPEs under testing. PPE1 consists of a neck-to-ankle outfit and includes a hood covering the neck. PPE2 is a head-to-ankle overall, and is a PPE ensemble frequently used in overseas settings to prevent Ebola transmission [3, 10, 11]. However, PPE removal is complicated because

Table 2 Sites of contamination during doffing of personal protective equipment

Location	Small sized contaminated patches (< 1 cm²), median				Extra large sized contaminated patches (≥ 5 cm²), median			
	PPE1	PPE2	PPE3	p-value	PPE1	PPE2	PPE3	p-value
Hair and head	1.00	2.00	2.50	0.68	0.00	17.00	0.00	N/A
Face	1.00	4.00	2.00	0.602	0.00	0.00	8.00	N/A
Neck (anterior)	2.50	5.00	11.00	0.095	0.00	0.00	24.00	N/A
Neck (posterior)	2.00	1.00	18.50	0.824	0.00	0.00	0.00	N/A
Arms (right)	3.50	1.00	4.00	0.414	0.00	0.00	28.00	N/A
Arms (left)	2.00	2.00	1.00	0.909	0.00	0.00	49.00	N/A
Hands or wrists	1.00	1.00	6.00	0.414	8.00	61.00	0.00	N/A
Working clothes (upper)	8.50	9.00	7.00	0.997	21.00	48.50	42.00	0.690
Working clothes (lower)	2.00	2.50	6.00	0.111	12.00	46.00	17.50	0.276
Clogs	3.00	5.00	13.50	< 0.001*	121.00	55.00	133.00	0.397
Environment (rubbish bin cover)	2.00	7.00	2.50	0.254	20.00	14.00	23.00	0.737
Environment (chair)	3.00	6.50	2.00	0.053	0.00	36.00	0.00	N/A
Faucet	2.00	2.00	1.50	0.659	0.00	16.00	14.00	N/A
Sink	12.50	14.00	10.00	0.072	75.50	66.50	44.00	0.649
Overall	5.00	7.00	7.00	0.05*	39.00	43.00	47.00	< 0.001*

*significant p values

N/A: There are fewer than two groups for the dependent variables, so no inferential statistics are computed using ANOVA

PPE1: Hospital Authority Standard Ebola PPE set

PPE2: DuPont™ Tyvek®, Model 1422A

PPE3: Hospital Authority isolation gown for routine patient care and performing aerosol-generating procedures

of the head-to-ankle, one-piece design and the elastication in the facial opening, wrists and ankles. HCWs have to take off the hood, unzip the front zipper, remove the overall and outer gloves together and place the trousers on the chair, thereby resulting in easy contamination of the hair and head, hands, working clothes, clogs and chair [17]. The elasticated one-piece coverall hood creates a potential contamination risk because the elastic contracts and pulls the outer part of the hood inwards and towards the participants' hair and neck during removal [22]. The zipper and its flap are also placed along the PPE2 centre front. Therefore, a plastic apron is worn to minimise the risk of body fluids being trapped in the zipper region. Herlihey et al. [22] also reported that when the subjects unzip the coverall, the zipper is stuck in the surrounding fabric or the gloves are stuck to the adhesive of the PPE, while unsealing the flaps covering the zipper results in ripping [22].

The WHO protocol requires the overall to be removed from top to bottom, followed by the removal of outer gloves whilst pulling the arms out of the sleeves of the overall. Special caution is needed to prevent self-contamination. PPE3 is recommended by HA for routine patient care, in which the neck, lower part of the legs and shoes are incompletely covered. Compared with PPE 1, additional sites, including the neck, arms, working clothes and clogs, were heavily contaminated when wearing PPE3 because it cannot provide adequate protection for HCWs caring for patients with EVD. These contaminated regions may be caused by self-contamination during doffing and contamination when the fluorescent solution was sprayed. Considering the possible underclothing contamination during doffing, the working clothes worn under the PPE ensembles should be frequently changed, especially when contamination is suspected.

During PPE1 or PPE2 doffing, the participants have to wear the clean clogs after removing their boots. However, the clogs may be possibly contaminated by the gowns or the environment in some cases. Hence, using footwear covers is an unideal option. During boot cover removal, HCWs struggle to balance their legs in the air [20]. Shoe covers are also difficult to doff, thereby often requiring assistance and increasing the risk of cross-contamination among workers [22].

The CDC and WHO recommend the use of double gloving with at least the outer pair possessing an extended cuff that reaches beyond the wrist [6] to decrease the incidence of hand contamination and provide improved protection for HCWs during PPE removal [16, 23]. Although double gloving is incorporated into the protocols for PPE use, the removal of the outer and inner gloves should be done with caution, followed by proper hand hygiene.

Previous studies defined contamination as small fluorescent stains (<1cm²) and large patches (>1cm²) [8, 13, 14] and revealed that fluorescent stain sizes are affected

Table 3 The deviation rate (%) during donning and doffing of personal protective equipment

Steps	Donning of PPE1		Donning of PPE2		Donning of PPE3	
	Procedure	Error (%)	Procedure	Error (%)	Procedure	Error (%)
1.	Visually inspect the PPE ensemble	0.00	Visually inspect the PPE ensemble	0.00	Visually inspect the PPE ensemble	0.00
2.	Perform hand hygiene	1.67	Perform hand hygiene	6.67	Perform hand hygiene	1.67
3.	Put on N95 respirator and perform fit test	3.33	Put on inner gloves	1.67	Put on N95 respirator and perform fit test	3.33
4.	Perform hand hygiene	5.00	Put on coverall & inspect for integrity	**8.33**	Perform hand hygiene	**6.67**
5.	Put on hood	**20.00**	Put on rubber boots	1.67	Put on cap	3.33
6.	Put on full face-shield	**11.67**	Put on N95 respirator and perform fit test	3.33	Put on full face-shield	**6.67**
7.	Put on gown	8.33	Put on face shield	**15.00**	Put on gown	1.67
8.	Perform hand hygiene	**13.33**	Put on hood	3.33	Perform hand hygiene	**10.00**
9.	Put on boots	0.00	Put on outer apron	**13.33**	Put on gloves	0.00
10.	Perform hand hygiene	3.33	Put on outer gloves	6.67		
11.	Put on gloves	0.00				
	Overall deviation rate	6.06		6.00		3.70
	Doffing of PPE1		**Doffing of PPE2**		**Doffing of PPE3**	
1.	Remove gloves	1.67	Disinfect outer gloves	**13.33**	Remove gloves	0.00
2.	Perform hand hygiene	0.00	Remove apron	11.67	Perform hand hygiene	1.67
3.	Remove gown	5.00	Disinfect outer gloves	**13.33**	Remove gown	**6.67**
4.	Perform hand hygiene	0.00	Remove hood	8.33	Perform hand hygiene	1.67
6.	Put clogs on the floor	5.00	Disinfect outer gloves	6.67	Remove full face-shield	**10.00**
7.	Take off the boots and put on clogs	**10.00**	Remove coverall and outer gloves together	**58.33**	Remove cap	**8.33**
8.	Perform hand hygiene	1.67	Disinfect inner gloves	1.67	Perform hand hygiene	0.00
	Remove full face-shield	**6.67**	Remove face shield	11.67	Remove N95 respirator	3.33
9.	Perform hand hygiene	0.00	Disinfect inner gloves	3.33	Perform Hand Hygiene	0.00
10.	Remove hood	**5.00**	Remove N95 respirator	3.33		
11.	Perform hand hygiene	0.00	Disinfect inner gloves	1.67		
12.	Remove N95 respirator	3.33	Put clogs on the floor	3.33		
13.	Perform hand hygiene	0.00	Remove boots and put on clogs	8.33		
14.			Disinfect inner gloves	5.00		
15.			Remove inner gloves	1.67		
16.			Perform hand hygiene	0.00		
	Overall deviation rate (%)	2.95		9.48		3.52

The top three highest deviation percentages in each type of PPE were bold
PPE1:Hospital Authority Standard Ebola PPE set
PPE2: DuPont™ Tyvek®, Model 1422A
PPE3: Hospital Authority isolation gown for routine patient care and performing aerosol-generating procedures

during gown removal [8]. In the present study, a precise estimation of the contaminated regions was performed in terms of the size of patches, that is, small ($\leq 1cm^2$), medium ($1cm^2$ to $<3cm^2$), large ($\geq 1cm^2$ to $5cm^2$), or extra large ($\geq 5cm^2$). The stain sizes can be associated with either inadequate PPE coverage or because of self-contamination during PPE removal. For example,

PPE3 cannot fully cover the neck of the participants, which resulted in many small or extra-large patches in the anterior and posterior neck region after spraying of the fluorescent solution onto the face shield and anterior surfaces of the gown. Meanwhile, PPE2 offers a high coverage area during fluorescent solution spraying. However, the hair/head, hands or wrists of the participants were heavily

Table 4 Time (in minutes) required for donning and doffing of personal protective equipment

	All participants Mean (sd) n = 59	High-risk group Mean (sd) n = 28	Low-risk group Mean (sd) n = 31	p-value # (t-test, high risk vs low risk)
Time required for donning (min)				
PPE1	6.59 (1.67)	6.19 (1.13)	6.94 (1.99)	0.086
PPE2	7.26 (2.06)	6.63 (1.77)	7.83 (2.16)	< 0.05*
PPE3	3.28 (1.15)	2.90 (0.98)	3.63 (1.25)	< 0.05*
	P < 0.001*			
Time required for doffing (min)				
PPE1	6.95 (2.59)	6.79 (2.42)	7.10 (2.77)	0.659
PPE2	10.31 (3.93)	10.24 (3.85)	10.38 (4.07)	0.893
PPE3	4.44 (1.87)	4.30 (1.38)	4.56 (2.23)	0.594
	P < 0.001*			

#t-test, participants working in units with higher infection risk versus working with lower infection risk
*significant p values PPE1: Hospital Authority Standard Ebola PPE set PPE2: DuPont™ Tyvek®, Model 1422A
PPE3: Hospital Authority isolation gown for routine patient care and performing aerosol-generating procedures

contaminated with extra-large patches during PPE removal. Similarly, medium-sized patch contamination can be due to either the PPE design or self-contamination. Therefore, a PPE with a high coverage area and simple ergonomic features that can minimise the risk of recontamination during doffing should be designed.

In this study, the older staff showed significantly less small-sized contaminated patches on their working clothes than the younger staff. This result may be due to the additional cautiousness of the older staff, whilst working than the younger staff. However, this finding cannot be generalised because of the low number of older staff (n = 4) who participated in this study.

Environmental contamination

In addition to self-contamination of HCWs during PPE doffing, environmental contaminations, such as those in the lid of the rubbish bin, chair, faucet and sink, were observed. Human-to-human transmission of EVD is also possible via indirect contact with the environment contaminated with such fluids [24]. The virus can survive for several hours on dry surfaces, such as doorknobs and countertops, to several days at room temperature in body fluids, such as blood [25]; virus-positive samples were still observed 7 days post-mortem [16].

Considering that hand hygiene methods using alcohol hand sanitiser fail to remove the fluorescent solution, handwashing with soap and water was performed by the participants. Thus, the sink may be contaminated because of handwashing, and the working clothes that came in contact with the sink may be contaminated because of the repeated handwashing. These results suggested that the height and width of the sink must be at a good working level of HCWs to prevent self-contamination during handwashing. Although alcohol gel is commonly used nowadays during PPE donning/doffing, hand cleansing with soap and water is recommended in cases of visible contamination in various situations, such as when areas are contaminated by vomitus, respiratory secretions, or fecal matter. Discarding used PPEs should be given much attention because of frequent contamination of rubbish bin covers [13].

Protocol deviations and importance of training

Deviations of the donning procedure may increase the risk of self-contamination whilst doffing [20]. Although the participants watched a video on PPE donning and doffing to familiarise themselves with the steps on the day of testing, they can also refer to the posters related to the procedures available in the venue. PPE1 exhibited the lowest overall deviation rate among the three PPE ensembles during doffing (2.95, 9.48 and 3.52% for PPE1, PPE2 and PPE3, respectively). This finding was expected because of the complexity of PPE2, as described above. The highest deviation rate (58.33%) was observed during the simultaneous removal of the overall and outer gloves in PPE2. As mentioned above, this result agrees with the WHO protocol for doffing overall [12]. This protocol requires the participants to remove the inner gloves, which were covered by the coverall. This procedure is difficult for many participants because they can only 'feel' the inner gloves during removal and cannot see them. Therefore, several participants cannot remove the overall and outer gloves together, or in certain situations, they removed both the inner and outer gloves simultaneously. Apart from the emphasis on regular training for HCWs to perform the procedure smoothly, the doffing procedure should be evaluated to increase its practicability for the users.

Being an international aviation hub, Hong Kong is frequently visited by travellers from all around the world. Moreover, contacts between Mainland China and African countries are becoming increasingly frequent. Although most HCWs in Hong Kong possess inadequate experience in handling EVD cases, providing regular training for HCWs is necessary to fill the gap between the desired PPE performance and actual practice. Contamination errors caused by unfamiliarity with the procedures, complexity with PPE ensembles and unconscious habits can be prevented through repeated practice and training. Evidence shows that traditional learning methods (e.g., watching educational videos and learning PPE guidelines) are inferior to immersive learning methods, including audio-visual devices and active learning involvement using simulation training that includes feedback on performance for clinical management of EVD cases, in guiding the PPE procedures [3, 17, 26, 27].

On the average, participants used the longest time for donning and doffing PPE2, followed by PPE1 and PPE3. A study reported that HCWs may show poor compliance with proper PPE removal protocol because of time constraints [28]. The most time-consuming processes include removing the shoe covers, putting on gloves and removing the outer gloves [3]. Thus, a short duration of doffing PPE is important for the faultless completion of removal protocol. Familiarisation of the HCWs with the procedures via frequent training and improved ergonomic features is necessary for the PPE design not only to prevent HCWs from self-contamination but also to shorten PPE donning and doffing time.

Limitations of study

This study has several limitations. Results showed the possibility of Hawthorne effect because the participants knew that they were being observed during the study. Therefore, compared with previous findings, real-life contamination rates or protocol deviations can be poorer than the findings presented in this study. Result generalisation is limited given the small number of participants, most of which are relatively young staff. A larger sample size with a better balance of staff seniority than that of the present study should be considered in future trials to evaluate whether clinical experiences influence the PPE performance.

The fluorescent solution used in this study was intended to mimic the mechanical effects of body fluids or secretions of patients with EVD. Although this method can provide a visualisation of contamination, it cannot provide information about viral load and shows no response to alcohol-based hand sanitiser, similar to EVD. Future studies may consider using surrogate viruses, such as MS2 (a surrogate for non-enveloped human viruses) and bacteriophage φ6 (a surrogate for enveloped viruses such as Ebola) to allow researchers to obtain quantitative data on virus transfer events and risks to HCWs without exposing participants to the risk of infection [16, 19, 23].

Conclusion

Our study demonstrated considerable self-contamination during PPE doffing of HCWs. Use of the head-to-ankle one-piece overall (PPE2) may result in a higher contamination risk than that of the neck-to-ankle outfit with a hood covering the neck (PPE1). Environmental contaminations, such as those in rubbish bin cover, chair, faucet and sink were detected. Procedure deviations during donning and doffing of the PPEs were observed, with PPE1 exhibiting the lowest overall deviation rate (%) among the three PPE ensembles during doffing. Although PPE1 showed the best performance in terms of low risk of self-contamination compared with PPE2 and PPE3 during doffing and protocol deviations, the design of PPE1 can be still further improved. Future directions should focus on designing a PPE with a high coverage area and simple ergonomic features. Evaluating the doffing procedure is also necessary to minimise the risk of recontamination during doffing. Regular training for users should be emphasised to minimise protocol deviations and in turn guarantee the best protection of HCWs.

Additional files

Additional file 1: Figure S1. Hospital Authority Standard Ebola PPE set (PPE1).

Additional file 2: Figure S2. DuPont™ Tyvek®, Model 1422A (PPE2).

Additional file 3: Figure S3. Hospital Authority isolation gown for routine patient care and performing aerosol-generating procedures (PPE 3).

Additional file 4: Figure S4. After putting on hood and full face-shield (PPE1).

Additional file 5: Figure S5. After wearing the outer plastic apron (PPE2).

Additional file 6: Figure S6. After putting on cap and full face-shield (PPE3).

Abbreviations
CDC: Centers for disease control and prevention; EVD: Ebola virus disease; HA: Hospital Authority; HCWs: Health care workers; PPE: Personal protective equipment; WHO: World Health Organisation

Acknowledgements
The authors extend their appreciation to the subjects for their sincere support and participation in this study.

Funding
This study was funded by the Infection Control Research Fund, Squina International Centre for Infection Control, School of Nursing, The Hong Kong Polytechnic University (Project Code: 4-ZZFR).

Authors' contributions
LS was the principal investigator. LS, YPG, DT, PL DL, WY, MN and TL were involved in conception and design of the study. TL, YPG, KL and CAY collected the data. LS and YPG were responsible for data analysis. LS and YPG drafted the manuscript supported by all authors. All authors read and approved the final manuscript.

Consent for publication
Were taken from each person in the photos.

Competing interests
The authors declare that they have no competing interests.

Author details
[1]School of Nursing, The Hong Kong Polytechnic University, Hung Hom, Hong Kong, Special Administrative Region of China, China. [2]Hospital Authority, Hong Kong, Special Administrative Region of China, China. [3]Department of Health Technology and Informatics, The Hong Kong Polytechnic University, Hung Hom, Hong Kong, Special Administrative Region of China, China. [4]Department of Clinical Pathology, Tuen Mun Hospital, Tuen Mun, Hong Kong, Special Administrative Region of China, China. [5]Infectious Disease Centre, Princess Margaret Hospital, Hong Kong, Special Administrative Region of China, China. [6]Institute of Textiles & Clothing, The Hong Kong Polytechnic University, Hung Hom, Kowloon, Hong Kong, Special Administrative Region of China, China.

References
1. World Health Organization: Ebola Virus Disease. 2018. http://www.who.int/mediacentre/factsheets/fs103/en/.
2. Centre for Health Protection: Ebola Virus Disease. 2017. https://www.chp.gov.hk/en/features/34199.html.
3. Lim SM, Cha WC, Chae MK, Jo IJ. Contamination during doffing of personal protective equipment by healthcare providers. Clin Exp Emerg Med. 2015; 2(3):162–7.
4. Bell T, Smoot J, Patterson J, Smalligan R, Jordan R. Ebola virus disease: the use of fluorescents as markers of contamination for personal protective equipment. ID Cases. 2015;2:27–30.
5. Centers for Disease Control and Prevention: Guidance on Personal Protective Equipment (PPE) To Be Used By Healthcare Workers during Management of Patients with Confirmed Ebola or Persons under Investigation (PUIs) for Ebola who are Clinically Unstable or Have Bleeding, Vomiting, or Diarrhea in U.S. Hospitals, Including Procedures for Donning and Doffing PPE. 2015. https://www.cdc.gov/vhf/ebola/healthcare-us/ppe/guidance.html.
6. Casanova LM, Rutala WA, Weber DJ, Sobsey MD. Effect of single- versus double-gloving on virus transfer to health care workers' skin and clothing during removal of personal protective equipment. Am J Infect Control. 2012;40:369–74.
7. Hospital Authority. 2018. http://www.ha.org.hk/visitor/ha_index.asp.
8. Guo YP, Li Y, Wong PL. Environment and body contamination: a comparison of two different removal methods in three types of personal protective clothing. Am J Infect Control. 2014;42(4):e39–45.
9. Wong TKS, Chung JWY, Li Y, Chan WF, Ching PTY, Lam CHS, Chow CH. Effective personal protective clothing (PPC) for healthcare workers attending patients with severe acute respiratory syndrome (SARS). Am J Infect Control. 2004;32:90–6.
10. Louis CS. Hospitals in the U.S. Get Ready for Ebola. 2014. https://www.nytimes.com/2014/08/16/health/hospitals-in-the-us-get-ready-for-ebola.html.
11. Bolden L. Central Florida Hospitals Prepare for Possible Ebola Cases. 2014. https://www.clickorlando.com/news/central-florida-hospitals-prepare-for-possible-ebola-cases.
12. World Health Organization: Steps to Take Off Personal Protective Equipment (PPE) Including Coverall. WHO/HIS/SDS/2015.4. 2015. http://apps.who.int/iris/handle/10665/150118.
13. Lai JY, Guo YP, Or PP, Li Y. Comparison of hand contamination rates and environmental contamination levels between two different glove removal methods and distances. Am J Infect Control. 2011;39(2):104–11.
14. Zamora JE, Murdoc J, Simchison B, Day AG. Contamination: a comparison of 2 personal protective systems. CMAJ. 2006;175:249–53.
15. Edmond MB, Diekema DJ, Perencevich EN. Ebola virus disease and the need for new personal protective equipment. JAMA. 2014;312(23):2495–6.
16. Fischer WA 2d, Weber DJ, Wohl DA. Personal protective equipment: protecting health care providers in an Ebola outbreak. Clin Ther. 2015;37:2402–10.
17. Kang JK, O'Donnell JM, Colaianne B, Bircher N, Ren D, Smith KJ. Use of personal protective equipment among health care personnel: results of clinical observations and simulations. Am J Infect Control. 2017;45:17–23.
18. Casanova L, Alfano-Sobsey E, Rutala WA, Weber DJ, Sobsey M. Virus transfer from personal protective equipment to healthcare employees' skin and clothing. Emerg Infect Dis. 2008;14(8):1291–3.
19. Tomas ME, Kundrapu S, Thota P, Sunkesula VCK, Cadnum JF, Mana TSC, Jencson A, O'Donnell M, Zabarsky TF, Hecker MT, Ray AJ, Wilson BM, Donskey CJ. Contamination of health care personnel during removal of personal protective equipment. JAMA Intern Med. 2015;175(12):1904–10.
20. Kwon JH, Burnham CD, Reske KA, Liang SY, Hink T, Wallace MA, Shupe A, Seiler S, Cass C, Fraser VJ, Dubberke ER. MSPH for the CDC prevention epicenters. Assessment of healthcare worker protocol deviations and self-contamination during personal protective equipment donning and doffing. Infect Control Hosp Epidemiol. 2017;38(9):1077–83.
21. Hall S, Poller B, Bailey C, Gregory S, Clark R, Roberts P, Tunbridge A, Poran V, Evans C, Crook B. Use of ultraviolet-fluorescence-based simulation in evaluation of personal protective equipment worn for first assessment and care of a patient with suspected high-consequence infectious disease. J Hosp Infect. 2018;99(2018):218–28.
22. Herlihey TA, Gelmi S, Flewwelling CJ, Hall TNT, BEng CB, Morita PP, Beverley P, Cafaxxo JA, Hota S. Personal protective equipment for infectious disease preparedness: a human factors evaluation. Infect Control Hosp Epidemiol. 2016;37:1022–8.
23. Casanova LM, Teal LJ, Sickbert-Bennett EE, Anderson DJ, Sexton DJ, Rutala WA, Weber DJ. The CDC prevention epicenters program: assessment of self-contamination during removal of personal protective equipment for Ebola patient care. Infect Control Hosp Epidemiol. 2016;37(10):1156–61.
24. Centre for Health Protection. Infection Control Recommendation for Ebola Virus Disease (EVD) in Healthcare Settings. Hong Kong: Centre for Health Protection; 2014 (Last updated on 11 July 2016).
25. Centers for Diseases Control and Prevention: CDC 24/7: Saving Lives. Protecting People. Persistence of the virus. https://www.cdc.gov/vhf/ebola/transmission/index.html. Accessed 20 Apr 2018.
26. Clay KA, O'Shea MK, Fletcher T, Moore AJ, Burns DS, Craig D, Adam M, Johnston AM, Bailey MS, Gibson C. Use of an ultraviolet tracer in simulation training for the clinical management of Ebola virus disease. J Hosp Infect. 2015;91(3):275–7.
27. Poller B, Hall S, Bailey C, Gregory S, Clark R, Roberts P, Tunbridge A, Poran V, Crook B, Evans C. 'VIOLET': a fluorescence-based simulation exercise for training healthcare workers in the use of personal protective equipment. J Hosp Infect. 2018;99(2018):229–35.
28. Zellmer C, Van Hoof S, Safdar N. Variation in health care worker removal of personal protective equipment. Am J Infect Control. 2015;43:750–1. https://doi.org/10.1016/j.ajic.2015.02.005.

Permissions

All chapters in this book were first published in ARIC, by BioMed Central; hereby published with permission under the Creative Commons Attribution License or equivalent. Every chapter published in this book has been scrutinized by our experts. Their significance has been extensively debated. The topics covered herein carry significant findings which will fuel the growth of the discipline. They may even be implemented as practical applications or may be referred to as a beginning point for another development.

The contributors of this book come from diverse backgrounds, making this book a truly international effort. This book will bring forth new frontiers with its revolutionizing research information and detailed analysis of the nascent developments around the world.

We would like to thank all the contributing authors for lending their expertise to make the book truly unique. They have played a crucial role in the development of this book. Without their invaluable contributions this book wouldn't have been possible. They have made vital efforts to compile up to date information on the varied aspects of this subject to make this book a valuable addition to the collection of many professionals and students.

This book was conceptualized with the vision of imparting up-to-date information and advanced data in this field. To ensure the same, a matchless editorial board was set up. Every individual on the board went through rigorous rounds of assessment to prove their worth. After which they invested a large part of their time researching and compiling the most relevant data for our readers.

The editorial board has been involved in producing this book since its inception. They have spent rigorous hours researching and exploring the diverse topics which have resulted in the successful publishing of this book. They have passed on their knowledge of decades through this book. To expedite this challenging task, the publisher supported the team at every step. A small team of assistant editors was also appointed to further simplify the editing procedure and attain best results for the readers.

Apart from the editorial board, the designing team has also invested a significant amount of their time in understanding the subject and creating the most relevant covers. They scrutinized every image to scout for the most suitable representation of the subject and create an appropriate cover for the book.

The publishing team has been an ardent support to the editorial, designing and production team. Their endless efforts to recruit the best for this project, has resulted in the accomplishment of this book. They are a veteran in the field of academics and their pool of knowledge is as vast as their experience in printing. Their expertise and guidance has proved useful at every step. Their uncompromising quality standards have made this book an exceptional effort. Their encouragement from time to time has been an inspiration for everyone.

The publisher and the editorial board hope that this book will prove to be a valuable piece of knowledge for researchers, students, practitioners and scholars across the globe.

List of Contributors

Frieder Pfäfflin
Department of Gastroenterology, Hepatology and Infectious Diseases (DGHID), Heinrich Heine University, Düsseldorf, Germany
Hirsch Institute of Tropical Medicine, research and training centre of DGHID, operated in cooperation with Arsi University, Asella, Ethiopia
Department of Infectious Diseases and Pulmonary Medicine, Charité – Universitätsmedizin Berlin, Augustenburger Platz 1, 13353 Berlin, Germany

Andreas Schönfeld, Dieter Häussinger and Torsten Feldt
Department of Gastroenterology, Hepatology and Infectious Diseases (DGHID), Heinrich Heine University, Düsseldorf, Germany
Hirsch Institute of Tropical Medicine, research and training centre of DGHID, operated in cooperation with Arsi University, Asella, Ethiopia

Tafese Beyene Tufa, Million Getachew and Tsehaynesh Nigussie
Hirsch Institute of Tropical Medicine, research and training centre of DGHID, operated in cooperation with Arsi University, Asella, Ethiopia
Arsi University, Asella, Ethiopia

Nicole Schmidt
Institute of Tropical Medicine and International Health, Charité – Universitätsmedizin Berlin, Berlin, Germany
Department for Infectious Disease Epidemiology, Robert Koch Institute, Berlin, Germany

Gebre Kibru, Lule Teshager and Mulatu Gashaw
School of Medical laboratory Science, Institute of Health, School of Medical laboratory Science, Jimma University, Jimma, Ethiopia

Solomon Ali
School of Medical laboratory Science, Institute of Health, School of Medical laboratory Science, Jimma University, Jimma, Ethiopia
WHO-TDR clinical research former fellow at AERAS Africa and Rockville, Rockville, MD, USA

Melkamu Birhane
Department of paediatrics and child health, Jimma University, Jimma, Ethiopia

Sisay Bekele
Department of ophthalmology, Jimma University, Jimma, Ethiopia

Yonas Yilma
Department of Surgery, Jimma University, Jimma, Ethiopia

Yesuf Ahmed
Department of Obstetrics and Gynaecology, Jimma University, Jimma, Ethiopia

Netsanet Fentahun
Department of Health education and behavioural health, Jimma University, Jimma, Ethiopia

Henok Assefa
Department of Epidemiology, Jimma University, Jimma, Ethiopia

Esayas Kebede Gudina
Department of Internal Medicine, Jimma University, Jimma, Ethiopia

Joost Hopman, Alma Tostmann, Heiman Wertheim, Maria Bos and Eva Kolwijck
Department of Medical Microbiology, Radboud university medical center, Geert Grooteplein 10, Postbus 9101, 6500, HB, Nijmegen, The Netherlands

Andreas Voss
Department of Medical Microbiology, Radboud university medical center, Geert Grooteplein 10, Postbus 9101, 6500, HB, Nijmegen, The Netherlands
Department of Medical Microbiology and Infectious Diseases, Canisius-Wilhelmina Hospital, Nijmegen, The Netherlands

Patrick Sturm
Department of Medical Microbiology, Radboud university medical center, Geert Grooteplein 10, Postbus 9101, 6500, HB, Nijmegen, The Netherlands
Department of Medical Microbiology, Laurentius hospital, Roermond, The Netherlands

Reinier Akkermans
Department of Primary and Community Care, Radboud university medical center, Nijmegen, The Netherlands

Peter Pickkers and Hans vd Hoeven
Department of Intensive Care, Radboud university medical center, Nijmegen, The Netherlands

Suhui Ko and Hye-sun An
Infection Control Office, Boramae Medical Center, Seoul, Republic of Korea

Sang-Won Park and Ji Hwan Bang
Infection Control Office, Boramae Medical Center, Seoul, Republic of Korea
Department of Internal Medicine, Boramae Medical Center, Seoul National University College of Medicine, 20 Boramae-ro 5-Gil, Dongjak-gu, Seoul 07061, Republic of Korea

Woo-Young Chung
Department of Internal Medicine, Boramae Medical Center, Seoul National University College of Medicine, 20 Boramae-ro 5-Gil, Dongjak-gu, Seoul 07061, Republic of Korea
Intensive Care Units, Boramae Medical Center, Seoul, Republic of Korea

Walter Zingg, Isabelle Soulake and Didier Pittet
Infection Control Program and WHO Collaborating Center for Patient Safety,|University of Geneva Hospitals, 4 Rue Gabrielle Perret-Gentil, 1211, 14 Geneva, Switzerland

Benedikt Huttner
Infection Control Program and WHO Collaborating Center for Patient Safety, University of Geneva Hospitals, 4 Rue Gabrielle Perret-Gentil, 1211, 14 Geneva, Switzerland
Division of Infectious Diseases, University of Geneva Hospitals and Faculty of Medicine, Geneva, Switzerland

Damien Baud
Genomic Research Laboratory, Division of Infectious Diseases, University of Geneva Hospitals, Geneva, Switzerland

Jacques Schrenzel and Patrice Francois
Genomic Research Laboratory, Division of Infectious Diseases, University of Geneva Hospitals, Geneva, Switzerland

Bacteriology Laboratory, Department of Genetics and Laboratory Medicine, University of Geneva Hospitals, Geneva, Switzerland

Riccardo Pfister
Neonatal Intensive Care Unit, Department of Paediatrics, University of Geneva Hospitals, Geneva, Switzerland

Gesuele Renzi
Bacteriology Laboratory, Department of Genetics and Laboratory Medicine, University of Geneva Hospitals, Geneva, Switzerland

Anna K. Barker and Kelli Brown
Department of Population Health Sciences, University of Wisconsin-Madison, School of Medicine and Public Health, Madison, WI, USA

Dawd Siraj
Department of Medicine, University of Wisconsin-Madison, School of Medicine and Public Health, Madison, WI, USA

Nasia Safdar
Department of Medicine, University of Wisconsin-Madison, School of Medicine and Public Health, Madison, WI, USA
William S. Middleton Memorial Veterans Affairs Hospital, Madison, WI, USA

Muneeb Ahsan
Medanta Institute of Eduation and Research, Medanta the Medicity Hospital, Gurgaon, Haryana, India

Sharmila Sengupta
Department of Clinical Microbiology & Infection Control, Medanta the Medicity Hospital, Gurgaon, Haryana, India

Claas Baier, Ella Ebadi and Franz-Christoph Bange
Institute for Medical Microbiology and Hospital Epidemiology, Hannover Medical School, Carl-Neuberg-Straße 1, 30625 Hannover, Germany

Sibylle Haid, Richard J. P. Brown and Thomas Pietschmann
Institute for Experimental Virology; Twincore-Centre for Experimental and Clinical Infection Research; a joint venture of Hannover Medical School (MHH) and Helmholtz Centre for Infection Research (HZI), Hannover, Germany

Andreas Beilken and Astrid Behnert
Department of Paediatric Haematology and
Oncology, Hannover Medical School (MHH),
Hannover, Germany

Martin Wetzke and Gesine Hansen
Department for Paediatric Pneumology, Allergy
and Neonatology, Hannover Medical School
(MHH), Hannover, Germany

Corinna Schmitt and Thomas F. Schulz
Institute of Virology, Hannover Medical School
(MHH), Hannover, Germany

Rebekah H. Borse and Shuvayu S. Sen
Merck & Co., Inc., Kenilworth, NJ, USA

Vimalanand S. Prabhu
Merck & Co., Inc., Kenilworth, NJ, USA
Center for Observational and Real World Evidence
(CORE), Merck & Co., Inc., 2000 Galloping Hill
Road, Kenilworth, NJ 07033, USA

Joseph S. Solomkin
University of Cincinnati College of Medicine,
Cincinnati, OH, USA

Goran Medic and Jason Foo
Mapi Group, Houten, The Netherlands

Teresa Kauf
Baxalta US Inc., Boston, MA, USA

Benjamin Miller
Shire, Lexington, MA, USA

Anirban Basu
Pharmaceutical Outcomes Research and Policy
Program, University of Washington, Seattle, WA,
USA

Manish Kakkar
Public Health Foundation of India, Plot 47, Sector
44, Gurgaon, Haryana 122002, India

Abhimanyu Singh Chauhan
Public Health Foundation of India, Plot 47, Sector
44, Gurgaon, Haryana 122002, India
Department of Public Health Sciences, Faculty of
Medicine, University of Liège - Hospital District,
Hippocrates Avenue 13 - Building 234000, Liège,
Belgium

Pranab Chatterjee
Public Health Foundation of India, Plot 47, Sector
44, Gurgaon, Haryana 122002, India
Indian Council of Medical Research, Division of
Epidemiology, National Institute of Cholera and
Enteric Diseases, Kolkata 700010, India

Mathew Sunil George
Indian Institute of Public Health, Gurgaon, Haryana
122002, India
Centre for Research and Action in Public Health
(CeRAPH), University of Canberra, Building 22,
Floor B, University Drive, Bruce ACT 2617, Australia

Delia Grace
International Livestock Research Institute, Nairobi
30709-00100, Kenya

Johanna Lindahl
International Livestock Research Institute, Nairobi
30709-00100, Kenya
Zoonosis Science Laboratory, Uppsala University,
Uppsala SE-751 23, Sweden
Department of Clinical Sciences, Swedish University
of Agricultural Sciences, Uppsala SE-750 07, Sweden

Marvin A. H. Berrevoets and Bart-Jan Kullberg
Department of Internal Medicine and Infectious
Diseases, Radboudumc, Nijmegen, the Netherlands

**Johannes (Hans) L. W. Pot, Anne E. Houterman
and Hanneke W. H. A. Fleuren**
Department of Clinical Pharmacy, Canisius-
Wilhelmina Hospital, Nijmegen, the Netherlands

Anton (Ton) S. M. Dofferhoff and Tom Sprong
Department of Internal Medicine, Canisius-
Wilhelmina Hospital, Nijmegen, the Netherlands

Marrigje H. Nabuurs-Franssen
Department of Medical Microbiology and Infectious
Diseases, Canisius-Wilhelmina Hospital, Nijmegen,
the Netherlands

Jeroen A. Schouten
Department of Intensive Care, Canisius-Wilhelmina
Hospital, Nijmegen, the Netherlands

**Missiani Ochwoto, Lucy Muita, Keith Talaam,
Cecilia Wanjala, Frank Ogeto, Faith Wachira,
Saida Osman and James Kimotho**
Production Department, Kenya Medical Research
Institute, Nairobi, Kenya

Linus Ndegwa
Centers for Disease Control and Prevention, Nairobi, Kenya

Michael Pulia and Rebecca J. Schwei
BerbeeWalsh Department of Emergency Medicine, University of Wisconsin-Madison School of Medicine and Public Health, Madison, WI, USA

Manish N. Shah
BerbeeWalsh Department of Emergency Medicine, University of Wisconsin-Madison School of Medicine and Public Health, Madison, WI, USA Department of Medicine, University of Wisconsin-Madison School of Medicine and Public Health, Madison, WI, USA

Michael Kern
University of Wisconsin-Madison School of Medicine and Public Health, Madison, WI, USA

Emmanuel Sampene
Department of Biostatistics and Medical Informatics, University of Wisconsin-Madison School of Medicine and Public Health, Madison, WI, USA

Christopher J. Crnich
Department of Medicine, University of Wisconsin-Madison School of Medicine and Public Health, Madison, WI, USA

Thomas-Jörg Hennig and Andreas Arndt
B. Braun Medical AG, Centre of Excellence Infection Control, Seesatz 17, 6204 Sempach, Switzerland

Sebastian Werner and Kathrin Naujox
HygCen Germany GmbH, Bornhövedstrasse 78, 19055 Schwerin, Germany

Sanae Lanjri, Jean Uwingabiye, Mohammed Frikh, Lina Abdellatifi, Jalal Kasouati, Adil Maleb, Abdelouahed Bait, Abdelhay Lemnouer and Mostafa Elouennass
Department of Clinical Bacteriology, Mohammed V Military teaching hospital, research team of Epidemiology and Bacterial resistance, Faculty of Medicine and Pharmacy, Mohammed V University, Rabat, Morocco

Hiroki Saito
Japan Ministry of Health, Labour and Welfare, Health Bureau, Tokyo, Japan

Kyoko Inoue
Institute of Tropical Medicine, Nagasaki University, Nagasaki, Japan

James Ditai
Sanyu Africa Research Institute, Mbale, Uganda

Benon Wanume, Julian Abeso and Jaffer Balyejussa
Mbale Regional Referral Hospital, Departments of Community Medicine, Paediatrics and Surgery, Mbale, Uganda

Andrew Weeks
University of Liverpool, Sanyu Research Unit, Liverpool, UK

Stefanie Kampmeier, Annelene Kossow and Alexander Mellmann
Institute of Hygiene, University Hospital Münster, Robert-Koch-Strasse 41, 48149 Münster, Germany

Stefanie Willems and Frank Kipp
Institute of Hygiene, University Hospital Münster, Robert-Koch-Strasse 41, 48149 Münster, Germany Institute of Hygiene, DRK Kliniken Berlin, Drontheimer Str. 39–40, 13359 Berlin, Germany

Dennis Knaack
Institute of Medical Microbiology, University Hospital Münster, Domagkstrasse 10, 48149 Münster, Germany

Christoph Schliemann and Wolfgang E. Berdel
Department of Medicine A, Haematology and Oncology, University Hospital Münster, Albert-Schweitzer-Campus 1, 48149 Münster, Germany

Ping Yang, Saiping Jiang and Xiaoyang Lu
Department of Pharmacy, the First Affiliated Hospital of Medicine School, Zhejiang University, Hangzhou, China

Yunbo Chen, Ping Shen and Yonghong Xiao
State Key Laboratory for Diagnosis and Treatment of Infectious Diseases, the First Affiliated Hospital of Medicine School, Zhejiang University, 79 Qingchun Road, Hangzhou, China

Miranda Suchomel and Markus Brillmann
Institute for Hygiene and Applied Immunology, Medical University of Vienna, Kinderspitalgasse 15, 1090 Vienna, Austria

Elisabeth Presterl
Department for Hospital Epidemiology and Infection Control, Medical University of Vienna, Vienna, Austria

Ojan Assadian
Department for Hospital Epidemiology and Infection Control, Medical University of Vienna, Vienna, Austria
Institute for Skin Integrity and Infection Prevention, University of Huddersfield, Huddersfield, UK

Karen J. Ousey
Institute for Skin Integrity and Infection Prevention, University of Huddersfield, Huddersfield, UK

Susanne Barnett, Warren Rose, Theresa Emmerling and Keng Hee Peh
University of Wisconsin-Madison School of Pharmacy, 777 Highland Ave, Madison, WI 53705, USA

Laurel Legenza
University of Wisconsin-Madison School of Pharmacy, 777 Highland Ave, Madison, WI 53705, USA
University of the Western Cape School of Pharmacy, Robert Sobukwe, Cape Town 7535, South Africa

Renier Coetzee
University of the Western Cape School of Pharmacy, Robert Sobukwe, Cape Town 7535, South Africa

Nasia Safdar
University of Wisconsin School of Medicine and Public Health, 750 Highland Ave, Madison, WI 53726, USA

Jonas Keller, Aline Wolfensberger, Lauren Clack, Stefan P. Kuster, Mesida Dunic and Hugo Sax
Division of Infectious Diseases and Hospital Epidemiology, University Hospital Zurich, University of Zurich, Rämistrasse 100, CH-8091 Zurich, Switzerland

Yvonne Flammer
Division of Infectious Diseases and Hospital Epidemiology, University Hospital Zurich, University of Zurich, Rämistrasse 100, CH-8091 Zurich, Switzerland
Baraka Health Centre, German Doctors Nairobi, Nairobi, Kenya

Doris Eis and Dagmar I. Keller
Emergency Department, University Hospital Zurich, University of Zurich, Zurich, Switzerland

Pa Saidou Chaw
PhD Programme, Epidemiology"Braunschweig-Hannover, Department of Epidemiology, Helmholtz Centre for Infection Research, 38124 Braunschweig, Germany
Institute for Medical Epidemiology, Biometry, and Informatics (IMEBI), Medical Faculty of the Martin-Luther University Halle-Wittenberg, 06112 Halle (Saale), Germany

Kristin Maria Schlinkmann
PhD Programme, Epidemiology"Braunschweig-Hannover, Department of Epidemiology, Helmholtz Centre for Infection Research, 38124 Braunschweig, Germany
Department of Epidemiology, Helmholtz Centre for Infection Research, 38124 Braunschweig, Germany

André Karch
PhD Programme, Epidemiology Braunschweig-Hannover, Department of Epidemiology, Helmholtz Centre for Infection Research, 38124 Braunschweig, Germany
Department of Epidemiology, Helmholtz Centre for Infection Research, 38124 Braunschweig, Germany
German Center for Infection Research (DZIF), Hannover-Braunschweig site, 30625 Hannover, Germany

Rafael Mikolajczyk
Institute for Medical Epidemiology, Biometry, and Informatics (IMEBI), Medical Faculty of the Martin-Luther University Halle-Wittenberg, 06112 Halle (Saale), Germany
Department of Epidemiology, Helmholtz Centre for Infection Research, 38124 Braunschweig, Germany
German Center for Infection Research (DZIF), Hannover-Braunschweig site, 30625 Hannover, Germany
Hannover Medical School, 30625 Hannover, Germany

Heike Raupach-Rosin
Department of Epidemiology, Helmholtz Centre for Infection Research, 38124 Braunschweig, Germany

Mathias W. Pletz
Center for Infectious Diseases and Infection Control, Jena University Hospital, Am Klinikum 1, 07747 Jena, Germany

Johannes Huebner
Division of Paediatric Infectious Diseases, Dr. Von Hauner Children's Hospital, Ludwig Maximilian University Munich, 80337 Munich, Germany

Ousman Nyan
Department of Medicine, School of Medicine and Allied Health Sciences, University of the Gambia, Edward Francis Small Teaching Hospital, Banjul, The Gambia

Caitlinn B. Lineback, Carine A. Nkemngong, Sophie Tongyu Wu and Haley F. Oliver
Department of Food Science, Purdue University, 745 Agriculture Mall Drive, West Lafayette, IN 47907, USA

Xiaobao Li and Peter J. Teska
Diversey Inc., Charlotte, NC 28273, USA

Lorna K. P. Suen, Yue Ping Guo, Timothy K. H. Lai, Kiki Y. K. Lo and Cypher H. Au-Yeung
School of Nursing, The Hong Kong Polytechnic University, Hung Hom, Hong Kong, Special Administrative Region of China, China

Danny W. K. Tong
Hospital Authority, Hong Kong, Special Administrative Region of China, China

Polly H. M. Leung
Department of Health Technology and Informatics, The Hong Kong Polytechnic University, Hung Hom, Hong Kong, Special Administrative Region of China, China

David Lung
Department of Clinical Pathology, Tuen Mun Hospital, Tuen Mun, Hong Kong, Special Administrative Region of China, China

Mandy S. P. Ng
Infectious Disease Centre, Princess Margaret Hospital, Hong Kong, Special Administrative Region of China, China

Winnie Yu
Institute of Textiles & Clothing, The Hong Kong Polytechnic University, Hung Hom, Kowloon, Hong Kong, Special Administrative Region of China, China

Index

www.ingramcontent.com/pod-product-compliance
Lightning Source LLC
Chambersburg PA
CBHW082018190326
41458CB00010B/3223